Intrahepatic Cholangiocarcinoma

Timothy M. Pawlik • Jordan M. Cloyd
Mary Dillhoff
Editors

Intrahepatic Cholangiocarcinoma

Diagnosis and Management

Springer

Editors
Timothy M. Pawlik
Wexner Medical Center
The Ohio State University
Columbus, OH
USA

Jordan M. Cloyd
Wexner Medical Center
The Ohio State University
Columbus, OH
USA

Mary Dillhoff
Wexner Medical Center
The Ohio State University
Columbus, OH
USA

ISBN 978-3-030-22260-4 ISBN 978-3-030-22258-1 (eBook)
https://doi.org/10.1007/978-3-030-22258-1

This Springer imprint is published by the registered company Springer Nature Switzerland AG
The registered company address is: Gewerbestrasse 11, 6330 Cham, Switzerland

Preface

The up-to-date management of intrahepatic cholangiocarcinoma (ICC) is growing increasingly complex as advances in basic and translational sciences highlight the unique genetic and molecular features that distinguish it from other biliary tract cancers. These advances called to attention the need for a single comprehensive resource focused specifically on ICC. *Intrahepatic Cholangiocarcinoma: Diagnosis and Management* was written to provide a comprehensive review of the epidemiology, molecular pathogenesis, diagnosis, and treatment of ICC. The textbook brings together an impressive group of international experts in cholangiocarcinoma research and clinical care. The book was organized and written to aid the clinician's understanding of emerging research in cholangiocarcinoma and its application to the clinical care of patients with ICC. Each chapter details the scientific evidence to support clinical decisions that are needed to care for these complex patients. The text is a concise but thorough guide to clinical care.

While the long-term outcomes of patients with cholangiocarcinoma have largely remained poor, recent developments in translational sciences have offered hope for treatment breakthroughs. Indeed, our understanding of the molecular pathogenesis of ICC is rapidly evolving which should lead to the development of targeted therapies and/or immunotherapies. For example, mutations in IDH1/2, BAP1, and FGFR2 are common in ICC and make for attractive targets for novel therapies. The wealth of basic science knowledge is being rapidly translated to the bedside into novel clinical trials with new agents that interfere with these pathways. At the same time, there has been a recent explosion of large prospective clinical trials evaluating adjuvant therapies for patients with resected biliary tract cancers. These trials are pivotal to understanding the optimal components of multimodality therapy. Although the survival for patients with ICC remains poor, these advances bring hope for prolonging life and increasing quality of life.

Multidisciplinary care in ICC is crucial in improving outcomes in this deadly disease, and this textbook is truly a collaborative transdisciplinary effort. Focused chapters detail the epidemiology, diagnostic evaluation, as well as staging and prognosis of this disease. In addition to dedicated chapters on surgical management of ICC, a broad emphasis on locoregional therapies, including percutaneous ablation and transarterial therapies, is included. An up-to-date overview of the molecular pathogenesis and pathological assessment of ICC is detailed prior to chapters focusing on systemic chemotherapy and emerging novel therapy options. Our sincere appreciation is owed to the authors for their contributions not only to this textbook but also to the science, advancement of research, and improvement of care for patients with cholangiocarcinoma. We hope that this textbook is not only an invaluable resource for many as they seek to provide the best multidisciplinary cancer care to patients with ICC but also an opportunity to identify new avenues of scientific discovery that lead to significant advances in the diagnosis and management of ICC.

Columbus, OH, USA

Timothy M. Pawlik, MD, MPH, MTS, PhD, FACS, FRACS
Jordan M. Cloyd, MD
Mary Dillhoff, MD, MS

Contents

Contributors

Arezou Abbasi, MD Department of Surgery, University of Washington Medical Center, Seattle, WA, USA

Daniel E. Abbott, MD, FACS Department of Surgery, Division of Surgical Oncology, University of Wisconsin School of Medicine and Public Health, Madison, WI, USA

Reham Abdel-Wahab, MD, PhD Department of Gastrointestinal Medical Oncology, The University of Texas MD Anderson Cancer Center, Houston, TX, USA

Clinical Oncology Department, Faculty of Medicine, Assiut University, Asyut, Egypt

Laith Abushahin, MD Division of Medical Oncology, Department of Internal Medicine, Columbus, OH, USA

Department of Oncology, The Ohio State University Wexner Medical Center, Columbus, OH, USA

Fabio Bagante, MD Department of Surgery, University of Verona, Verona, Italy

Massimiliano Cadamuro, PhD Department of Molecular Medicine, University of Padua, Padua, Italy

International Center for Digestive Health (ICDH), University of Milano-Bicocca, Milano, Italy

Tommaso Campagnaro, MD, PhD Department of Surgery, University of Verona, Verona, Italy

Yun Shin Chun, MD Department of Surgical Oncology, The University of Texas MD Anderson Cancer Center, Houston, TX, USA

Simone Conci, MD, PhD Department of Surgery, University of Verona, Verona, Italy

Luca Fabris, MD, PhD Department of Molecular Medicine, University of Padua, Padua, Italy

International Center for Digestive Health (ICDH), University of Milano-Bicocca, Milano, Italy

Section of Digestive Diseases, Department of Internal Medicine, Yale University, New Haven, CT, USA

Alfredo Guglielmi, MD Department of Surgery, University of Verona, Verona, Italy

Theodore S. Hong, MD Department of Radiation Oncology, Massachusetts General Hospital, Boston, MA, USA

Calogero Iacono, MD Department of Surgery, University of Verona, Verona, Italy

Milind Javle, MD Department of Gastrointestinal Medical Oncology, The University of Texas MD Anderson Cancer Center, Houston, TX, USA

Ning Jin, MD, MS Department of Oncology, The Ohio State University Wexner Medical Center, Columbus, OH, USA

Ihab R. Kamel, MD, PhD Russell H. Morgan Department of Radiology and Radiological Sciences, Johns Hopkins Hospital, Baltimore, MD, USA

Riham Katkhuda, MD Department of Molecular Pathology, The University of Texas MD Anderson Cancer Center, Houston, TX, USA

Florence K. Keane, MD Department of Radiation Oncology, Massachusetts General Hospital, Boston, MA, USA

Pegah Khoshpouri, MD Russell H. Morgan Department of Radiology and Radiological Sciences, Johns Hopkins Hospital, Baltimore, MD, USA

Georgios Antonios Margonis, MD, PhD John L. Cameron Division of Pancreatic and Hepatobiliary Surgery, Department of Surgery, The Johns Hopkins Hospital, Baltimore, MD, USA

Eleonora Milani, MD Department of Molecular Medicine, University of Padua, Padua, Italy

Jonathan D. Mizrahi, MD Division of Cancer Medicine, The University of Texas MD Anderson Cancer Center, Houston, TX, USA

Timothy M. Pawlik, MD, MPH, MTS, PhD, FACS, FRACS Wexner Medical Center, The Ohio State University Wexner Medical Center, Columbus, OH, USA

George A. Poultsides, MD, MS, FACS Department of Surgery, Stanford University Hospital, Stanford, CA, USA

Guojun Qian, MD Department of Ultrasound Interventional Therapy, Eastern Hepatobiliary Surgery Hospital, Naval Medical University, Shanghai, China

Amir A. Rahnemai-Azar, MD Department of Surgery, Division of Surgical Oncology, University of Wisconsin School of Medicine and Public Health, Madison, WI, USA

Janelle F. Rekman, MD, MAEd, FRCSC Section of General, Thoracic and Vascular Surgery, Virginia Mason Medical Center, Seattle, WA, USA

Flavio G. Rocha, MD Section of General, Thoracic and Vascular Surgery, Virginia Mason Medical Center, Seattle, WA, USA

Sean M. Ronnekleiv-Kelly, MD Department of Surgery, Division of Surgical Oncology, University of Wisconsin School of Medicine and Public Health, Madison, WI, USA

Andrea Ruzzenente, MD, PhD Department of Surgery, University of Verona, Verona, Italy

Susan Shamimi-Noori, MD Division of Interventional Radiology, Department of Radiology, Hospital of the University of Pennsylvania, Philadelphia, PA, USA

Feng Shen, MD Department of Hepatic Surgery, Eastern Hepatobiliary Surgery Hospital, Naval Medical University, Shanghai, China

Michael C. Soulen, MD Department of Radiology, Abramson Cancer Center, University of Pennsylvania, Philadelphia, PA, USA

Division of Interventional Radiology, Department of Radiology, Hospital of the University of Pennsylvania, Philadelphia, PA, USA

Mario Strazzabosco, MD, PhD International Center for Digestive Health (ICDH), University of Milano-Bicocca, Milano, Italy

Section of Digestive Diseases, Department of Internal Medicine, Yale University, New Haven, CT, USA

Benjamin J. Swanson, MD, PhD Department of Pathology and Microbiology, University of Nebraska Medical Center, Omaha, NE, USA

Sharon M. Weber, MD Department of Surgery, Division of Surgical Oncology, University of Wisconsin School of Medicine and Public Health, Madison, WI, USA

Jinglei Zhang, MMed Department of Ultrasound Interventional Therapy, Eastern Hepatobiliary Surgery Hospital, Naval Medical University, Shanghai, China

Chapter 1
Epidemiology and Risk Factors

Riham Katkhuda and Yun Shin Chun

Introduction

Cholangiocarcinoma arises from the epithelial lining of the intrahepatic or extrahepatic biliary tract. In the United States (USA), extrahepatic bile duct cancers located in the perihilar and distal bile duct account for 50–60% and 20–30% of all cholangiocarcinomas, respectively. Intrahepatic cholangiocarcinoma comprises 20% of all cholangiocarcinomas and is the second most common primary liver cancer, following hepatocellular carcinoma [1, 2]. The incidence of intrahepatic cholangiocarcinoma is rising, partly due to improved diagnosis, and is highly dependent upon geographic location. In the USA, approximately 5000 to 8000 patients are affected with intrahepatic cholangiocarcinoma annually [2]. In contrast, the prevalence is tenfold higher in Southeast Asia, due to endemic liver fluke infection [3].

Epidemiology

In the USA, the incidence of intrahepatic cholangiocarcinoma parallels advancing age, with a progressive increase starting in the sixth decade of life. The annual age-adjusted incidence of intrahepatic cholangiocarcinoma is 0.7–1.5 cases per 100,000 population [2]. Worldwide, there is variation in incidence rates related to

R. Katkhuda
Department of Molecular Pathology, The University of Texas MD Anderson Cancer Center, Houston, TX, USA
e-mail: rkatkhuda@mdanderson.org

Y. S. Chun (✉)
Department of Surgical Oncology, The University of Texas MD Anderson Cancer Center, Houston, TX, USA
e-mail: yschun@mdanderson.org

T. M. Pawlik et al. (eds.), *Intrahepatic Cholangiocarcinoma*,
https://doi.org/10.1007/978-3-030-22258-1_1

risk factors. The highest recorded incidence is in Thailand because of endemic liver fluke infection, leading to chronic injury and inflammation of the bile ducts. In Thailand, the age-adjusted incidence rate is greater than 80 per 100,000 population [4].

Several studies have reported a rising global incidence of intrahepatic cholangiocarcinoma and corresponding increased mortality. In England and Wales, from 1968 to 1996, Taylor-Robinson et al. reported a 15-fold increase in age-adjusted death rate from intrahepatic cholangiocarcinoma per 100,000 population aged 45 years and older [5]. The age-adjusted incidence rate for men in England and Wales rose from 0.11 per 100,000 population in 1971–1973 to 1.33 in 1999–2001; the rate in women also rose from 0.09 to 1.06 [6]. A study by Patel et al., based on the Surveillance, Epidemiology, and End Results (SEER) database in the USA, reported a rise in age-adjusted death rate from 0.07 per 100,000 in 1973 to 0.69 in 1997 (Fig. 1.1) [7]. Another SEER analysis by Shaib et al. found that age-adjusted incidence rates rose from 0.32 in 1975–1979 to 0.85 in 1995–1999, reflecting a 165% increase [8]. Men had higher age-adjusted incidence rates than women.

Although the reported increasing incidence of intrahepatic cholangiocarcinoma may reflect a true rise in the disease, it may also be attributable to improved diagnosis and coding misclassification. The International Classification of Disease for

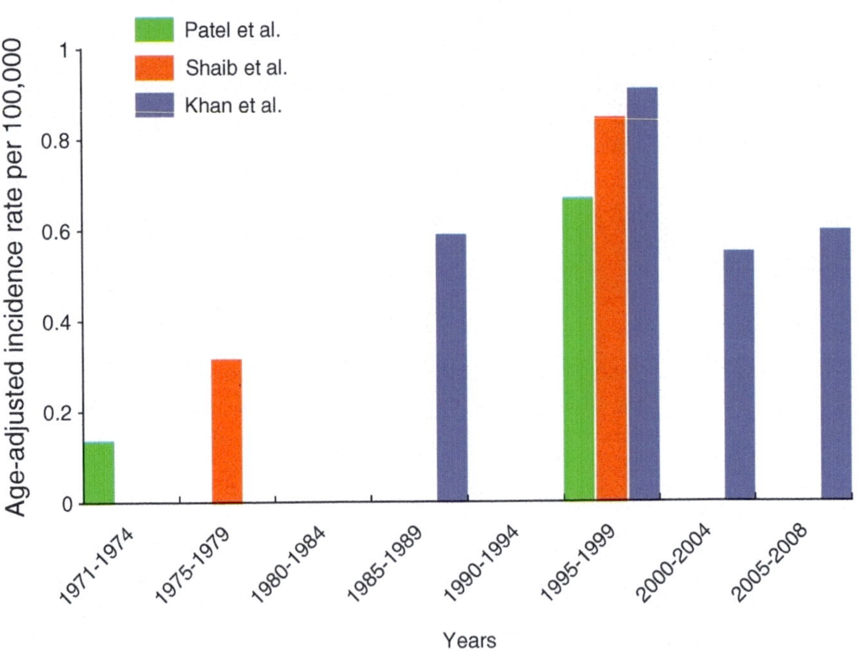

Fig. 1.1 Trends in age-adjusted incidence rates of intrahepatic cholangiocarcinoma per 100,000 population in the USA according to 3 analyses of the Surveillance, Epidemiology, and End Results (SEER) database

Oncology (ICD-O) editions are revised every few years and adopted by countries at different times. ICD-O comprises 2 coding systems to describe a tumor: a topographical code based on anatomic site and a morphological code based upon histology. The term "Klatskin tumor" is an eponym for perihilar cholangiocarcinoma, named after an American physician who described unique features of cholangiocarcinoma at the confluence of the right and left hepatic ducts. The second edition of the ICD-O designated a unique morphological code for Klatskin tumors which was cross-referenced to the topographical code for intrahepatic cholangiocarcinoma. The third edition of the ICD-O cross-referenced Klatskin tumors to either intra- or extrahepatic cholangiocarcinoma. In the USA, the third edition of the ICD-O (ICD-O-3) was adopted in 2001.

An analysis of the SEER database by Khan et al. showed an increase in age-adjusted incidence rate for intrahepatic cholangiocarcinoma from 0.59 per 100,000 population in 1990 to 0.91 in 2000 [9]. However, in 2001, coincident with adoption of the ICD-O-3, the rate fell and plateaued at 0.60 in 2007 (Fig. 1.1). Another SEER analysis found that, between 1992 to 2000, 91% of perihilar cholangiocarcinomas were incorrectly coded as intrahepatic cholangiocarcinoma, leading to an overestimation of intrahepatic cholangiocarcinoma by 13% [10]. However, even after excluding Klatskin tumors, the age-adjusted incidence rate of intrahepatic cholangiocarcinoma increased between 1992 and 2000. Taken together, these data suggest a true rise in incidence of intrahepatic cholangiocarcinoma between the 1970s and 1990s, followed by possibly a plateau in the 2000s.

Risk Factors

Risk factors for intrahepatic cholangiocarcinoma in Western countries include viral hepatitis, cirrhosis, and obesity, which are rising in incidence. The magnitude of risk of developing cholangiocarcinoma depends upon the factor and population studied (Table 1.1). Most patients diagnosed with intrahepatic cholangiocarcinoma do not have any identifiable risk factors. Environmental exposure to toxic chemicals, such as radon and Thorotrast, are primarily of historical interest and not applicable to patients today. In parts of Asia, liver fluke infection remains endemic, leading to high prevalence rates of intrahepatic cholangiocarcinoma.

Liver Flukes

The highest recorded incidence of cholangiocarcinoma is in northeast Thailand, where the liver fluke *Opisthorchis viverrini* is endemic. Here, approximately, 5000 cases are diagnosed annually, and the incidence rate among adults aged 35–64 is more than 100 per 100,000 population annually [11]. Another liver fluke, *Clonorchis sinensis*, is implicated in cholangiocarcinoma carcinogenesis

Table 1.1 Studies on risk factors for intrahepatic cholangiocarcinoma. Data presented as odds ratios (95% confidence interval)

Risk factor	Author, country, years of study				
	Petrick, USA, 2000–2011 [38]	Palmer, 1990–2011[a] [33]	Welzel, USA, 1993–2005 [30]	Zhou, China, 2004–2006 [40]	Kamsa-ard, Thailand, 1985–2014 [18]
Bile duct cyst	15.66 (11.58–21.18)		43.03 (29.16–63.49)		
Cirrhosis	8.26 (6.83–9.99)	22.92 (18.24–26.79)	22.11 (16.47–29.68)		
Opisthorchis viverrini infection					6.35 (2.87–14.05)
Hepatolithiasis				5.77 (1.97–16.85)	
Hepatitis C	4.67 (3.57–6.11)	4.84 (2.41–9.71)	8.05 (5.08–12.75)		
Hepatitis B	2.97 (1.97–4.46)	5.10 (2.91–8.95)	3.07 (1.43–6.58)	8.88 (5.97–13.19)	
Excess alcohol	3.72 (3.17–4.35)	2.81 (1.52–5.21)	5.69 (3.65–8.86)		3.01 (2.00–4.54)
Diabetes	1.54 (1.41–1.68)	1.89 (1.74–2.07)	1.82 (1.56–2.11)		
Obesity	1.42 (1.21–1.66)	1.56 (1.26–1.94)	1.71 (1.30–2.23)		
Cigarette smoking	1.46 (1.28–1.66)	1.31 (0.95–1.82)	2.21 (1.74–2.81)		1.46 (1.10–1.94)

[a]Meta-analysis of studies from Japan, Korea, the USA, Italy, China, and Denmark

in China and Korea. Both parasites are classified by the World Health Organization as group 1 carcinogens for cholangiocarcinoma. Unlike the distribution of cholangiocarcinoma in Western countries, where extrahepatic cancers predominate, up to 60% percent of cholangiocarcinomas associated with liver fluke infection are intrahepatic [12].

Liver fluke infections are endemic in areas where raw or poorly cooked fish is consumed. Human beings represent the definitive host of *O. viverrini*, which travels from the infected person's duodenum into the ampulla of Vater and bile duct. The adult fluke can live up to 20 years in the bile duct, mainly intrahepatic bile ducts, and lay eggs, which are passed with the infected person's feces [11]. The eggs are ingested by snails and metamorphose into free-swimming larvae, which then penetrate between the scales of freshwater fish, mostly cyprinoids such as carp. *C. sinensis* has a similar life cycle. Inside bile ducts, the liver flukes lead to DNA damage, periductal fibrosis, and periportal inflammation. Chronic injury and inflammation of the bile duct lead to cholangiocarcinoma development [13].

Among patients chronically infected with liver flukes, an estimated 8–10% will develop intrahepatic cholangiocarcinoma [14]. *O. viverrini* is prevalent not only in Thailand, but also in Laos, Vietnam, and Cambodia. In these countries, approximately 700 million people are at risk of liver fluke infection [15]. In Thailand, an estimated 6 million people are infected, with the highest prevalence in the Northeast region, where the prevalence of *O. viverrini* infection is as high as 67%, compared with only 0.1% in South Thailand [16]. Consequently, the incidence of cholangiocarcinoma in 2013 was significantly higher in Northeast Thailand than in the South (28.83 per 100,000 population, Northeast Thailand vs. 2.98, South).

Efforts to eradicate endemic liver fluke infection include education on eating raw fish, treatment with the antiparasitic praziquantel, and improvements in hygiene and sewage systems to interrupt disease transmission [11, 17]. With these measures, the incidence of *O. viverrini* infection in Thailand has fallen from greater than 60% in 1984 to less than 10% after 1997 [18]. However, infection rates remain high in the Mekong River where uncooked or improperly fermented fish remains a staple in the diet, particularly among the elderly. Treatment with praziquantel is effective, but reinfection often occurs [13].

C. sinensis is endemic in China, Korea, Vietnam, and East Russia. The highest prevalence is in China, where an estimated 15 million people are infected [19]. Worldwide, an estimated 5500 cases of cholangiocarcinoma annually are attributed to *C. sinensis* infection. Clonorchiasis is associated with two precancerous lesions, intraductal papillary neoplasm of the bile duct (IPNB) and biliary intraepithelial neoplasia. [20] IPNB is characterized by prominent intraductal papillary growth, mucin production, and potential to transform into invasive cholangiocarcinoma (Fig. 1.2). The incidence of IPNB is higher in Asia, where it accounts for up to 30% of bile duct tumors, in contrast to only 7–11% in Western countries [21].

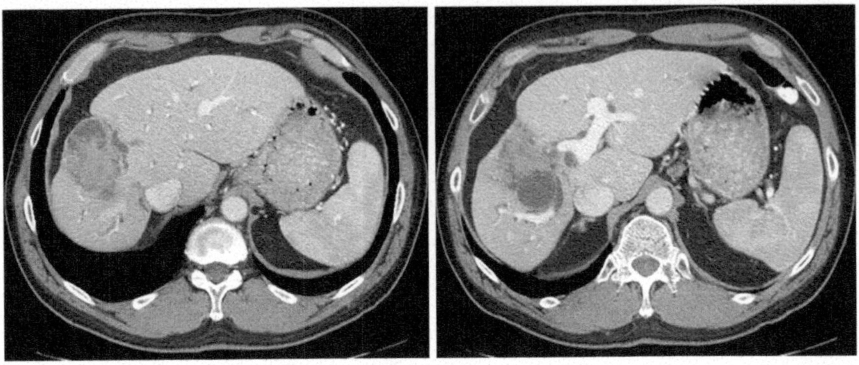

Fig. 1.2 Computed tomography images of intraductal papillary neoplasm of the bile duct that transformed to invasive intrahepatic cholangiocarcinoma

Hepatolithiasis

Hepatolithiasis, the formation of stones in the intrahepatic biliary tree, is more common in Asian countries than the West and leads to the development of intrahepatic cholangiocarcinoma in 7% of patients [22]. The stones are pigmented calcium bilirubinate stones and thought to arise from factors associated with poor hygiene and malnutrition [23]. Up to 30% of patients with hepatolithiasis also suffer from liver fluke infection [24]. Hepatolithiasis results in biliary strictures, bacterial infection, and secondary sclerosing cholangitis. The resultant chronic inflammation leads to hyperplasia and dysplasia, including precancerous lesions IPNB and biliary epithelial neoplasia, which can undergo malignant transformation.

Primary Sclerosing Cholangitis

Primary sclerosing cholangitis (PSC) is a chronic disease of unclear etiology characterized by progressive inflammation and fibrosis of the bile ducts. Patients with PSC have a 5–10% lifetime risk of developing cholangiocarcinoma, primarily perihilar cholangiocarcinoma [14]. Patients with PSC present with cholangiocarcinoma earlier, between the third and fifth decades of life, compared with patients with sporadic cholangiocarcinoma, whose mean age at presentation is the seventh decade [22].

Bile Duct Cysts

Bile duct cysts are congenital cystic dilatations of the biliary tree, classified by their location, shape, and extent [25]. The most common types are type I, solitary, extrahepatic cyst, and type IV, multiple extrahepatic, or extra- and intrahepatic cysts. A meta-analysis of 2904 patients with bile duct cysts reported a 7.3% prevalence of malignancy [26]. Cyst drainage had a higher risk of malignancy compared with complete cyst excision, with an odds ratio of 3.97. Bile duct cysts are more prevalent in Asia than in Western countries. Furthermore, the incidence of cholangiocarcinoma is higher in Asian patients with bile duct cysts, approximately 18%, compared with 5% in the US patients [14, 27]. Average age at diagnosis with cholangiocarcinoma is 33, and incidence increases with age.

Type V bile duct cysts, also known as Caroli's disease, are rare and characterized by saccular ectasia of intrahepatic bile ducts. Caroli's disease can be associated with congenital hepatic fibrosis and autosomal recessive disease as Caroli's syndrome. Patients with Caroli's disease reportedly harbor a 100-fold greater risk of developing cholangiocarcinoma than the general population [28].

Viral Hepatitis

Two studies based on the SEER database demonstrated an increased risk of intrahepatic cholangiocarcinoma with hepatitis C infection, but not with hepatitis B [29, 30]. In contrast, a study from Italy reported a hepatitis B rate of 13% among patients with intrahepatic cholangiocarcinoma, compared with 6.7% in controls without cholangiocarcinoma [31]. Hepatitis C is consistently found to be a stronger risk factor for intrahepatic cholangiocarcinoma than hepatitis B [22]. The risk of developing intrahepatic cholangiocarcinoma with hepatitis C is 3.5% at 10 years, which is significantly lower than the risk of developing hepatocellular carcinoma [32]. With both hepatitis B and C, it is unclear if the viral infection itself or the cirrhotic, diseased liver plays a greater role in the development of intrahepatic cholangiocarcinoma.

Cirrhosis

Cirrhosis is a strong risk factor for development of both hepatocellular carcinoma and intrahepatic cholangiocarcinoma. In a meta-analysis of risk factors for intrahepatic cholangiocarcinoma, cirrhosis had the highest combined odds ratio of 22.92, compared with other risk factors including viral hepatitis, diabetes, and obesity [33]. Cirrhosis confers a 30-fold increased risk of hepatocellular carcinoma and a 10- to 20-fold increase in intrahepatic cholangiocarcinoma [34]. The mechanisms leading to cirrhosis, including hepatocyte cell death, proliferation, and fibrosis, promote hepatocarcinogenesis. Shared risk factors for both hepatocellular carcinoma and intrahepatic cholangiocarcinoma support the hypothesis of a common pathogenesis. The term "combined hepatocellular-cholangiocarcinoma" includes a heterogeneous group of tumors that have varying degrees of hepatocytic and cholangiocytic differentiation [35]. Stem cell features are observed histologically and by immunohistochemistry, suggesting a single precursor population that can give rise to both hepatocellular carcinoma and intrahepatic cholangiocarcinoma [33].

Obesity

Lifestyle is increasingly recognized as a risk factor for malignancy and higher cancer-related mortality [36]. Obesity is an epidemic in the USA, with one third of the adult population classified as obese. Nonalcoholic fatty liver disease (NAFLD) occurs in 30% of US adults due to the prevalence of the metabolic syndrome, marked by obesity, diabetes, hypertension, and/or hyperlipidemia. NAFLD can progress to nonalcoholic steatohepatitis, cirrhosis, and primary liver cancer [37]. In addition, NAFLD may exert synergistic effects with viral hepatitis in the development of intrahepatic cholangiocarcinoma.

A study of the SEER database found that 29.7% of patients who developed intrahepatic cholangiocarcinoma had the metabolic syndrome compared with 17.1% in the control group [30]. Another SEER analysis reported that NAFLD conferred a threefold increased risk of intrahepatic cholangiocarcinoma [38]. In addition, a meta-analysis by Palmer et al. identified diabetes and obesity as major risk factors for intrahepatic cholangiocarcinoma, with odds ratios of 1.89 and 1.56, respectively [33].

Smoking and Alcohol

Studies on the association between smoking and risk of intrahepatic cholangiocarcinoma have demonstrated inconsistent results [22]. In contrast, excess alcohol intake was shown in a meta-analysis to be a risk factor, with an odds ratio of 2.81 [33]. Petrick et al. analyzed pooled data from a consortium of 14 US-based prospective cohort studies and found that consuming ≥5 alcoholic beverages a day was associated with a 68% increased risk of developing intrahepatic cholangiocarcinoma [39].

Conclusion

The highest prevalence of intrahepatic cholangiocarcinoma is in Southeast Asia and is attributed to endemic liver fluke infection. Rates are also high in China and Korea due to clonorchiasis and hepatolithiasis, which give rise to premalignant neoplasms that can transform into invasive cancer. In Western countries, most patients do not have an identifiable risk factor. The most prevalent risk factors associated with intrahepatic cholangiocarcinoma in the USA are cirrhosis, obesity, and viral hepatitis. Due to the epidemic of obesity in the USA, the incidence of intrahepatic cholangiocarcinoma may rise, paralleling the rise in hepatocellular carcinoma related to NAFLD. Lifestyle changes in the East and West can reduce the prevalence of risk factors and potentially reduce the incidence of intrahepatic cholangiocarcinoma.

References

1. Rizvi S, Khan SA, Hallemeier CL, Kelley RK, Gores GJ. Cholangiocarcinoma – evolving concepts and therapeutic strategies. Nat Rev Clin Oncol. 2018;15(2):95–111.
2. Sia D, Tovar V, Moeini A, Llovet JM. Intrahepatic cholangiocarcinoma: pathogenesis and rationale for molecular therapies. Oncogene. 2013;32(41):4861–70.
3. Javle M, Lowery M, Shroff RT, Weiss KH, Springfeld C, Borad MJ, et al. Phase II study of BGJ398 in patients with FGFR-altered advanced cholangiocarcinoma. J Clin Oncol. 2018;36(3):276–82.
4. Lafaro KJ, Cosgrove D, Geschwind JF, Kamel I, Herman JM, Pawlik TM. Multidisciplinary care of patients with intrahepatic cholangiocarcinoma: updates in management. Gastroenterol Res Pract. 2015;2015:860861.
5. Taylor-Robinson SD, Foster GR, Arora S, Hargreaves S, Thomas HC. Increase in primary liver cancer in the UK, 1979–94. Lancet. 1997;350(9085):1142–3.
6. West J, Wood H, Logan RF, Quinn M, Aithal GP. Trends in the incidence of primary liver and biliary tract cancers in England and Wales 1971–2001. Br J Cancer. 2006;94(11):1751–8.
7. Patel T. Increasing incidence and mortality of primary intrahepatic cholangiocarcinoma in the United States. Hepatology. 2001;33(6):1353–7.
8. Shaib YH, Davila JA, McGlynn K, El-Serag HB. Rising incidence of intrahepatic cholangiocarcinoma in the United States: a true increase? J Hepatol. 2004;40(3):472–7.
9. Khan SA, Emadossadaty S, Ladep NG, Thomas HC, Elliott P, Taylor-Robinson SD, et al. Rising trends in cholangiocarcinoma: is the ICD classification system misleading us? J Hepatol. 2012;56(4):848–54.
10. Welzel TM, McGlynn KA, Hsing AW, O'Brien TR, Pfeiffer RM. Impact of classification of hilar cholangiocarcinomas (Klatskin tumors) on the incidence of intra- and extrahepatic cholangiocarcinoma in the United States. J Natl Cancer Inst. 2006;98(12):873–5.
11. Sripa B, Bethony JM, Sithithaworn P, Kaewkes S, Mairiang E, Loukas A, et al. Opisthorchiasis and Opisthorchis-associated cholangiocarcinoma in Thailand and Laos. Acta Trop. 2011;120(Suppl 1):S158–68.
12. Luvira V, Nilprapha K, Bhudhisawasdi V, Pugkhem A, Chamadol N, Kamsa-ard S. Cholangiocarcinoma patient outcome in northeastern Thailand: single-center prospective study. Asian Pac J Cancer Prev. 2016;17(1):401–6.
13. Yongvanit P, Pinlaor S, Loilome W. Risk biomarkers for assessment and chemoprevention of liver fluke-associated cholangiocarcinoma. J Hepatobiliary Pancreat Sci. 2014;21(5):309–15.
14. Gupta A, Dixon E. Epidemiology and risk factors: intrahepatic cholangiocarcinoma. Hepatobiliary Surg Nutr. 2017;6(2):101–4.
15. Cai Q. Infectious agents associated cancers : epidemiology and molecular biology. New York: Springer Berlin Heidelberg; 2017.
16. Chaiteerakij R, Pan-Ngum W, Poovorawan K, Soonthornworasiri N, Treeprasertsuk S, Phaosawasdi K. Characteristics and outcomes of cholangiocarcinoma by region in Thailand: a nationwide study. World J Gastroenterol. 2017;23(39):7160–7.
17. Kaewpitoon SJ, Rujirakul R, Loyd RA, Panpimanmas S, Matrakool L, Tongtawee T, et al. Re-examination of Opisthorchis viverrini in Nakhon Ratchasima Province, northeastern Thailand, indicates continued needs for health intervention. Asian Pac J Cancer Prev. 2016;17(1):231–4.

18. Kamsa-Ard S, Luvira V, Suwanrungruang K, Kamsa-Ard S, Luvira V, Santong C, et al. Cholangiocarcinoma trends, incidence, and relative survival in Khon Kaen, Thailand from 1989 through 2013: a population-based cancer registry study. J Epidemiol. 2018;29(5):197–204.
19. Qian MB, Chen YD, Liang S, Yang GJ, Zhou XN. The global epidemiology of clonorchiasis and its relation with cholangiocarcinoma. Infect Dis Poverty. 2012;1(1):4.
20. Lim JH. Liver flukes: the malady neglected. Korean J Radiol. 2011;12(3):269–79.
21. Park HJ, Kim SY, Kim HJ, Lee SS, Hong GS, Byun JH, et al. Intraductal papillary neoplasm of the bile duct: clinical, imaging, and pathologic features. AJR Am J Roentgenol. 2018;211(1):67–75.
22. Razumilava N, Gores GJ. Cholangiocarcinoma. Lancet. 2014;383(9935):2168–79.
23. Tsui WM, Lam PW, Lee WK, Chan YK. Primary hepatolithiasis, recurrent pyogenic cholangitis, and oriental cholangiohepatitis: a tale of 3 countries. Adv Anat Pathol. 2011;18(4):318–28.
24. Tyson GL, El-Serag HB. Risk factors for cholangiocarcinoma. Hepatology. 2011;54(1):173–84.
25. Todani T, Watanabe Y, Narusue M, Tabuchi K, Okajima K. Congenital bile duct cysts: classification, operative procedures, and review of thirty-seven cases including cancer arising from choledochal cyst. Am J Surg. 1977;134(2):263–9.
26. Ten Hove A, de Meijer VE, Hulscher JBF, de Kleine RHJ. Meta-analysis of risk of developing malignancy in congenital choledochal malformation. Br J Surg. 2018;105(5):482–90.
27. Bridgewater J, Galle PR, Khan SA, Llovet JM, Park JW, Patel T, et al. Guidelines for the diagnosis and management of intrahepatic cholangiocarcinoma. J Hepatol. 2014;60(6):1268–89.
28. Mabrut JY, Kianmanesh R, Nuzzo G, Castaing D, Boudjema K, Letoublon C, et al. Surgical management of congenital intrahepatic bile duct dilatation, Caroli's disease and syndrome: long-term results of the French Association of Surgery Multicenter Study. Ann Surg. 2013;258(5):713–21; discussion 21.
29. Shaib YH, El-Serag HB, Davila JA, Morgan R, McGlynn KA. Risk factors of intrahepatic cholangiocarcinoma in the United States: a case-control study. Gastroenterology. 2005;128(3):620–6.
30. Welzel TM, Graubard BI, Zeuzem S, El-Serag HB, Davila JA, McGlynn KA. Metabolic syndrome increases the risk of primary liver cancer in the United States: a study in the SEER-Medicare database. Hepatology. 2011;54(2):463–71.
31. Donato F, Gelatti U, Tagger A, Favret M, Ribero ML, Callea F, et al. Intrahepatic cholangiocarcinoma and hepatitis C and B virus infection, alcohol intake, and hepatolithiasis: a case-control study in Italy. Cancer Causes Control. 2001;12(10):959–64.
32. Bridgewater JA, Goodman KA, Kalyan A, Mulcahy MF. Biliary tract cancer: epidemiology, radiotherapy, and molecular profiling. Am Soc Clin Oncol Educ Book. 2016;35:e194–203.
33. Palmer WC, Patel T. Are common factors involved in the pathogenesis of primary liver cancers? A meta-analysis of risk factors for intrahepatic cholangiocarcinoma. J Hepatol. 2012;57(1):69–76.
34. Massarweh NN, El-Serag HB. Epidemiology of hepatocellular carcinoma and intrahepatic cholangiocarcinoma. Cancer Control. 2017;24(3):1073274817729245.
35. Brunt E, Aishima S, Clavien PA, Fowler K, Goodman Z, Gores G, et al. cHCC-CCA: consensus terminology for primary liver carcinomas with both hepatocytic and cholangiocytic differentation. Hepatology. 2018;68(1):113–26.
36. Calle EE, Rodriguez C, Walker-Thurmond K, Thun MJ. Overweight, obesity, and mortality from cancer in a prospectively studied cohort of U.S. adults. N Engl J Med. 2003;348(17):1625–38.
37. Page JM, Harrison SA. NASH and HCC. Clin Liver Dis. 2009;13(4):631–47.
38. Petrick JL, Yang B, Altekruse SF, Van Dyke AL, Koshiol J, Graubard BI, et al. Risk factors for intrahepatic and extrahepatic cholangiocarcinoma in the United States: a population-based study in SEER-Medicare. PLoS One. 2017;12(10):e0186643.
39. Petrick JL, Campbell PT, Koshiol J, Thistle JE, Andreotti G, Beane-Freeman LE, et al. Tobacco, alcohol use and risk of hepatocellular carcinoma and intrahepatic cholangiocarcinoma: the liver cancer pooling project. Br J Cancer. 2018;118(7):1005–12.
40. Zhou YM, Yin ZF, Yang JM, Li B, Shao WY, Xu F, et al. Risk factors for intrahepatic cholangiocarcinoma: a case-control study in China. World J Gastroenterol. 2008;14(4):632–5.

Chapter 2
Clinical Presentation and Diagnosis

Arezou Abbasi, Amir A. Rahnemai-Azar, Sean M. Ronnekleiv-Kelly, Daniel E. Abbott, and Sharon M. Weber

Introduction

Cholangiocarcinoma (CCA) is a diverse group of malignancies arising from the epithelial lining of the biliary tract and encompasses three distinct anatomic categories, namely intrahepatic (ICC), perihilar (pCCA), and distal (dCCA) cholangiocarcinoma. Each of the categories demonstrates different clinical, morphologic, and epidemiologic features [1]. The ICC variant develops from the malignant transformation of the cholangiocytes located proximal to the second-degree bile ducts.

In the classic model of ICC pathogenesis, chronic biliary inflammation and cholestasis triggered by external stimuli (e.g., liver fluke or hepatitis viral infection) instigate malignant transformation of cholangiocytes [2]. However, recent findings have challenged the classic model of a single cholangiocyte progenitor to explain both intratumoral heterogeneity and subtype phenotypic heterogeneity in ICC. Malignant transformation of multiple peribiliary stem cell niches as well as hepatic progenitor cells has been proposed as potential progenitors rather than a single cholangiocyte [3].

The majority of cholangiocarcinomas are adenocarcinomas (>90%), with the rare occurrence of other histologic subtypes such as squamous cell carcinoma,

A. Abbasi
Department of Surgery, University of Washington Medical Center, Seattle, WA, USA

A. A. Rahnemai-Azar · S. M. Ronnekleiv-Kelly · D. E. Abbott · S. M. Weber (✉)
Department of Surgery, Division of Surgical Oncology, University of Wisconsin School of Medicine and Public Health, Madison, WI, USA
e-mail: rahnemaiazar@wisc.edu; ronnekleiv-kelly@surgery.wisc.edu; abbott@surgery.wisc.edu; webers@surgery.wisc.edu

T. M. Pawlik et al. (eds.), *Intrahepatic Cholangiocarcinoma*,
https://doi.org/10.1007/978-3-030-22258-1_2

signet-ring carcinoma, papillary adenocarcinoma, clear cell, and lymphoepithelial types [4]. The mixed hepatocellular-cholangiocarcinoma subtype is a histologically distinct presentation, especially in patients with chronic liver disease, and is associated with poor prognosis. In contrast to the described histologic subtypes, ICC is also classified according to pathologic growth pattern. Under this system, morphologic subtypes of cholangiocarcinoma have been described: mass-forming, periductal infiltrating, intraductal growth, and mixed type (periductal infiltrating and mass-forming) ICC [5]. In addition to distinct characteristics in cross-sectional imaging, these three subtypes are associated with different proliferative activity and biologic behavior. Mass-forming subtype is the most common type of ICC, which usually spreads to the liver parenchyma via the portal system at early stages followed by invasion of the lymphatic vessels [6–8]. In contrast, the periductal infiltrating subtype grows longitudinally along and within the biliary tract with resultant ductal dilatation. Finally, the intraductal type grows into the bile duct with a papillary growth pattern. As a result of different biologic behavior and spreading patterns, the mass-forming subtype typically develops intrahepatic metastasis, while periductal subtype presents with pedicular lymph node metastasis.

Due to silent nature of the disease in early stages, especially in patients without a previous history of liver disease, the majority of patients present at advanced stages when the tumor has already metastasized or progressed locally to involve adjacent vital structures. Unfortunately, delayed clinical diagnosis limits the benefit of surgical treatment and curative management options, contributing to the poor outcome of ICC patients. Similarly, due to the tumor burden and complex biologic heterogeneity, the currently available systemic and targeted therapies pose a limited therapeutic benefit. Therefore, early diagnosis and screening of high-risk patients play a crucial role in optimizing the outcomes of patients with ICC.

Epidemiology and Risk Factors

ICC is the second most common primary liver tumor after hepatocellular carcinoma (HCC) [9]. Despite its lower frequency compared to other biliary tract carcinomas and HCC, there has been an increasing trend in incidence and mortality rate of ICC globally in recent years [10–14]. In the United States, the age-adjusted incidence rate has increased by 165% from 0.32 per 100,000 (95% CI 0.28–0.36) in 1975–1979 to 0.85 per 100,000 (95% CI 0.80–0.90) in 1995–1999 [10]. Likewise, the age-adjusted mortality rate increased from 0.07 per 100,000 in 1973 to 0.69 per 100,000 in 1997, with an estimated annual percent change of 9.44% (95% CI, 8.46–10.41) [15].

Primary sclerosing cholangitis (PSC), hepatolithiasis, biliary tract cysts, hepatobiliary flukes (*Clonorchis sinensis, Opisthorchis viverrini)*, cirrhosis, chronic hepatitis B and C, diabetes, alcohol, obesity and nonalcoholic fatty liver disease, and toxins such as nitrosamines and vinyl chloride are some of the known risk factors of ICC [16]. The chronic biliary inflammatory process caused by some of these risk factors has been identified as a trigger of increased cholangiocyte turnover and subsequent tumorigenesis [17]. However, most ICC cases occur de novo in otherwise healthy individuals without a known underlying liver disease.

Clinical Presentation

Most patients with ICC remain asymptomatic until advanced stages of the disease [18]. In 28% of cases, the tumor is detected incidentally during a physical examination or cross-sectional imaging, which is performed for other reasons. Furthermore, in some cases, abnormal liver function tests may initiate clinical suspicion. Vague nonspecific abdominal pain or constitutional symptoms such as malaise, fatigue, night sweats, and weight loss are some of the most common complains of the patient at the time of presentation [19]. Unlike other biliary tract and hepatic malignancies, jaundice is an infrequent presentation, involving only 11–16% of patients with ICC [20, 21]. Compression of the biliary duct confluence by tumor located in an adjacent location or malignant infiltration of the Glissonian sheath, mostly in periductal ICC, is the leading cause of jaundice in ICC patients. The presence of hepatomegaly or ascites at the time of presentation is an ominous sign of advanced disease.

Diagnosis

Due to the nonspecific presenting symptoms, history taking and physical examination have a limited role in the diagnosing of ICC. Once there is a clinical suspicion, thorough diagnostic investigations are mandatory to confirm the diagnosis and plan for the treatment.

Laboratory Biomarkers

Although liver function tests and tumor markers are routinely assessed in the context of suspicious liver masses, there is low sensitivity and specificity for a conclusive diagnosis. Serum bilirubin level usually is not elevated in patients with ICC, unless there is biliary confluence compression or infiltration of the Glissonian pedicle by the tumor. The elevated serum aminotransferases are mostly observed in advanced disease due to extensive liver parenchyma replacement by the tumor and associated hepatocytes damage [22].

CA 19-9 is a sialylated Lewis blood group antigen that is naturally produced by normal human pancreatic cells, biliary ductal cells, and gastric and colonic epithelial cells. Hence, it may be elevated in a variety of benign biliary diseases (e.g., cholangitis, primary biliary cirrhosis) as well as other gastrointestinal malignancies (e.g., pancreatic and gastric cancers). Therefore, the majority of studies examining CA 19-9 as a biomarker for detection of CCA have noted suboptimal accuracy with a wide variation of reported sensitivity (38–93%) and specificity (67–98%) [23, 24]. Furthermore, CA 19-9 is not detectable in 7% of the general population due to the absence of the Lewis antigen. Notwithstanding these limitations, utilization of CA 19-9 may still have a role. A recent meta-analysis of 31 articles including 1264 CCA patients and 2039 controls concluded that serum CA 19-9 was a useful diagnostic biomarker for CCA with 72% and 84% diagnostic sensitivity and specificity, respectively [24]. Shen et al. demonstrated that serum concentrations of CA19-9 were elevated in 57% of 429 patients with ICC and that high levels of CA19-9 (>37 U/mL) effectively predicted the incidence of lymph node metastasis (LNM) and survival [25]. A separate meta-analysis by Liu et al. also demonstrated that elevated preoperative CA19-9 levels correlated with a poor prognosis [26].

Carcinoembryonic antigen (CEA), an effective marker for colorectal cancer, is also frequently elevated in the setting of other gastrointestinal and gynecologic malignancies, but with demonstrated low diagnostic yield in the diagnosis of ICC. Serum alpha-fetoprotein (AFP), a well-known and commonly used biomarker for HCC, can sometimes be used to differentiate between HCC and ICC. Tao et al. used a combination of AFP and CA242 to increase the specificity of AFP to differentiate between ICC and HCC [27]. Recent advances have elucidated molecular and genetic characteristics of ICC and offered the potential for molecular-based diagnosis of ICC. Several genomic (e.g., secreted phosphoprotein 1 (SPP1), *KRAS* and *PIK3CA mutations,* expression of SMAD4 and TGF-β) and proteomic markers (e.g., IL-6, 14-3-3 protein, serum cytokeratin 19 fragments) have been demonstrated to play a role in the diagnosis and prediction of the prognosis of ICC [28]. However, the clinical applicability of most existing markers is limited due to a lack of adequate sensitivity and specificity.

Imaging Modalities

Ultrasonography (US) is frequently the initial abdominal imaging in the investigation of patients with vague abdominal pain. The mass-forming ICC presents as an irregular lesion with intermediate to increased echogenicity and a peripheral hypoechoic halo with or without intrahepatic biliary ductal dilation. However, these findings are not specific and cannot be used to differentiate ICC from other liver malignancies. Recently, contrast-enhanced US (CEUS) has been used with increasing frequency to investigate liver lesions. Different morphologic types of ICC show distinct diagnostic features on CEUS (Fig. 2.1). On CEUS images, hyperenhancing areas are indicative of increased cancer cells density, whereas hypoenhancing parts are correlated with the presence of fibrous stroma. In the arterial phase, the mass-forming ICC might present as four different enhancement

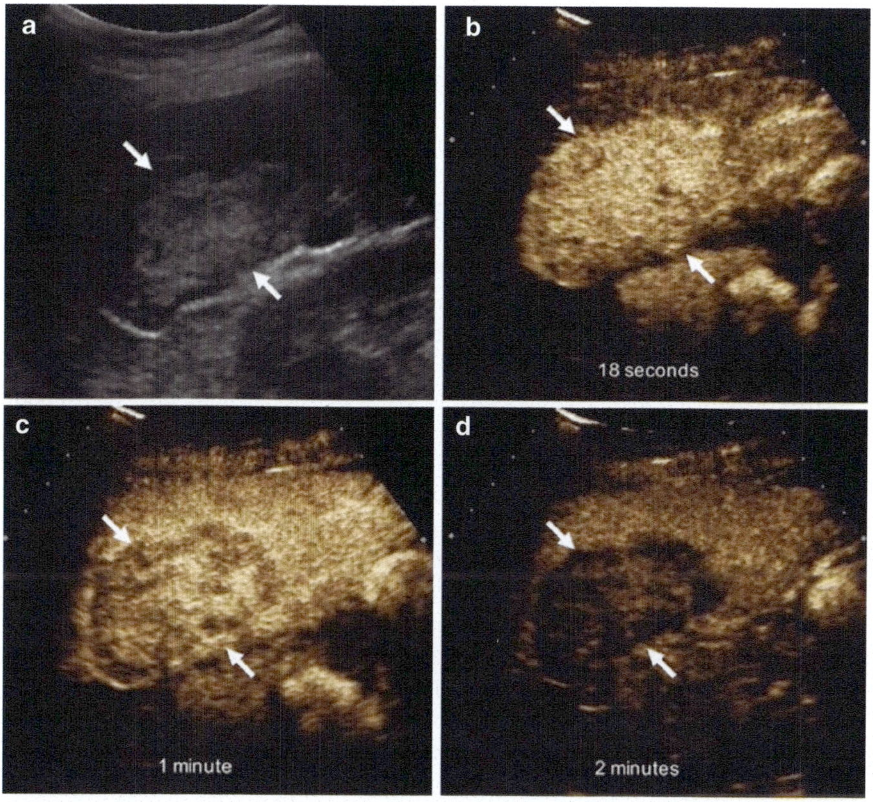

Fig. 2.1 Ultrasonographic studies of intrahepatic cholangiocarcinoma: Sagittal B-mode image (**a**) shows a heterogeneous predominantly hyperechoic lesion with a hypoechoic halo (arrows) in the right liver lobe. Contrast-enhanced ultrasound (**b**–**d**) demonstrates that the lesion (arrows) has homogenous arterial phase enhancement (**b**), followed by early and heterogeneous washout in the portal venous phase within 60 s (**c**) as well as hypoenhancement in the late phase (**d**). (Reprinted by permission from SpringerNature: Durot et al. [37])

patterns: (1) peripheral irregular rim-like enhancement, (2) heterogeneous hyperenhancement, (3) homogeneous hyperenhancement, or (4) heterogeneous hypoenhancement. These patterns have been demonstrated to correspond with the histopathological characteristics of the tumor [29]. Peripheral irregular rim-like enhancement corresponds with a central fibrous stroma surrounded by cancerous cells. Hyperenhancing ICC, both homogenous and heterogeneous, are associated with malignant cells located both centrally and peripherally. Ultimately, heterogeneous hypoenhancing tumors have a scarce number of cancerous cells. Furthermore, the size of the tumor correlates with either homogeneous or heterogeneous enhancement as well [30]. Small ICC with less fibrous tissue and abundant cancerous cells has homogeneous pattern, while large ICC that mostly comprised of fibrous tissue enhances heterogeneously. Periductal infiltrating ICC appears as a heterogeneously enhancing lesion in the arterial phase and stays hypoenhancing in both the portal and late phases [30]. Intraductal ICC has a pattern of homogenous hyperenhancement in the arterial phase and hypoenhancement in both the portal and late phases. As CEUS contrast materials are blood pool tracers without extravasation to the stroma, delayed enhancement pattern cannot be detected on delayed phase. Therefore, on CEUS, ICC may resemble HCC with early enhancement and subsequent washout. The delayed enhancement pattern on computed tomography (CT) scan with intravenous contrast images is a sign of contrast material washout from the blood pool and retention in the fibrous stroma. Of note, rim-like enhancement pattern might also be visualized in other primary liver cancers and further investigations are required prior to definitive diagnosis [29].

Cross-sectional imaging studies such as CT scan and magnetic resonance imaging (MRI) are diagnostic modalities used to improve assessment of the type of tumor, the extent of the tumor invasion locally, for the presence of metastatic disease, and the tumor's resectability. On the other hand, ICC imaging features on CT scan often are not specific enough to render tissue biopsy unnecessary [16]. ICC typically presents as a hypo- to isodense mass with irregular and infiltrative margins on noncontrast CT [31]. Mild peripheral rim enhancement with central hypodensity is the dominant feature in the arterial phase, which may become iso- or hypodense in the portal venous phase (Fig. 2.2). The central hypodensity progressively hyperattenuates during the delayed phase, unless there is abundant central mucin or necrosis. The central fibrous stroma retaining the slowly diffused contrast material is the reason for delayed and progressive enhancing of the ICC lesions. This pattern can differentiate ICC from HCC, which presents as an enhancing lesion in the arterial phase with rapid washout during the venous and delayed phases, mainly due to the hypercellular characteristic of HCC with scarce fibrous tissue. However, small size ICC might have a similar presentation to HCC on CT scan images due to hypercellularity of the tumor.

On MRI, ICC mass presents as a hypo- to isointense lesion compared to the liver parenchyma on the T1-weighted study [32]. In the presence of abundant fibrosis, T2-weighted study tends to show slight hyperintensity along with pooling of the contrast on delayed images, while strong hyperintensity is a sign of necrosis or mucous secretion [33]. Similar to contrast-enhanced CT, gadolinium-enhanced MRI shows a hypovascular mass with progressive concentric filling. Additionally, MRI with cholangiopancreatography (MRI/ MRCP) permits an improved visualization of the intra- and extrahepatic bile ducts, vascular structures, and anatomic extent of the tumor.

Unlike other imaging techniques, [18] F-fluorodeoxyglucose positron emission tomography (FDG-PET) is regarded as a staging modality rather than a diagnostic tool. The role of FDG-PET in management of biliary tract cancers is ill-identified. However, there is emerging evidence that, in patients with potentially resectable tumors based on conventional imaging, FDG-PET can identify occult metastatic disease that may alter treatment decision making [34, 35].

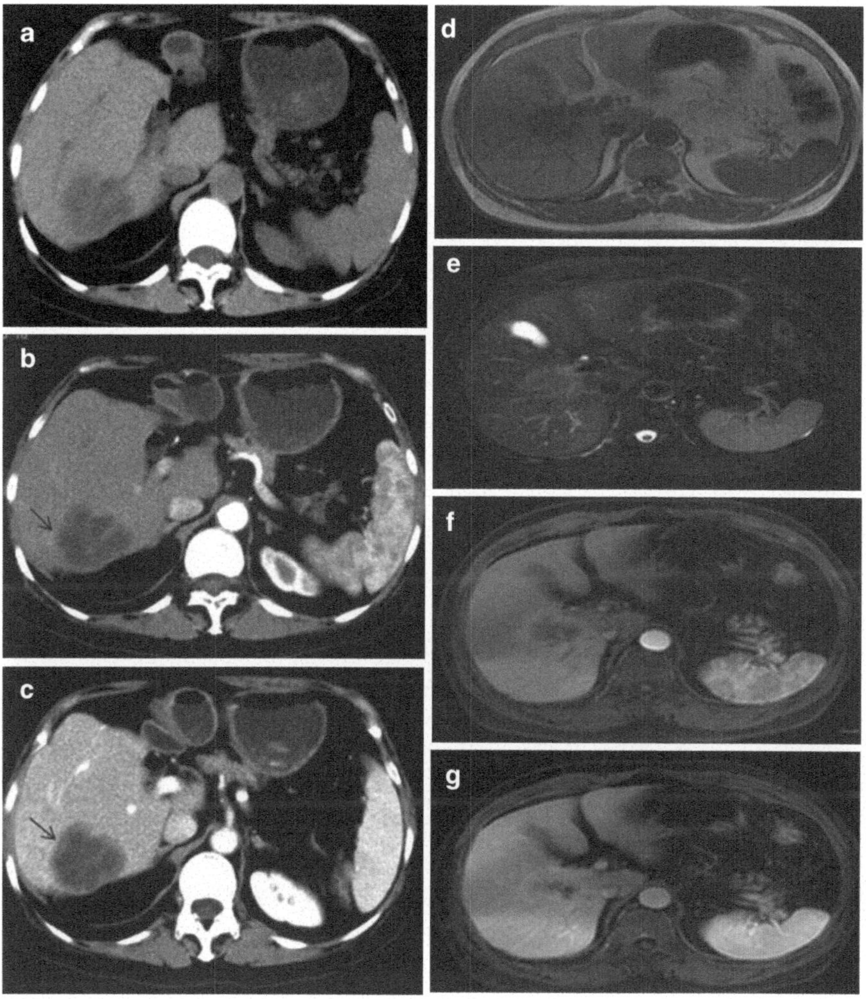

Fig. 2.2 CompuRadiographic features of intrahepatic cholangiocarcinoma: (**a–c**) Computed tomography showing a low-density mass with a regular and distinct boundary on arterial (**b**) and portal venous phases (**c**). (**d–g**) Magnetic resonance imaging showing a mass low signal on T1-W1 (**d**) and a heterogeneous high signal on T2-W1 (**e**) with a regular and distinct boundary. The same features are present on the enhanced T1-W1, with a sharp ring-like enhancement, during the arterial (**f**) and portal venous phases (**g**). (From Jiang et al. [38], by permission of Oxford University Press)

Tissue Diagnosis

Although clinical presentation, laboratory analyses, and radiologic studies raise the clinical suspicion, the definitive diagnosis of ICC is possible only via tissue biopsy. In the case of high clinical suspicion, even a negative biopsy does not rule out the disease due to sampling error. The pathologic confirmation is mandatory in patients who are unresectable due to underlying liver disease. Furthermore, tissue biopsy is recommended in patients who are being considered for clinical trials or neoadjuvant therapy [31].

The most common pathologic feature of ICC is adenocarcinoma showing tubular and/or papillary structures with variable fibrous stroma [16]. Histologically, ICC and metastatic adenocarcinoma from other primary tumors, especially foregut malignancies, have similar features and further immunohistochemical evaluation warrants a definitive diagnosis [31]. Similarly, differentiating between ICC and mixed hepatocellular tumors requires further investigation using specific markers of hepatocellular progenitor cells (e.g., Hep-Par-1, GPC3, HSP70, EpCAM, etc.) [36]

Conclusion

In summary, the majority of patients with ICC present as either an incidental finding or with vague abdominal symptoms. Several serum lab tests and/or radiographic features are suggestive of ICC, but tissue biopsy is needed to confirm the diagnosis. Despite recent advances in the development of novel diagnostic modalities, the majority of patients with ICC present at an advanced stage when the tumor is locally advanced or has already metastasized. Therefore, novel methods that permit earlier diagnosis of ICC are imperative to improve patient outcomes from this aggressive malignancy. Future studies are required to focus on improved understanding of the molecular pathogenesis of ICC with the hope of identifying novel molecular biomarkers with higher diagnostic and prognostic accuracy.

References

1. Razumilava N, Gores GJ. Cholangiocarcinoma. Lancet. 2014;383(9935):2168–79.
2. Hill MA, Alexander WB, Guo B, Kato Y, Patra KC, O'Dell MR, et al. Kras and Tp53 mutations cause cholangiocyte-and hepatocyte-derived cholangiocarcinoma. Cancer Res. 2018;78(16):4445–51.
3. Andersen JB. Molecular pathogenesis of intrahepatic cholangiocarcinoma. J Hepatobiliary Pancreat Sci. 2015;22(2):101–13.
4. Nakanuma Y, Sato Y, Harada K, Sasaki M, Xu J, Ikeda H. Pathological classification of intrahepatic cholangiocarcinoma based on a new concept. World J Hepatol. 2010;2(12):419.
5. Banales JM, Cardinale V, Carpino G, Marzioni M, Andersen JB, Invernizzi P, et al. Expert consensus document: cholangiocarcinoma: current knowledge and future perspectives consensus statement from the European Network for the Study of Cholangiocarcinoma (ENS-CCA). Nat Rev Gastroenterol Hepatol. 2016;13(5):261.
6. Blechacz B, Komuta M, Roskams T, Gores GJ. Clinical diagnosis and staging of cholangiocarcinoma. Nat Rev Gastroenterol Hepatol. 2011;8:512.
7. Nathan H, Aloia TA, Vauthey J-N, Abdalla EK, Zhu AX, Schulick RD, et al. A proposed staging system for intrahepatic cholangiocarcinoma. Ann Surg Oncol. 2009;16(1):14–22.
8. Sasaki A, Aramaki M, Kawano K, Morii Y, Nakashima K, Yoshida T, et al. Intrahepatic peripheral cholangiocarcinoma: mode of spread and choice of surgical treatment. Br J Surg. 1998;85(9):1206–9.

9. Olnes MJ, Erlich R. A review and update on cholangiocarcinoma. Oncology. 2004;66(3): 167–79.
10. Shaib YH, Davila JA, McGlynn K, El-Serag HB. Rising incidence of intrahepatic cholangiocarcinoma in the United States: a true increase? J Hepatol. 2004;40(3):472–7.
11. Khan S, Toledano M, Taylor-Robinson S. Epidemiology, risk factors, and pathogenesis of cholangiocarcinoma. HPB. 2008;10(2):77–82.
12. Alvaro D, Crocetti E, Ferretti S, Bragazzi MC, Capocaccia R. Descriptive epidemiology of cholangiocarcinoma in Italy. Dig Liver Dis. 2010;42(7):490–5.
13. von Hahn T, Ciesek S, Wegener G, Plentz RR, Weismüller TJ, Wedemeyer H, et al. Epidemiological trends in incidence and mortality of hepatobiliary cancers in Germany. Scand J Gastroenterol. 2011;46(9):1092–8.
14. Taylor-Robinson S, Toledano M, Arora S, Keegan T, Hargreaves S, Beck A, et al. Increase in mortality rates from intrahepatic cholangiocarcinoma in England and Wales 1968–1998. Gut. 2001;48(6):816–20.
15. Patel T. Increasing incidence and mortality of primary intrahepatic cholangiocarcinoma in the United States. Hepatology. 2001;33(6):1353–7.
16. Bridgewater J, Galle PR, Khan SA, Llovet JM, Park J-W, Patel T, et al. Guidelines for the diagnosis and management of intrahepatic cholangiocarcinoma. J Hepatol. 2014;60(6):1268–89.
17. Jaiswal M, LaRusso N, Gores GJ. Cholangiocarcinoma and pro-inflammatory cytokines. Cancer Alert. 2000;1:141–4.
18. Alvaro D, Bragazzi MC, Benedetti A, Fabris L, Fava G, Invernizzi P, et al. Cholangiocarcinoma in Italy: a national survey on clinical characteristics, diagnostic modalities and treatment. Results from the “cholangiocarcinoma” committee of the Italian Association for the Study of liver disease. Dig Liver Dis. 2011;43(1):60–5.
19. Weber SM, Jarnagin WR, Klimstra D, DeMatteo RP, Fong Y, Blumgart LH. Intrahepatic cholangiocarcinoma: resectability, recurrence pattern, and outcomes1. J Am Coll Surg. 2001;193(4):384–91.
20. Yedibela S, Demir R, Zhang W, Meyer T, Hohenberger W, Schönleben F. Surgical treatment of mass-forming intrahepatic cholangiocarcinoma: an 11-year Western single-center experience in 107 patients. Ann Surg Oncol. 2009;16(2):404.
21. Shimada K, Sano T, Sakamoto Y, Esaki M, Kosuge T, Ojima H. Surgical outcomes of the mass-forming plus Periductal infiltrating types of intrahepatic cholangiocarcinoma: a comparative study with the typical mass-forming type of intrahepatic cholangiocarcinoma. World J Surg. 2007;31(10):2016–22.
22. Bartella I, Dufour JF. Clinical diagnosis and staging of intrahepatic cholangiocarcinoma. J Gastrointestin Liver Dis (JGLD). 2015;24(4):481–9.
23. Leelawat K, Narong S, Wannaprasert J, Ratanashu-ek T. Prospective study of MMP7 serum levels in the diagnosis of cholangiocarcinoma. World J Gastroenterol. 2010;16(37):4697–703.
24. Singh S, Tang SJ, Sreenarasimhaiah J, Lara LF, Siddiqui A. The clinical utility and limitations of serum carbohydrate antigen (CA19-9) as a diagnostic tool for pancreatic cancer and cholangiocarcinoma. Dig Dis Sci. 2011;56(8):2491–6.
25. Shen WF, Zhong W, Xu F, Kan T, Geng L, Xie F, et al. Clinicopathological and prognostic analysis of 429 patients with intrahepatic cholangiocarcinoma. World J Gastroenterol. 2009;15(47):5976–82.
26. Liu SL, Song ZF, Hu QG, Shan D, Hu SB, Li J, et al. Serum carbohydrate antigen (CA) 19-9 as a prognostic factor in cholangiocarcinoma: a meta-analysis. Front Med China. 2010;4(4):457–62.
27. Tao LY, Cai L, He XD, Liu W, Qu Q. Comparison of serum tumor markers for intrahepatic cholangiocarcinoma and hepatocellular carcinoma. Am Surg. 2010;76(11):1210–3.
28. Rahnemai-Azar AA, Weisbrod A, Dillhoff M, Schmidt C, Pawlik TM. Intrahepatic cholangiocarcinoma: molecular markers for diagnosis and prognosis. Surg Oncol. 2017;26(2): 125–37.
29. Xu HX, Chen LD, Liu LN, Zhang YF, Guo LH, Liu C. Contrast-enhanced ultrasound of intrahepatic cholangiocarcinoma: correlation with pathological examination. Br J Radiol. 2012;85(1016):1029–37.

30. D'Onofrio M, Crosara S, De Robertis R, Canestrini S, Mucelli RP. Contrast-enhanced ultrasound of focal liver lesions. AJR Am J Roentgenol. 2015;205(1):W56–66.
31. Weber SM, Ribero D, O'reilly EM, Kokudo N, Miyazaki M, Pawlik TM. Intrahepatic cholangiocarcinoma: expert consensus statement. HPB. 2015;17(8):669–80.
32. Miller G, Schwartz LH, D'Angelica M. The use of imaging in the diagnosis and staging of hepatobiliary malignancies. Surg Oncol Clin N Am. 2007;16(2):343–68.
33. Vilgrain V, Van Beers BE, Flejou J-F, Belghiti J, Delos M, Gautier A-L, et al. Intrahepatic cholangiocarcinoma: MRI and pathologic correlation in 14 patients. J Comput Assist Tomogr. 1997;21(1):59–65.
34. Corvera CU, Blumgart LH, Akhurst T, DeMatteo RP, D'Angelica M, Fong Y, et al. 18F-fluorodeoxyglucose positron emission tomography influences management decisions in patients with biliary cancer. J Am Coll Surg. 2008;206(1):57–65.
35. Lee SW, Kim HJ, Park JH, Park DI, Cho YK, Sohn CI, et al. Clinical usefulness of 18F-FDG PET-CT for patients with gallbladder cancer and cholangiocarcinoma. J Gastroenterol. 2010;45(5):560–6.
36. Maithel SK, Gamblin TC, Kamel I, Corona-Villalobos CP, Thomas M, Pawlik TM. Multidisciplinary approaches to intrahepatic cholangiocarcinoma. Cancer. 2013;119(22):3929–42.
37. Durot I, Wilson SR, Willmann JK. Contrast-enhanced ultrasound of malignant liver lesions. Abdom Radiol. 2018;43(4):819–47.
38. Jiang W, Zeng ZC, Tang ZY, Fan J, Sun HC, Zhou J, et al. A prognostic scoring system based on clinical features of intrahepatic cholangiocarcinoma: the Fudan score. Ann Oncol. 2011;22(7):1644–52.

Chapter 3
Staging and Prognosis

Janelle F. Rekman and Flavio G. Rocha

Introduction

The incidence of intrahepatic cholangiocarcinoma (ICC) has been steadily increasing worldwide. It is the second most common primary liver cancer, next to hepatocellular carcinoma (HCC), currently accounting for approximately 5–30% of all primary hepatic malignancies [1, 2]. While the clinical presentation in patients may vary, the ultimate goal is to make a timely diagnosis and determine eligibility for hepatic resection, the treatment of choice. Unfortunately, only a small proportion of patients are eligible for surgical resection, and even those who undergo curative-intent hepatectomy often experience recurrent disease. In order to better prepare patients for the expected outcomes of treatment, and to provide information to treating physicians regarding the likelihood of recurrence and need for adjuvant therapy, there has been a recent interest to identify and validate prognostic factors specific to ICC.

Until recently, the staging of ICC was combined with HCC given its relative rarity and the difficulty of establishing strong evidence derived from small patient cohorts. Over the last two decades, there has been a significant effort to form multi-institution, international database collaborations to study this uncommon tumor, providing a higher volume of patients for statistical data analysis. In addition to the challenge of creating a prognostic system for primary liver cancer, the

J. F. Rekman · F. G. Rocha (✉)
Section of General, Thoracic and Vascular Surgery, Virginia Mason Medical Center, Seattle, WA, USA
e-mail: Janelle.rekman@virginamason.org; flavio.rocha@virginiamason.org

T. M. Pawlik et al. (eds.), *Intrahepatic Cholangiocarcinoma*,
https://doi.org/10.1007/978-3-030-22258-1_3

patient's projected course is also intimately related to their underlying liver function. Many patients in Eastern countries, where primary liver cancer is more common, have underlying hepatitis and liver dysfunction that must be taken into account [3].

A Brief History of ICC Staging

Until the 7th edition of the American Joint Committee on Cancer/Union for International Cancer Control (AJCC/UICC) TMN staging system in 2010, all primary liver tumors fell under the same staging system in Western countries. Distinct staging systems for ICC, providing the foundation for current staging systems, were first proposed and used in Japan where cholangiocarcinoma is more prevalent. The National Cancer Center of Japan (NCCJ) and the Liver Cancer Study Group of Japan (LCSGJ) staging systems each investigated factors predicting prognosis in order to guide clinical care (see Table 3.1) [4, 5].

The NCCJ presented a staging system specific for mass-forming intrahepatic cholangiocarcinoma based on a small cohort of 60 patients. Multivariate modeling, including 14 clinical and 12 postoperative surgical and pathologic parameters, identified several independent factors associated with worse long-term survival including: multiple tumors, vascular invasion, symptomatic disease, and regional lymph node metastasis. Based on these data, this staging system was proposed: Stage 1 disease, solitary tumor without vascular invasion; Stage 2 disease, solitary tumor with vascular invasion; Stage 3a disease, multiple tumors with or without vascular invasion; Stage 3b disease, any tumor with regional lymph node metastasis; and Stage 4 disease, ICC with distant metastasis [4]. This staging system was criticized for both its small population base ($N = 60$) and for its lack of generalizability given that the patient population had only mass-forming ICC and one third of them were Hepatitis B or C positive [6, 7].

In contrast to the NCCJ, the LCSGJ staging system included tumor size as a factor and highlighted all three morphological subtypes of ICC (mass-forming, periductal-infiltrating, and intraductal-growth type). Specifically, the system stratified patients based on: number of tumors, presence of vascular or serosal invasion, and tumor size >2 cm. One point was assigned to each of these factors and staging was a summation of the points [5]. Lymph nodes and distant metastases were included in a binary fashion similar to the subsequent AJCC/UICC 7th edition.

These two Japanese staging systems were first analyzed in a large Western cohort by Nathan et al. in 2009 [7] in a large Surveillance, Epidemiology, and End Results (SEER) database study of 598 patients having undergone surgery for ICC. Both the LCSGJ and the NCCJ exhibited poor correlation among the T stages and for survival prediction in this population. Specifically, the LCSGJ

Table 3.1 Comparison of TMN Staging Systems for Intrahepatic Cholangiocarcinoma

Stage Classification	AJCC/UICC 7th edition	Liver cancer study group of Japan	National Cancer Center Japan
		Criteria: 1 – tumor size ≤2 cm	
		2 – tumor number = 1	
		3 – no portal vein, hepatic vein, or serosal involvement	
Primary tumor			
TX	Primary tumor cannot be assessed	–	–
Tis	Carcinoma in situ (intraductal tumor)	–	–
T0	No evidence of primary tumor	–	–
T1	Solitary tumor without vascular invasion	All three criteria	Solitary tumor without vascular invasion
T2a	Solitary tumor with vascular invasion	Two of three criteria	Solitary tumor with vascular invasion
T2b	Multiple tumors, with or without vascular invasion	–	–
T3	Tumors perforating the visceral peritoneum	One of three criteria	Multiple tumors with or without vascular invasion
T4	Tumors with periductal invasion	None of three criteria	–
Regional lymph nodes (LN)			
NX	Regional LN metastases cannot be assessed	–	–
N0	No regional LN metastases present	No regional LN metastases present	No regional LN metastases present
N1	Regional LN metastases present	Regional LN metastases present	Regional LN metastases present
Metastatic disease (M)			
M0	No distant metastases	No distant metastases	No distant metastases
M1	Distant metastases	Distant metastases	Distant metastases

failed to identify differences between patients for stages I-III in this Western cohort [7] (see Fig. 3.1).

Up until this point, ICC had been staged with HCC under 'primary liver tumors' in the AJCC/UICC 6th edition, ignoring clinicopathologic features specific to ICC. The SEER analysis used a Cox proportional hazard model to predict independent predictors of survival identified multiple tumors [hazard ratio (HR) 1.42, confidence interval (CI) 1.01–2.01], lymph node status in nonmetastatic

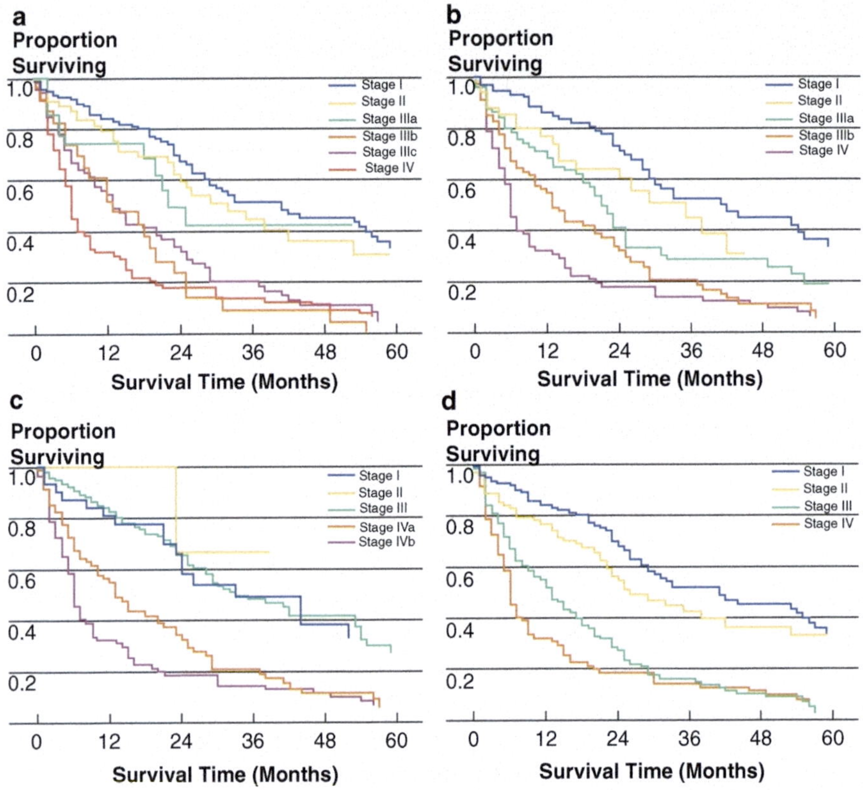

Fig. 3.1 Kaplan-Meier survival curves for all patients. (**a**) AJCC/UICC 6th edition TMN liver cancer staging system. (**b**) Okabayashi ICC staging system. (**c**) Liver Cancer Study Group of Japan ICC staging system. (**d**) AJCC 7th edition ICC staging system (proposed by National et al). (Used with permission from Springer: Nathan et al. [7])

patients (HR 3.21, CI 1.23–8.37), and vascular invasion (HR 1.53, CI 1.10–2.120), as previously reported by Okabayashi, to predict adverse outcomes. Size of the primary tumor was not an independent predictor of survival in the Nathan study (HR 0.97, CI 0.72–1.30). Interestingly, this study did not show an additive effect of tumor number and vascular invasion, with the impact of having both on survival being similar to either alone. However, it was limited by the confines of the SEER database itself. No morphologic details of the primary tumor were included (mass-forming, intraductal, etc.), and there was no information regarding serosal invasion of the primary tumor (meaning exact evaluation of the LCSGJ system was not possible). It is, therefore, possible that the true performance of the LCSGJ staging system was underestimated.

The predictive features for survival of patients with ICC described by Nathan et al. were confirmed in a multi-institutional, international study of 449 patients from 11 institutions who had undergone hepatic resection for ICC [8]. Overall, 5-year survival rates improved if final pathology showed: a single tumor, no vascular invasion, and no lymph node spread. Overall, survival dropped in an accumulated fashion if patients had 1, 2, or 3 of these factors (38.3%, 27.3%, and 18.1%, respectively). Lymph node status was found to be the worst prognostic indicator, in that multiple tumors and vascular invasion were only relevant for survival in N0 patients. In this study, although tumor size was relevant to survival in the univariate analysis, there was no prognostic significance on multivariate confirmation.

At this time, with the help of these studies, AJCC/UICC developed the first independent TMN staging system for ICC [9]. T-stage categories were broken down into the following: T1, solitary tumor without vascular invasion; T2a, solitary tumor with vascular invasion; T2b, multiple tumors with or without vascular invasion; T3, tumors perforating the visceral peritoneum or involving local hepatic structures by direct invasion; and T4, tumor with periductal invasion. N1 disease was considered stage IVa disease. See Table 3.2 for a comparison of 6th and 7th AJCC/UICC ICC staging system. Farges et al. [10] of the French Association of Surgery intrahepatic cholangiocarcinoma (AFC-IHCC) study group validated the 7th edition system on a resectable ICC patient population of 163, showing that the proposed TMN classification could be used to predict survival. Those with stage 1 disease did not

Table 3.2 Different AJCC staging definitions for intrahepatic cholangiocarcinoma based on the AJCC 6th edition (2004), AJCC 7th edition (2010), and AJCC 8th edition (2017) staging systems

AJCC staging classification (6th edition, 2004)		AJCC staging classification (7th edition, 2010)	
T1	Single tumor without vascular invasion	T1	Solitary tumor without vascular invasion
T2	Single tumor with vascular invasion or multiple tumors none more than 5 cm	T2a	Solitary tumor with vascular invasion
T3	Multiple tumors more than 5 cm or tumors involving major branch of portal or hepatic veins	T2b	Multiple tumors, with or without vascular invasion
T4	Tumors with direct invasion of adjacent organs other than the gallbladder or with perforation of visceral peritoneum	T3	Tumor perforating the visceral peritoneum or involving the local extra hepatic structures by direct invasion
		T4	Tumor with periductal invasion

(continued)

Table 3.2 (continued)

AJCC staging classification (6th edition, 2004)		AJCC staging classification (7th edition, 2010)	
N0	No regional lymph node metastasis	N0	No regional lymph node metastasis
N1	Regional lymph node metastasis	N1	Regional lymph node metastasis
M0	No distant metastasis	M0	No distant metastasis
M1	Distant metastasis	M1	Distant metastasis

AJCC staging classification (8th edition, 2017)	
T1a	Solitary tumor ≤5 cm without vascular invasion
T1b	Solitary tumor >5 cm without vascular invasion
T2	Solitary tumor with intrahepatic vascular invasion or multiple tumors, with or without vascular invasion
T3	Tumor perforating the visceral peritoneum
T4	Tumor involving the local extrahepatic structures by direct invasion
N0	No regional lymph node metastasis
N1	Regional lymph node metastasis present
M0	No distant metastasis
M1	Distant metastasis

AJCC (6th edition, 2004)				AJCC (7th edition, 2010)				AJCC (8th edition, 2017)			
Stage	T	N	M	Stage	T	N	M	Stage	T	N	M
I	T2	N0	M0	I	T1	N0	M0	Ia	T1a	N0	M0
II	T2	N0	M0	II	T2a	N0	M0	Ib	T1b	N0	M0
IIIa	T3	N0	M0		T2b	N0	M0	II	T2	N0	M0
IIIb	T4	N0	M0	III	T3	N0	M0	IIIa	T3	N0	M0
IIIc	Any T	N1	M0	IVa	T4	N0	M0	IIIb	T4	N0	M0
IV	Any T	Any N	M1		Any T	N1	M0		Any T	N1	M0
				IVb	Any T	Any N	M1	IV	Any T	Any N	M1

From Meng et al. [54]

reach the median survival cut-off at the median follow-up of 34 months, patients with stage 2 tumors had a median survival of 53 months (p = 0.01), and stage 3 patients had a median survival of 16 months ($p < 0.0001$), thus demonstrating prognostic stratification.

While the LCSGJ and AJCC/UICC 7th edition staging systems do stratify patients into categories, their discriminatory ability is still relatively poor. In Nathan et al.'s [7] comparison of the T-staging systems to date at that time (AJCC/UICC 6th edition, NCCJ/Okabayashi, LCSGJ, and their proposed system), the discriminatory abilities of these various systems were evaluated by calculating the c-indices for Cox proportional hazards models, both for the T classification systems and the overall stage groupings [7]. In fact, all the systems had comparable c-statistics in their

T-staged model (Nathan's proposed system c = 0.61, AJCC/UICC 6th edition c = 0.6, Okabayashi/NCCJ 0.59), except the LCSGJ (c = 0.51) which was difficult to evaluate using the SEER database. The overall stage groupings performed similarly and are shown in Fig. 3.1. If the model perfectly predicted the ICC patients who would experience diminished overall survival, the c-statistic would be equal to 1 [11]. These models provide a prediction that is moderate to good, but not strong [12], and therefore, continued work to discover discriminatory factors was felt to be necessary [13].

Transitioning from the 7th AJCC/UICC Edition to the 8th Edition

As soon as the AJCC 7th edition was published, some concerns began to surface. The SEER database that formed the backbone of its patient population had some notable missing information including status of the resection margins, tumor morphology, and serosal penetration of the tumor. In addition, most notably, half of the patients in the database had not undergone a lymphadenectomy [7]. The AFC-IHCC-2009 study group (French Association of Surgery) produced a registry of patients with resected ICC, including only patients who had undergone a curative operation and had complete clinical and pathologic data including lymphadenectomy. Of 522 patients resected for ICC, only 163 fit the inclusion criteria. Their analysis of the 7th edition, compared to historical systems achieved the most uniform distribution of patients among the stages and behaved in exactly the same way as Japanese patients, suggesting worldwide applicability [10].

The Mayo Clinic also sought to validate the AJCC 7th edition on their patient population and found differing results [14]. One hundred twenty-six patients with resected ICC were included and median length of follow-up was 4.5 years. In contrast to previous studies, the 7th edition did not stratify patients according to survival. Their univariate analysis showed worse prognosis with the following variables: tumor size >5 cm (HR 2.50, 95% CI 1.27–4.93), multiple tumors (HR 1.79, 95% CI 1.05–3.04), pN1 status (HR 3.14, 95% CI 1.84–5.38), presence of grade 4 disease (HR 3.72, 95% CI 1.74–7.95), and microvascular invasion (HR 1.87, CT 1.12–3.09). Final stepwise multivariate analysis showed similar results with significantly worse survival for high grade/dedifferentiated tumors, pN1 disease, and microvascular invasion (see Table 3.3).

The median overall survival for node-positive patients in the Mayo clinic study was 20 months, with 1- and 5-year survival rates of 61% and 13%, respectively. Interestingly, the more positive LNs, the worse the survival ($P < 0.001$). This leads to an analysis of what was called the 'lymph node ratio' (number of positive nodes/total number removed), and an impact on survival was seen with a ratio of >0.1 (HR 1.34, 95% CI 1.20–1.50). Therefore, it seemed that achieving a greater lymph node harvest would give a more accurate and discriminatory prognosis for the patient [14]. This was later reflected in the 8th edition of the AJCC/UICC staging [15].

Table 3.3 Univariate and multivariate hazard ratios for node-negative and metastasis-negative (N0 M0) patients and all patients

Variables	N0 M0 patients (n = 93)					All patients (n = 126)				
		n	Median survival, months	HR (95% CI)	P-value		n	Median survival, months	HR (95% CI)	P-value
Univariate analysis										
Tumor size of >5 cm	Yes	58	60	1.91 (0.87–4.20)	0.102	Yes	88	38	2.50 (1.27–4.93)	0.008
	No	35	99			No	38	99		
Grade 4 disease	Yes	6	14	4.23 (1.58–11.28)	0.004	Yes	10	6	3.72 (1.75–7.95)	<0.001
	No	87	81			No	116	49		
Periductal invasion	Yes	28	66	1.75 (0.85–3.61)	0.123	Yes	41	38	1.61 (0.96–2.69)	0.064
	No	65	84			No	85	60		
Direct invasion	Yes	11	70	0.85 (0.30–2.41)	0.762	Yes	18	43	1.21 (0.61–2.39)	0.582
	No	82	99			No	108	49		
Macrovascular invasion	Yes	9	49	1.36 (0.48–3.86)	0.561	Yes	11	44	1.32 (0.60–2.89)	0.491
	No	84	81			No	115	49		
Microvascular invasion	Yes	37	66	1.12 (0.57–2.17)	0.741	Yes	60	32	1.87 (1.13–3.09)	0.016
	No	56	79			No	66	70		
Multiple tumors	Yes	30	81	1.40 (0.67–2.92)	0.362	Yes	38	31	1.79 (1.05–3.04)	0.031
	No	63	79			No	88	57		
Positive lymph nodes	–	–	–	–	–	Yes	33	20	3.14 (1.83–5.39)	<0.001
						No	93	79		
Multivariate analysis										
Grade 4 disease						Yes	10	6	7.84(3.35–18.35)	<0.001
						No	116	49		
Positive lymph nodes						Yes	33	20	2.93 (1.65–5.21)	<0.001

						No	93	79		
Microvascular invasion						Yes	60	32	1.85 (1.06–3.22)	0.030
						No	66	70		
Multiple tumors						Yes	38	31	1.68 (0.96–2.92)	0.067
						No	88	57		
Periductal invasion						Yes	41	38	1.53 (0.87–2.68)	0.136
						No	85	60		
Tumor size of >5 cm						Yes	88	38	1.51 (0.75–3.06)	0.248
						No	38	99	1.51 (0.75–3.06)	0.248
Resection margin	–	–	–	–	–	R0	110	66	–	–
	–	–	–	–	–	Non-R0	16	25	–	–
Margin width	–	–	–	–	–	>5 mm	70	99		<0.001
						<5 mm	56	38		

Reprinted from Ali et al. [14], with permission from Elsevier
CI confidence interval, *HR* hazard ratio, *N0 M0* node-negative and metastasis-negative disease

Ali et al. at Mayo [14] constructed a new model using their data, which included a tumor size >5 cm as a negative prognostic factor. The concordance of their model reached 0.66 (95% CI 0.58–0.74), slightly improved from the $c = 0.61$ seen in the Nathan study 5 years earlier [7]. There had been considerable debate since before the 7th edition AJCC was written regarding the prognostic significance of tumor size for ICC. Although the 7th edition did not include tumor size in their criteria, it became evident that the impact of size was likely more nuanced and nonlinear in terms of its effect. For example, the survival of a patient with a 1 cm tumor did not seem to be significantly different than one with a 4 cm tumor, but if the tumor reached 10 cm, survival worsened. Differing size plateaus were suggested, from 2 cm to 7 cm [16]. There is some evidence that tumor size ≥5 cm had been associated with microscopic vascular invasion and worse tumor grade in patients with resected ICC, which may account for this difference in size [17].

In 2017, the 8th edition of the AJCC/UICC TMN staging was published and contained these changes described above, as well as a few additional factors based on evolution of knowledge in the intervening 8 years. ICC staging remains separate from both extrahepatic cholangiocarcinomas and HCCs, but rare mixed hepato-cholangiocarcinomas and intrahepatic primary hepatic neuroendocrine masses are now also included in the system. T1 disease has been broken up based on the size of the lesion (T1a, solitary tumor ≤5 cm vs. T1b, solitary tumor >5 cm), the T2 category has been modified to indicate the equivalent survival outcomes of patients with multiple lesions and vascular invasion (rather than separating them into T2a and 2b), and the T4 category has become defined by local peri-tumoral extension to adjacent organs rather than based on morphology and periductal infiltration. It seems that the significance of periductal infiltration was overstated in the initial studies (prompting its prominence in the 7th edition), and further studies have not shown this to be true.

T categories in the 8th edition of the AJCC were thus redefined as: T1, single large tumor (T1a <5 cm, T1b > 5 cm); T2, solitary tumor +/− vascular invasion or multiple tumors +/− vascular invasion; T3, tumor on the verge of local extrahepatic invasion; and T4, overt extrahepatic invasion. It is worth mentioning that 'multiple tumors' in the T2 category could refer to: multifocal disease, satellitosis, or intrahepatic metastases. Clinically, at this time it is challenging to determine on preoperative imaging, but from a staging perspective, it does not seem to affect outcomes [1]. See Table 3.4 for AJCC 8th edition staging system.

In addition to T-stage categories, N1 disease has been reclassified as stage IIIb rather than stage IV disease. This downstaging reflects findings that there is the possibility of prolonged survival in LN-positive patients, rarely mimicked in those with true metastatic spread [18]. Given that the number of harvested LNs and the number of positive LNs are highly predictive of survival [14, 19], an adequate nodal harvest is considered 6 LNs in the 8th edition. Although not officially part of the staging system, Ca19–9 level greater than 200 IU/mL is introduced as an additional risk factor, along with underlying liver fibrosis/cirrhosis and primary sclerosing cholangitis [15, 20].

Table 3.4 AJCC 8th edition staging classification for intrahepatic cholangiocarcinoma. Compiled from The AJCC Cancer Staging Manual, Eighth Edition (2017), Springer International Publishing

Classification	Description
T category	*T criteria*
Tis	Carcinoma in situ (intraductal tumor)
T1a	Solitary tumor ≤5 cm without vascular invasion
T1b	Solitary tumor >5 cm without vascular invasion
T2	Solitary tumor with intrahepatic vascular invasion or multiple tumors ± vascular invasion
T3	Tumor perforating visceral peritoneum
T4	Tumor involving local extrahepatic structures by direct invasion
N category	*N criteria*
N0	No regional lymph node metastasis
N1	Regional lymph node metastasis present
M category	*M criteria*
M0	No distant metastasis
M1	Distant metastasis
AJCC prognostic stage groups	
T1a/N0/M0	IA
T1b/N0/M0	IB
T2/N0/M0	II
T3/N0/M0	IIIA
T4/N0/M0	IIIB
Any T/N1/M0	IIIB
Any T/Any N/M1	IV

Validation of the AJCC 8th Edition

To date, two high volume studies have attempted to validate the prognostic impact of the 8th edition of the AJCC staging system. The first, an international study group, containing 14 hepatobiliary centers and 1154 patients with resected ICC between 1990 and 2015 staged each patient according to the 7th and 8th edition criteria [21]. The second was a study in the USA conducted on the SEER database including 1008 patients [22]. They both found similar results; that the prognostic power of the AJCC/UICC 8th edition is either just partially improved or comparable with that of the 7th edition.

Spolverato et al. [21] performed a validation analysis to compare the ability of the two editions (7th and 8th AJCC) to stratify patients. The 7th edition T-category had a C-index of 0.59 in their cohort and the 8th edition was only marginally improved at 0.609. Interestingly, although T3 patients had a high HR of death compared with T1 patients in the 8th edition (HR 1.65, 95% CI 1.22–2.24 $P = 0.001$), they survived longer than T1b and T2 patients in this cohort. A similar effect was noted when looking closer at the overall staging groups. Overall, stage IIIa patients had a higher risk of death (39.7% 5y OS) versus stage Ia (38.8% 5y OS) patients, but the difference was not statistically significant ($P > 0.05$). These data suggest that perforation of the visceral peritoneum may not carry as poor a prognostic impact as tumors with vascular invasion [20, 21].

The large, US-representative SEER database study by Kim et al. [22] also demonstrated only marginal discrimination improvements between the 7th and 8th AJCC/UICC staging systems. Previous studies [14, 23] indicated a c-index between 0.62 and 0.65 for the 7th edition, and this study was roughly the same with a c-index of 0.669 (see Fig. 3.2).

It did confirm the prognostic significance of >5 cm tumor size as the risk of death in this cohort was 36% higher than patients with ICC lesions measuring <5 cm (HR 1.36, 95% CI 1.14–1.62; $P = 0.001$). The data from this study also supported the alteration of LN positivity from stage IV disease to a separate stage IIIb definition, given that the median survival among patients with 8th edition stage IIIb disease was 16 months, significantly better than the 9 months seen for those with distant metastases (8th edition stage IV disease).

Role of Lymphadenectomy

Although recommended by International and National consensus guidelines [National Comprehensive Cancer Network (NCCN) [24], International Hepato-Pancreato Biliary Association (IHPBA) consensus statement [1], and the European Association for the Study of the Liver (EASL) statement [25]], the role of lymphadenectomy is still controversial, especially in the West. A multi-institutional study of 449 patients at 11 institutions indicated that only 55.2% of patients undergoing resection for ICC have at least 1 lymph node removed and pathologically evaluated [8], despite LN metastases being universally cited as a negative prognostic factor [8, 26, 27]. Of those who had LNs harvested in the previous study, the median number resected was 3 and the number with lymph node-positive disease was 29.8%. This incidence is as high as 40% in some studies [27]. Similar results were noted by Kim et al. [22] when they reported on 749 patients from the SEER database who underwent surgical resection between 1988 and 2011.

The AJCC 8th edition recommends a minimum of 6 LNs to be resected for adequate nodal staging [15] and the IHPBA Expert Consensus Statement recommends clearing all locoregional nodal stations. Locoregional nodal stations (N1), or what are also named the first echelon nodes, differ depending on the hemiliver involved. Clinical and pathologic data indicate that LNs in the porta hepatis and along the hepatic artery (see Fig. 3.3) are the first to become involved and should be removed in all patients. See Fig. 3.4 for an intraoperative picture of the result of a complete porta hepatis lymph node dissection. If the ICC originates in the right hemiliver (segments 5–8), resection of the retropancreatic nodes should occur. In contrast, a lymphatic drainage pathway along the lesser omentum from the left hemiliver (segments 2 and 3) to the lesser curve of the stomach is recognized. Therefore, left-sided

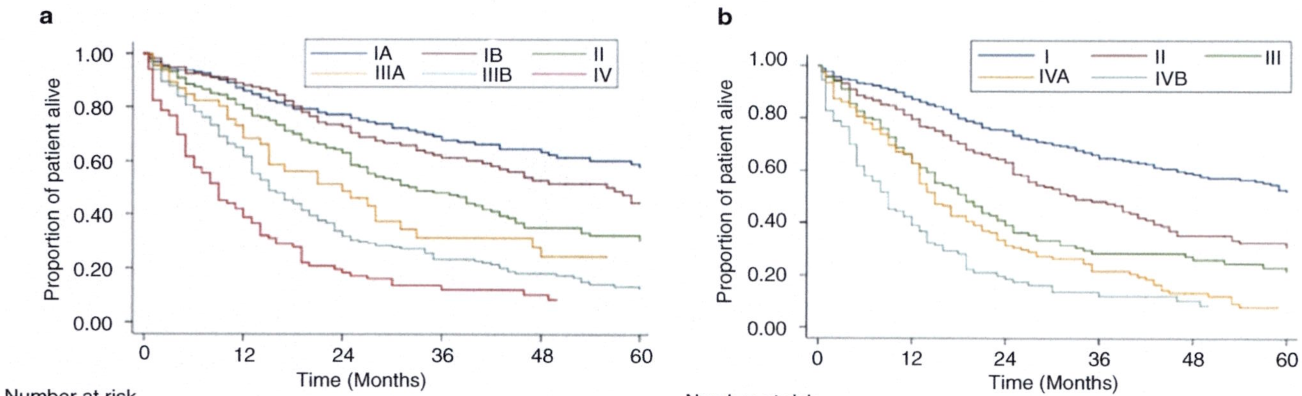

(a) Number at risk

	0	12	24	36	48	60
IA	192	145	112	90	63	49
IB	166	125	97	67	44	31
II	234	151	103	67	40	34
IIIA	48	31	20	9	8	5
IIIB	265	156	70	41	26	15
IV	103	39	16	9	6	4

	Median OS (months)	95% CI
IA	81	60-116
IB	57	42-87
II	33	27-41
IIIA	24	15-31
IIIB	15	13-19
IV	9	6-12

(b) Number at risk

	0	12	24	36	48	60
I	358	270	209	157	107	80
II	234	151	103	67	40	34
III	132	79	45	27	22	15
IVA	181	108	45	23	12	5
IVB	103	39	16	9	6	4

	Median OS (months)	95% CI
I	67	54-87
II	33	27-41
III	19	15-23
IVA	15	13-17
IVB	9	6-12

Fig. 3.2 Kaplan-Meier curves stratified by (**a**) AJCC/UICC 8th edition, and (**b**) AJCC/UICC 7th ed staging systems. (Used with permission from Kim et al. [22])

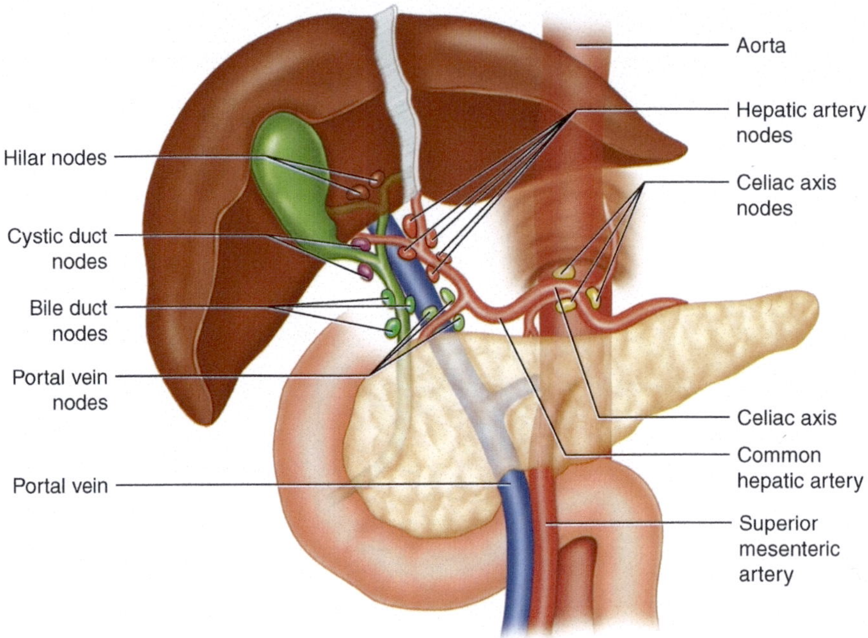

Fig. 3.3 Lymph node drainage patterns vary based on intrahepatic location of ICC. Segments 2 and 3 tumors can drain to lymph nodes (LNs) along the lesser curvature of the stomach and subsequently to the celiac nodal basin. ICCs of the right liver (segments 5–8) may preferentially drain to the hilar LNs and subsequently to the caval and periaortic LNs. (Used with the permission of the American College of Surgeons. Adapted from Compton et al. [55])

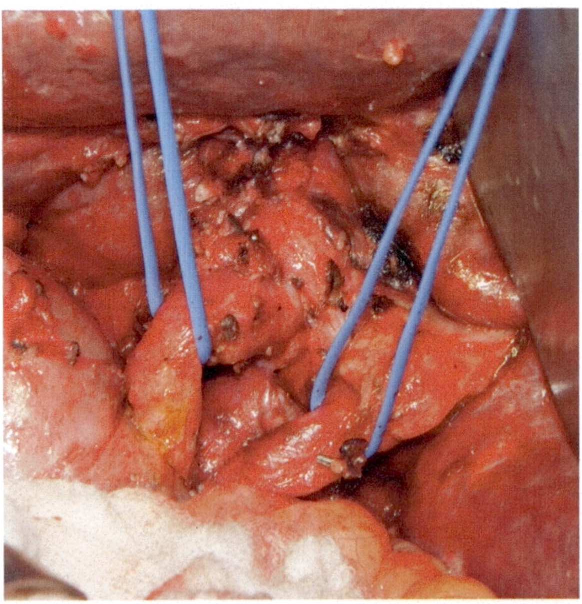

Fig. 3.4 Intraoperative picture following portal lymph node dissection for ICC. Blue vessel loops demonstrate the common bile duct on the left and the common hepatic artery looped on the right with the portal vein demonstrated between and lying behind

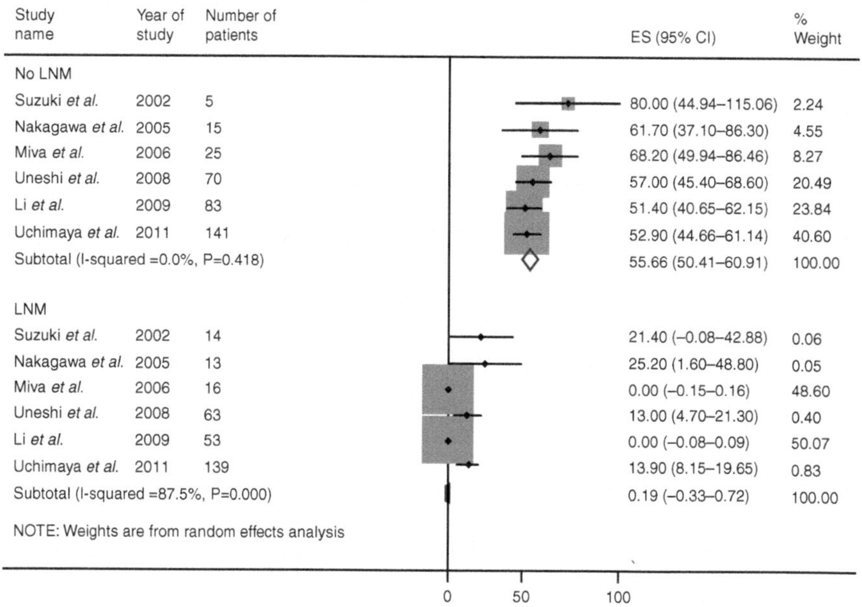

Fig. 3.5 Meta-analysis of 3-year survival among patients with intrahepatic cholangiocarcinoma stratified by lymph node (LN). Patients without LN involvement experienced 55.3% 3-year survival compared to 0.2% 3-year survival in those with LN metastases. (Used with permission from SpringerNature: Amini et al. [29])

ICC should also involve resection of LNs around the cardia and lesser curve of the stomach along the left gastric artery [1, 9]. Evidence of gross LN involvement outside of these first echelon LNs, such as celiac or para-aortic LNs, should be considered a contraindication to hepatic resection, representing metastatic disease [28].

There is no evidence that overall survival is improved when a lymphadenectomy is performed; however, important prognostic information and accurate staging have been shown in multiple studies following lymphadenectomy [8, 22, 27]. A recent meta-analysis of 3-year survival in patients with ICC stratified by LN status showed approximately 55.7% 3-year survival compared to 0.2% 3-year survival in those possessing lymph node metastases [29]. See Fig. 3.5 for the forest plot from the meta-analysis performed by Amini et al.

Lymph node involvement is one of the single most important prognostic pieces of information for patients with ICC. Even in patients with negative margins after resection, the presence of N1 disease appears to negate all the benefit of surgery [26]. DeJong et al. [8] found that N1 disease translated to a survival of 22.9 compared to 30.1 months in N0 patients, and that patients with N1 disease had the same overall survival regardless of number of tumors or vascular invasion in the liver. However, the presence of vascular and biliary invasion was strongly associated with the risk of LN positivity, and even those without vascular and biliary invasion had a 9.1% and 20.7% chance of LN metastases, respectively. Tumor number and size,

Table 3.5 Factors associated with increased risk of lymph node metastasis ($n = 258$)[a]

Prognostic factor	OR	95% CI	*P*
Size of largest lesion (continuous)	0.99	0.92 to 1.07	0.80
Multiple tumors	1.56	0.81 to 3.02	0.19
Vascular invasion	2.89	1.56 to 5.35	0.001
Direct invasion of adjacent organ	1.74	0.68 to 4.47	0.25
Perineural invasion	1.87	0.78 to 4.49	0.16
Biliary invasion	4.03	1.94 to 8.36	< 0.001
Morphologic subtype			
Mass-forming		Reference	
Papillary	0.65	0.15 to 2.74	0.55
Periductal-infiltrating	0.19	0.02 to 1.56	0.12
Mass-forming plus periductal-infiltrating	0.15	0.65 to 2.74	0.55

Reprinted from de Jong et al. [8]. Reprinted with permission
Abbreviation: *OR* odds ratio
[a]Univariate analysis

direct invasion of other organs, and mass-forming morphology were not associated with increased rates of LN positivity in this study (see Table 3.5).

Long-term survival is possible, although rare, in the setting of LN metastases. These long-term survivors likely had occult involved LNs on preoperative imaging rather than grossly positive nodes on exploration. Bagante et al. [30] attempted to answer the question of prognostic relevance of preoperative radiographic versus pathologic LN status on long-term outcomes following resection. In this multi-institutional, international cohort of 1154 patients, 44.6% of patients had a lymphadenectomy. On final pathology, 200 (17.3% of total) patients had positive LNs and 315 (27.3% of total) patients had negative LNs. Preoperative imaging used to identify LN status was assessed by EUS, CT, MRI, or PET and was found to be inaccurate in 40% of patients, suggesting it should not replace a formal lymphadenectomy. Despite this fact, for those patients who did have positive LNs on imaging, 5y OS was 25.8% or roughly half of the 5y OS (49.7%) among patients without LN disease on preoperative imaging (see Fig. 3.6).

In addition to studying predictive power of preoperative imaging for ICC LNs, Bagante et al. assessed the AJCC 8th edition recommendation for a minimum recovery of 6 LNs and whether this number was truly necessary. According to the AJCC 8th edition staging system, N1 disease patients have a 2.5-fold increased risk of death at 5 years [15]. The findings of Bagante et al. [30] support both the survival advantage and the quality of the LN harvest (6+ LNs). The 5y OS of N0 patients was 54.9% (IQR, 41.6–66.3) versus 15.2% (IQR, 8.7–23.4) for N1 patients ($p < 0.001$) (see Fig. 3.7). Hazard of death for N1 patients compared to N0 patients increased from 1.6 to 1.8 with radiologic assessment, to 2.4 with pathologic assessment, and using the AJCC 8th edition recommendations for nodal harvest, to 3-fold (HR 3.03; $p < 0.001$).

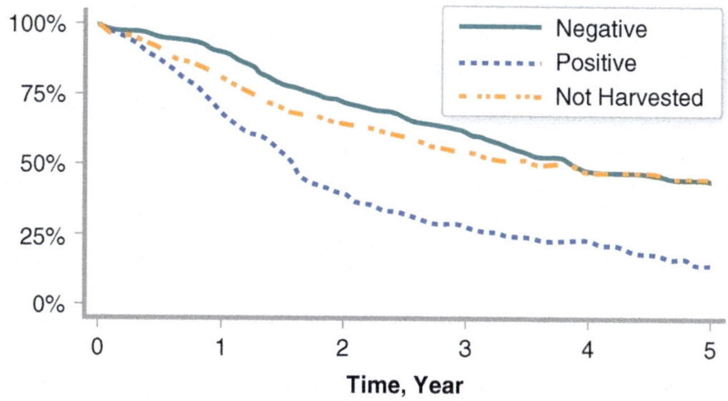

Number at risk

Negative	315	232	167	112	65	45
Positive	200	112	51	29	16	9
Not Harvested	638	474	311	212	143	88

Fig. 3.6 Kaplan-Meier overall survival curves for patients with intrahepatic cholangiocarcinoma stratified by pathologic nodal status. (Reprinted by permission from SpringerNature. Adapted from Bagante et al. [30])

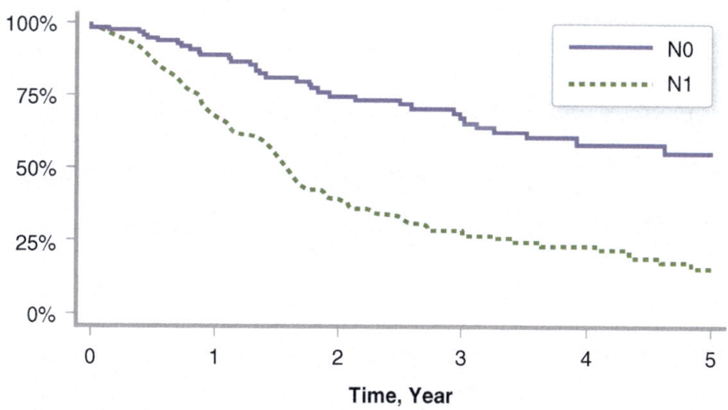

Number at risk

N0	117	86	60	42	24	16
N1	200	113	51	29	16	9

Fig. 3.7 Kaplan-Meier overall survival curves for patients with intrahepatic cholangiocarcinoma stratified by AJCC/UICC 8th edition nodal stages. (Reprinted by permission from SpringerNature. Adapted from Bagante et al. [30])

Some studies have suggested lymphadenectomy may have a therapeutic effect on local recurrence; however, prospective evidence to support this statement is lacking. Because of the poor outcome in patients with gross N1 disease in the porta hepatis on imaging (median survival 7–14 months), most authors advocate beginning with systemic chemotherapy as an initial treatment, with restaging prior to considering resection [1].

Role of Staging Laparoscopy

Staging laparoscopy for ICC is still controversial as consensus among surgeons is lacking. NCCN guidelines suggest considering staging laparoscopy, and the IHPBA guidelines suggest considering it if there are high-risk features (i.e., multicentric disease, high Ca19-9, possible peritoneal disease, or vascular invasion) in order to avoid unnecessary laparotomy [1]. The yield of staging laparoscopy for occult metastatic disease was 25–36% in two prospective studies [31, 32], and therefore, a substantial portion of ICC patients would benefit from this procedure (see Fig. 3.8). In addition to surveying for peritoneal deposits, N2 lymph node basins should be inspected, and laparoscopic ultrasound of the liver should be considered to look for extensive intrahepatic disease or vascular invasion precluding resection [28]. Although this is recommended, practice variation does occur.

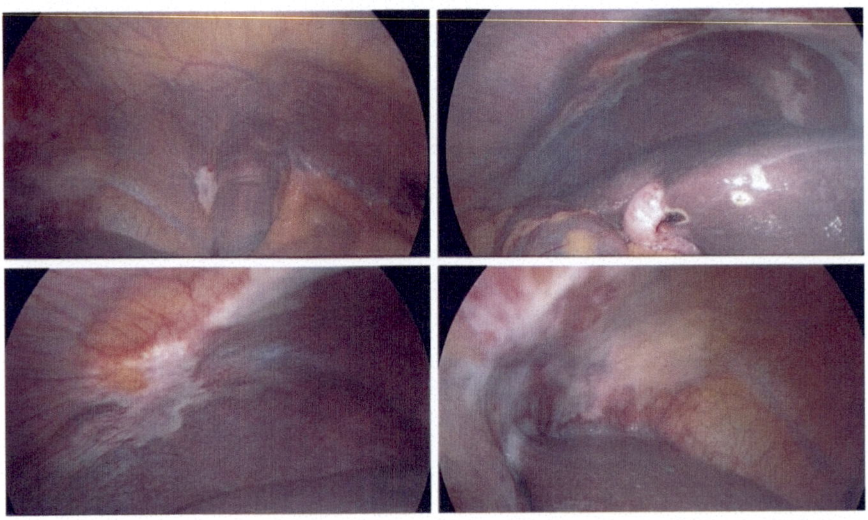

Fig. 3.8 Intraoperative photographs during staging laparoscopy for intrahepatic cholangiocarcinoma. Biopsies of white areas on peritoneal were positive for cholangiocarcinoma peritoneal carcinomatosis not visualized on preoperatively CT scan

Role of Tumor Markers

The AJCC/UICC has recently begun incorporating tumor markers into staging systems for tumors other than ICC. For example, the staging system for testicular cancer includes serum AFP measurements [9] and decreased survival in pancreatic cancer patients has recently been shown to be independently associated with increased Ca19-9 [33]. Both Ca 19-9 and CEA levels have been shown to have potential prognostic significance for ICC independent of the LN status and tumor morphologic characteristics in single-institution studies [23, 34].

Bergquist et al. [33] from the Mayo Clinic performed a review of 2816 patients in the National Cancer Database to investigate the prognostic significance of Ca19-9 levels in ICC. They hypothesized that any Ca19-9 elevation in a resectable ICC signifies a biologically aggressive phenotype and should indicate the need for multidisciplinary therapy. A Ca19-9 of 37 was considered the upper limit of normal in this study and a multivariate Cox proportions hazard model was used to estimate impact on survival. Elevated CA 19-9 was seen in 1878 (66.7%) of patients. Among those patients with elevated Ca19-9, stage-specific survival was decreased in every stage. In the resected cohort, elevated Ca19-9 resulted in similar perioperative outcomes, but decreased long-term survival (median OS 22.6 months in Ca19-9 elevated versus 47.8 months in Ca 19-9 normal patients, $P < 0.001$). In addition, they contrasted the survival analysis, after incorporating Ca19-9 into the AJCC 7th edition staging system; with the original stage, the patient would have been assigned in the original AJCC 7th TMN system. The new staging system had a concordance of 60.2%, as opposed to 54.6% for the AJCC 7th edition, with a Gamma statistic (measure of rank correlation) of 0.321 (improved from 0.144). This indicates a potential improvement in prognostic staging power [35].

Despite having good evidence that Ca19-9 is associated with survival in ICC, the optimal cut-off value has not yet been identified. Sasaki et al. [2] used a multi-institutional dataset to attempt to answer this question for both Ca19-9 and CEA levels. The association of Ca19-9 levels with long-term survival had a bimodal distribution. At a threshold level of 100 IU/mL, the hazard of death increased (HR 1.66 95%CI 1.29–2.12), and then it increased again at 500 IU/mL (HR 3.55 95%CI 2.44–5.15). CEA elevation also showed prognostic significance in this study, but it was not bimodal; prognostic power of CEA was noted only above a 5 ng/mL (HR 2.20 95%CI 1.57–2.81) threshold (see Fig. 3.9).

Based on these data, Ca19-9 cut-off values of 100 IU/mL and 500 IU/mL, and 5 ng/mL for CEA, were suggested as the best cut-off values for stratifying patients. Kaplan-Meier estimates show that these values are prognostic of survival. Patients with a Ca19-9 less than 100 IU/mL had a median OS of 50.0 months, whereas those with a preoperative Ca19-9 of 100-500 IU/mL were found to have a median of 28.1 months ($p < 0.001$). Those with a Ca19-9 > 500 IU/mL had an even worse prognosis, showing a median overall survival of only 15.5 months ($p < 0.001$). CEA values provided a similar prognostic stratification.

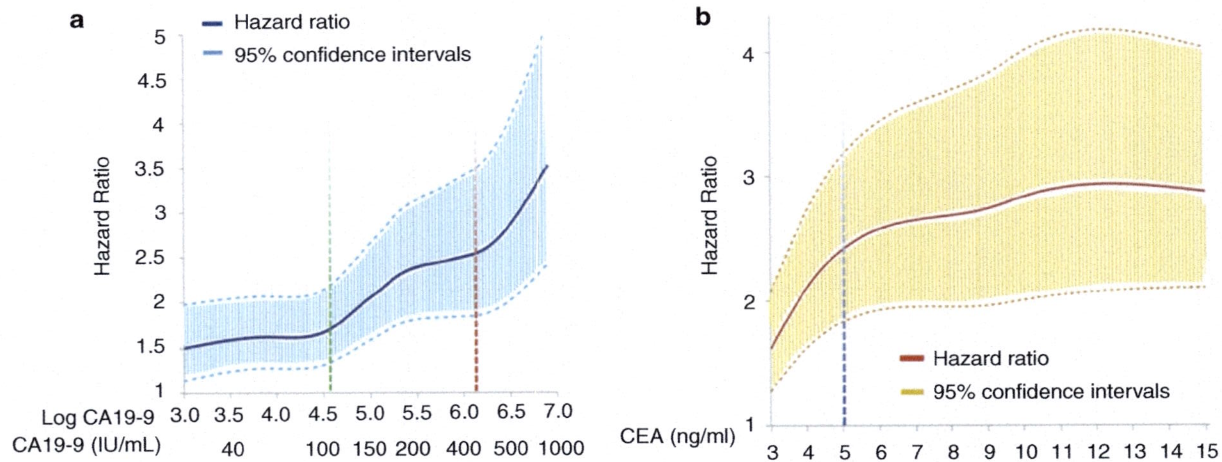

Fig. 3.9 (**a**) The hazard of death remained relatively unchanged among patients with a Ca19-9 ranging from 20 IU/mL to 100 IU/mL. Following a plateauing from 200 IU/mL to 500 IU/mL, there was a continuous increase in the hazard of death associated with Ca19-9 levels from 500 IU/mL to 1000 IU/mL (**b**) The risk of death increased as CEA levels rose from 3 ng/mL to 5 ng/mL. (Reprinted from Sasaki et al. [2], with permission from Elsevier)

Similar to Bergquist [35], Sasaki et al. noted that both Ca19-9 and CEA are associated with tumor biology. They are not simply surrogates for morphometric findings such as tumor size and number, but are independently associated with overall survival, even once controlling for these other factors using a multivariate model. Both CEA and 19–9 were independently associated with increased risk of death in their patient dataset. Using both markers, as compared to either alone, demonstrated increased prognostic power. They concluded that the addition of these biomarkers into the AJCC/UICC 8th edition and the LCSGJ schema improved prognostic stratification and increased the Harrell's C-index from 0.540 to 0.626 (p < 0.001) and from 0.553 to 0.626 (p < 0.001), respectively.

Effect of Morphologic Subtype on Prognosis

Perhaps, an often-overlooked clinicopathologic prognostic indicator for ICC is tumor morphology. The LCSGJ has classified cholangiocarcinoma into several categories based on gross appearance of the tumor: mass-forming (see Fig. 3.10), intraductal growth (or papillary cholangiocarcinomas as they are sometimes termed), and periductal-infiltrating (PI) type. The mass-forming type, as its name implies, presents as a defined mass in the liver parenchyma. The intraductal-growth subtype spreads inside the ducts by growing inward or within the lumen of the duct. PI types are seen spreading along outside the ducts longitudinally, often causing enhancement of the duct on cross-sectional imaging [5]. The precursor lesion to intraductal-growth cholangiocarcinoma, termed IPNBs (intraductal papillary neoplasm of the bile duct), is thought to represent a similar carcinogenic pathway of intraductal papillary neoplasms of the pancreas (IPMN) to pancreatic cancer. If an IPNB is found, it should be resected as they have been shown to harbor invasive carcinoma 70% of the time [36].

Among 1083 patients in an international cohort undergoing liver resection for ICC, 911 (84.1%) had mass-forming type, 30 (2.8%) intraductal growth, 54

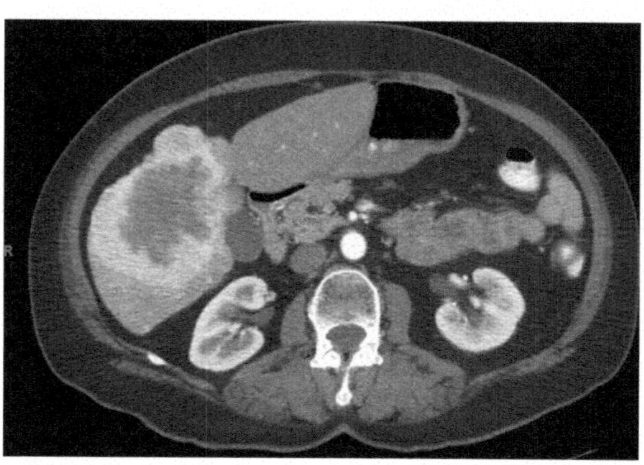

Fig. 3.10 Large mass-forming ICC in right liver on CT scan

(5.0%) had a periductal-infiltrating type, and 88 (8.1%) had a mixed mass-forming/periductal-infiltrating type. Compared with mass-forming and intraductal-growth patients, those tumors with a periductal-infiltrating component (even if they were the mixed type) had more major vascular invasion (26.8% vs. 9.5%, $p < 0.001$), lymphovascular invasion (46.1% vs. 28.8%, $p < 0.001$), perineural invasion (37.7% vs. 17.9%, $p < 0.001$), positive margin resection (23.4% vs. 10.8%, $p < 0.001$), and N1 disease (59.2% vs. 34.7%, $p < 0.001$). Applying the AJCC 8th edition, periductal-infiltrating (and mixed mass-forming and periductal-infiltrating) tumors had more advanced T categories and 95.0% of these patients were staged II/IIIa/IIIb versus 86.0% of mass-forming or intraductal-growth type tumor patients ($p = 0.017$). After propensity score matching, patients with mass-forming and intraductal-growth type tumors ICC had a significantly better 5 year OS of 35.7% (95% CI 24.0–47.6) compared with the 26.2% (95% CI 16.4–37.1, $p = 0.03$) in periductal-infiltrating masses ($p < 0.001$) (see Fig. 3.11 for Kaplan-Meier survival curves) [37]. These data are consistent with other studies reporting that patients with mass-forming ICC tumors have a more favorable prognosis [38] and that periductal-infiltrating tumors have increased association

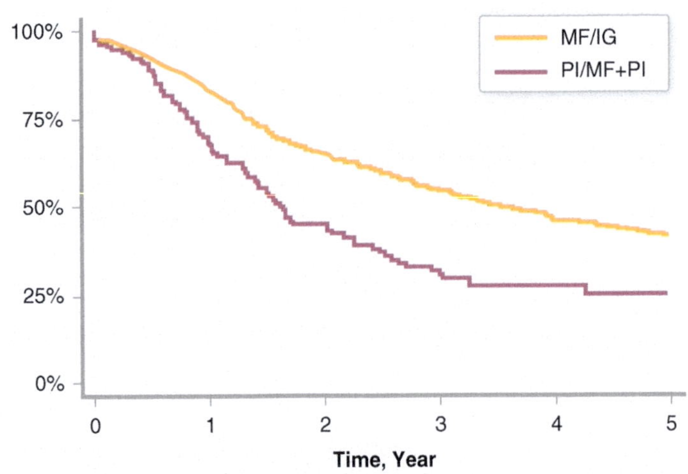

Number at risk

MF/IG	941	693	450	301	190	132
PI/MF+PI	142	85	50	29	16	10

Fig. 3.11 Kaplan-Meier overall survival curves stratified by morphological type classification. *MF* mass-forming, *IG* intraductal growth, *PI* periductal-infiltrating, *MF* + PI mixed mass-forming & periductal-infiltrating type. (Reprinted by permission from SpringerNature. Adapted from Bagante et al. [37])

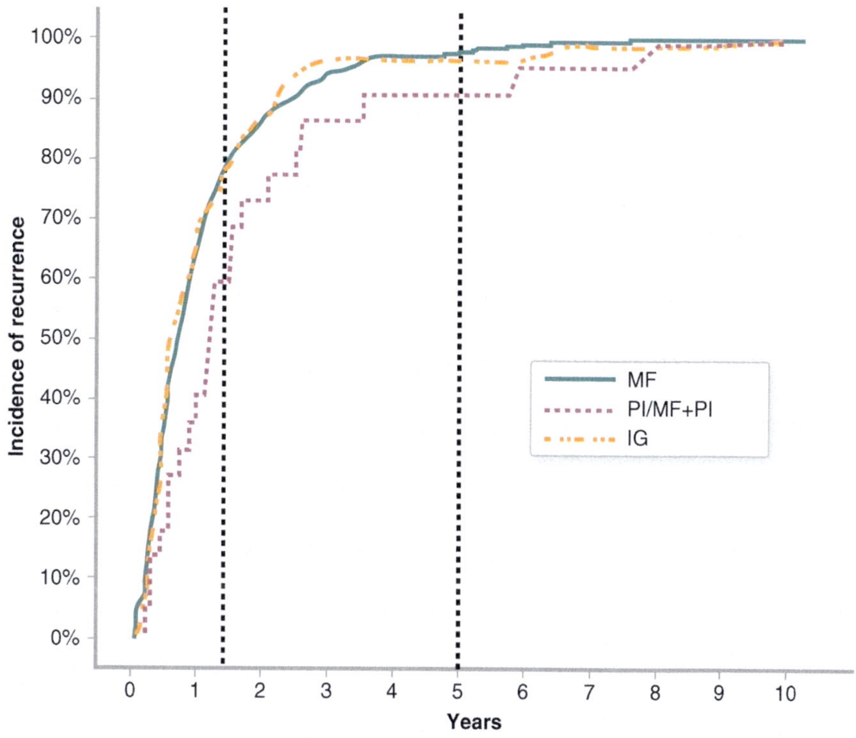

Fig. 3.12 Cumulative incidence of recurrence after surgery stratified by the morphological classification (mass-forming [MF], intraductal growth [IG], and periductal-infiltrating/mixed [PI/MF + PI]) . (Adapted from Bagante et al. [42], with permission from Elsevier)

with jaundice, bile duct invasion, portal vein invasion, lymph node metastases, and R1 margins [19]. There are also studies that have pointed to intraductal-growth tumors having improved survival [39–41] but the data cannot be considered complete.

It is possible that data are mixed given the trend found by Bagante et al. in 2018 [42] of differing patterns of recurrence. Mass-forming and periductal-infiltrating ICC patients are more likely to experience an early recurrence after surgery, whereas intraductal ICC requires long-term follow-up past 5 years given their tendency for late recurrence (see Fig. 3.12). Nearly 1 in 10 intraductal-growth ICC patients experienced a recurrence of 5 years after surgery (recurrence >5 years from surgery: mass-forming, 2%, periductal-infiltrating ICC, 3%, intraductal growth, 9%; $p = 0.03$). These recurrences occur both in intra- and extrahepatic. Until now, most studies have failed to consider, or even report, tumor morphologic subtype, but given recent evidence, this aspect of ICCs should likely be studied in depth prior to future staging system revisions [37].

Prognosis Post-Resection

Margin Status

Long-term survival after surgery for ICC is dependent on several factors, the majority of which have already been discussed in this chapter. One of those not yet discussed is how margin status affects survival and recurrence. Complete R0 resection is the only potential cure for ICC, but the optimal surgical margin is under debate. Some reports have described R0 margin status to be an important predictor of survival and recurrence [43–45]. Ribero et al. [45] from the Italian Intrahepatic Cholangiocarcinoma Study group found a significantly lower recurrence rate (53.9% vs. 73.6%) between R0 resections and those with a positive margin. The same study group also found that survival rates were significantly higher with negative margin rates (5 yr. survival 39.8% vs. 4.7%) with no impact on survival of margin width. Other groups have suggested that margin status is not a significant factor in outcome [10, 46]. Despite this, current recommendations (NCCN, IHPBA) opt for R0 resection margins if at all possible, aiming for a minimum of 0.5 cm.

Recurrence

Recurrences post-resection for ICC can occur in as many as 70% of patients [25, 27]. The prognosis after recurrence tends to be dismal (5-year survival ranging from 15% to 45% post-resection) and treatment strategies tend to be limited [27]. In contrast to hilar and distal extrahepatic cholangiocarcinoma, intrahepatic recurrence is a major issue for ICC. Systemic failure tends to be a secondary consideration. Following resection, 50–60% of patients experience recurrence in the liver, 20% in the peritoneum, and 20–30% in the portal LNs [1, 16].

In one single-institution study out of Korea, cumulative survival rates for 128 patients who underwent hepatic resection for ICC were 73% at 1 year, 52% at 3 years, and 43% at 5 years [47]. Recurrent ICC developed in 81 patients with a median time from resection to recurrence of 9 months (range, 0–124 months). The median survival time after recurrence was 8 months (range 0–108 months), with survival after documented recurrence noted to be 47% at 1 year, 23% at 3 years, and 15% at 5 years (see Kaplan-Meier survival curves for this population in Fig. 3.13). On univariate analysis, nine factors were significant: male gender, site of recurrence, DFS, LN metastasis, lymphatic invasion, perineural invasion, bile duct invasion, high initial CA 19-9 (>50 IU/mL), and high Ca19–9 at recurrence (>200 IU/mL). Interestingly, multivariate analysis of this small patient cohort showed disease-free survival time shorter than 1 year and bile duct invasion to be the only significant prognostic factor. Various treatment strategies were attempted for this patient population as shown in Table 3.6.

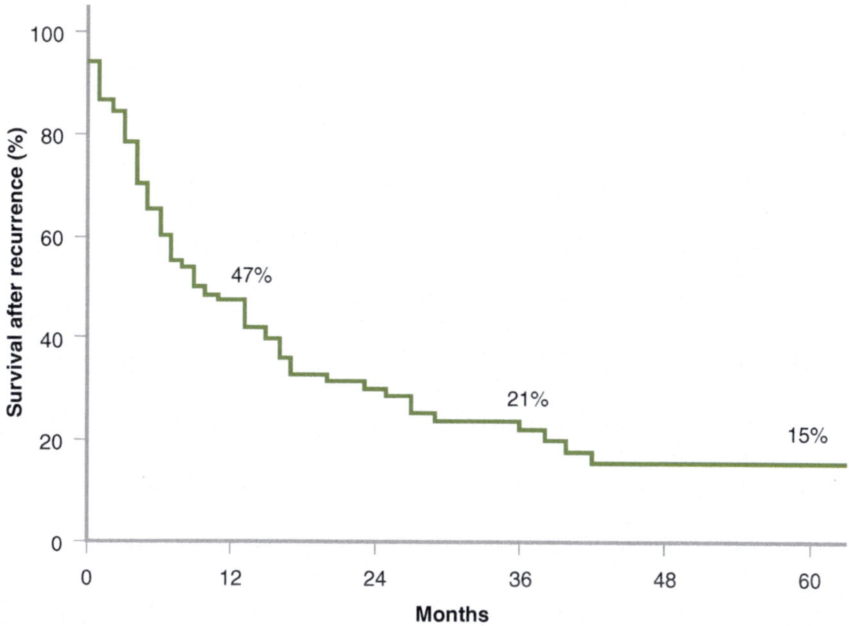

Number at risk

84	33	21	11	6	5

Fig. 3.13 Overall 1-, 3-, and 5-year survival rates after recurrence in ICC patients after resection ($n = 81$) by Kaplan-Meier method. (Reprinted by permission from SpringerNature: Adapted from Park et al. [47])

Table 3.6 Number of recurrences by type of treatment for recurrent intrahepatic cholangiocarcinoma ($n = 81$)

Type	No	Median DFS months (range)	Median survival after recurrence months (range)
Surgery	12	13 (1–54)	21 (1–66)
TACE	2	21 (9–32)	66 (38–94)
RFA	4	5 (2–22)	17 (13–108)
Chemotherapy	21	6 (1–28)	10 (2–54)
Radiotherapy	3	7 (1–9)	7 (4–23)
CCRT	5	6 (0–28)	9 (5–17)
Supportive care	34	5 (0–38)	4 (0–42)

Reprinted by permission from SpringerNature: Park et al. [47]
No number, *DFS* disease-free survival, *TACE* transarterial chemoembolization, *RFA* radiofrequency ablation, *CCRT* concurrent chemoradiotherapy

Prognosis for Locally Advanced Unresectable and Metastatic ICC

Unfortunately, patients with advanced unresectable and metastatic ICC have a very poor prognosis. Outcome is largely dictated by tumor extent at presentation, the underlying quality of the liver and patient comorbidities. Patients with disease confined to their liver have an overall better prognosis than those with metastatic disease at presentation [27]. There is limited data on adjuvant treatment for this population, and most trials to date have included patients with not only intra- and extrahepatic cholangiocarcinoma, but also gallbladder and ampullary cancers. One of these trials, the Advanced Biliary Cancer (ABC)-02 trial, was a randomized phase II-III trial that showed improvement in survival (11.7 months versus 8.1 months; $P < 0.001$) for this mixed population when treated with gemcitabine and cisplatin rather than just gemcitabine alone. Progression-free survival was also improved on the order of months (8 months versus 5 months; $P < 0.001$) [48].

There has been some study of anti-angiogenic therapy and disruption of the epidermal growth factor receptor (EGFR) pathway for biliary cancers with the addition of erlotinib 100 mg daily to a gemcitabine/oxaliplatin regime [49]. Although there was no statistical difference for the primary outcome of progression-free survival (PFS) for the entire cohort, a subgroup analysis showed patients with advanced cholangiocarcinoma experienced 5.9 months of PFS with chemo and erlotinib compared with just chemo alone (HR 0.73, 95% CI 0.53–1.00; $P = 0.049$). There is increasing evidence for local treatments for locally advanced ICC, including TACE (transarterial chemoembolization), DEB-TACE (doxorubicin eluting beads), and HAI (hepatic arterial infusion) therapy [50]. However, these are experimental without established prognostic estimates and will be discussed elsewhere in this textbook.

Prognostic Nomograms

A nomogram is a graphical representation of a complex statistical formula accepting multiple complex input variables to provide an easy to understand answer [11]. Nomograms tend to have a high discriminatory power since they can include more variables and have less need for simplicity. In addition, they tend to be patient-specific, without the need to be applicable to wide populations. The use of a nomogram to help answer patients' questions regarding individualized prognostication is becoming more common in clinical oncology management.

There are several nomograms available for ICC [16, 23, 51]. One of these, the Wang nomogram, exceeded the discriminatory ability of the AJCC 7th edition staging system in a large multicenter cohort of 1054 patients. The nomogram was developed to predict prognosis post-resection for ICC, using data from a single institution in China. Factors included were: serum CEA, vascular invasion, LN metastases,

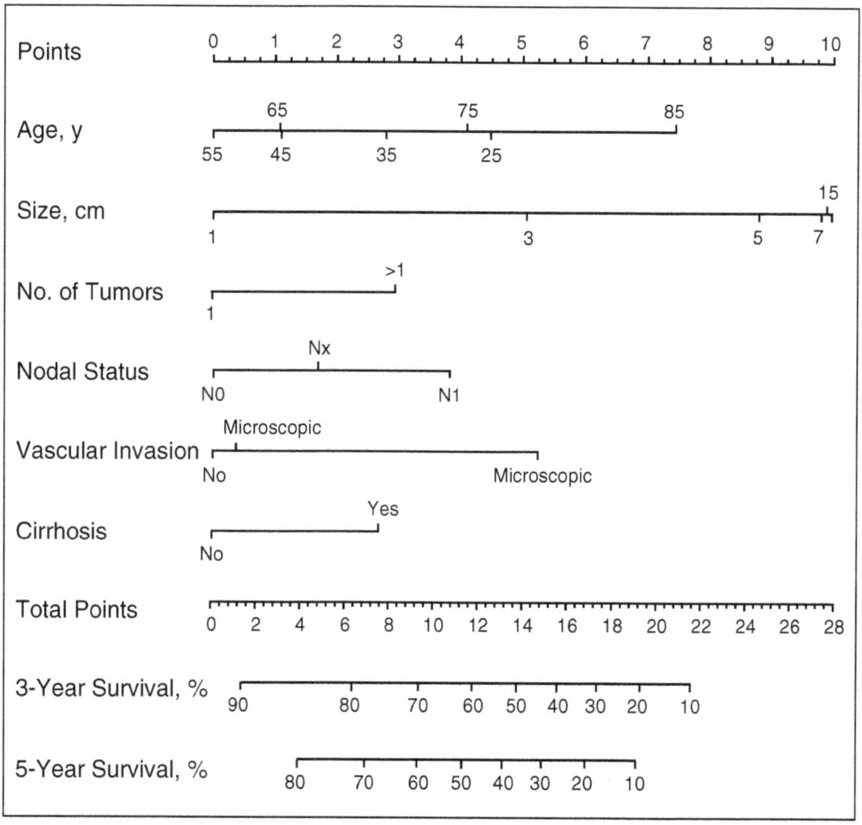

Fig. 3.14 A prognostic nomogram for predicting postsurgical survival of patients with resectable intrahepatic cholangiocarcinoma. (Reprinted from Burkhart and Pawlik [3]. https://doi.org/10.1177/1073274817729235)

direct invasion of other organs, and local extrahepatic metastasis. More recently, Hyder et al. [16] developed a refined nomogram, also for patients undergoing resection for ICC (Fig. 3.14) from an international multi-institutional cohort collaboration. Additional factors included were age at diagnosis and presence of cirrhosis. External validation of this nomogram has confirmed its discriminatory ability versus the AJCC/UICC 7th edition [52], but likely should be reevaluated in light of the new AJCC 8th edition.

Another prognostic score, called the MEGNA (Multifocality, Extrahepatic extension, Grade, Node positivity, and Age older than 60 years) prognostic score, based on evaluation of data from 275 patients listed in the California Cancer Registry undergoing resection for ICC between 2004 and 2011, was published recently [53]. The authors developed the prognostic score claiming all the factors in a nomogram should be available prior to resection if it is to be useful for surgical decision-making. Based on multivariate analysis, the simplified MEGNA prognostic score assigns 1 point each for the presence of: multifocality, extrahepatic contiguous organ involvement, grade (high), node positivity, and age older than 60 years. The score was validated in a SEER database cohort of ICC patients and offered an improved discrimination index (0.21; 95% CI, 0.11–0.33) compared with the AJCC 7th edition (0.18; 95% CI, 0.08–0.30). Again, this prognostic score should be validated using the new AJCC 8th edition.

Conclusion

The goal of a staging system is to provide "high prognostic contrast" between groups of patients to support patient education regarding long-term clinical outcomes, to help plan the frequency of postoperative surveillance, and to aid in selecting patients for adjuvant treatment. The AJCC/UICC is the most commonly used system worldwide for ICC, but arguably provides only moderate prognostic contrast. Continued active investigation based on the data provided in this chapter is necessary. In the near future, molecular and tumor markers indicative of disease biology will likely be used in clinicopathologic staging systems. Currently, more individualized prognostic information may come from the clinical use of a nomogram.

Outcomes for patients with ICC who have unresectable and metastatic disease are unfortunately dismal, and long-term results after hepatic resection continue to be plagued by frequent recurrence. This high recurrence rate should reinforce a multidisciplinary approach to ICC treatment. At present, however, hepatectomy is the standard of care for resectable ICC, and lymphadenectomy for every case, with consideration of diagnostic laparoscopy, should be part of every HPB surgeon's algorithm for accurate staging and prognosis.

References

1. Weber S, Ribero D, O'Reilly E, Kokudo N, Miyazaki M, Pawlik T. Intrahepatic cholangiocarcinoma: expert consensus statement. HPB. 2015;17:669–80.
2. Sasaki K, Margonis GA, Andreatos N, Chen Q, Barbon C, Bagante F, et al. Serum tumor markers enhance the predictive power of the AJCC and LCSGJ staging systems in resectable intrahepatic cholangiocarcinoma. HPB. 2018; https://doi.org/10.1016/j.hpb.2018.04.005.
3. Burkhart RA, Pawlik TM. Staging and prognostic models for hepatocellular carcinoma and intrahepatic cholangiocarcinama. Cancer Control. 2017;24(3):1–11.
4. Okabayashi T, Yamamoto J, Kosuge T, Shimada K, Yamasaki S, Takayama T, Makuuchi M. A new staging system for mass-forming intrahepatic cholangiocarcinoma: analysis of preoperative and postoperative variables. Cancer. 2001;92(9):2374–83.
5. Yamasaki S. Intrahepatic cholangiocarcinoma: macroscopic type and stage classification. J Hepato-Biliary-Pancreat Surg. 2003;10(4):288–91.
6. Blechacz B, Komuta M, Roskams T, Gores G. Clinical diagnosis and staging of cholangiocarcinoma. Nat Rev Gastroenterol Hepatol. 2011;8:512–22.

7. Nathan H, Aloia TA, Vauthey JN, Abdalla E, Zhu A, Schulick R, Choti M, Pawlik T. A proposed staging system for intrahepatic cholangiocarcinoma. Ann Surg Oncol. 2009;16(1):14–22.
8. de Jong M, Nathan H, Sotiropoulos G, Paul A, Alexandrescu S, Marques H, et al. Intrahepatic cholangiocarcinoma: an international multi-institutional analysis of prognostic factors and lymph node assessment. J Clinic Oncol. 2011;29:3140–5.
9. Edge S, Byrd DR, Compton CC, et al. Intrahepatic cholangiocarcinoma staging. In: Edge S, Byrd DR, Compton CC, et al., editors. AJCC cancer staging manual. 7th ed. New York: Springer; 2010.
10. Farges O, Fuks D, Le Treut YP, Azoulay D, Laurent A, Bachellier P, et al. AJCC 7th edition of TNM staging accurately discriminates outcomes of patients with resectable intrahepatic cholangiocarcinoma: by the AFC-IHCC-2009 study group. Cancer. 2011;117(10):2170–7.
11. Balachandran VP, Gonen M, Smith JJ, DeMatteo R. Nomograms in oncology: more than meets the eye. Lancet Oncol. 2015;16:e173–80.
12. Hosmer DW, Lemeshow S. Applied logistic regression. 2nd ed. New York: Wiley; 2000.
13. Buettner S, Galjart B, van Vugt JL, Bagante F, Alexandrescu S, Marques HP, et al. Performance of prognostic scores and staging systems in predicting long-term survival outcomes after surgery for intrahepatic cholangiocarcinoma. J Surg Oncol. 2017;116:1085–95.
14. Ali SM, Clark CJ, Mounajjed T, Wu T, Harmsen W, Reid-Lombardo K. Model to predict survival after surgical resection of intrahepatic cholangiocarcinoma: the Mayo Clinic experience. HPB. 2015;17:244–50.
15. Amin MB, Edge S, Greene F, Byrd DR, Brookland RK, Washington MK, et al. Intrahepatic cholangiocarcinoma staging. In: Amin MB, Edge S, Greene F, Byrd DR, Brookland RK, Washington MK, et al., editors. AJCC cancer staging manual. 8th ed. New York: Springer; 2017.
16. Hyder H, Marques H, Pulitano C, Marsh W, Alexandrescu S, Bauer TW, et al. A nomogram to predict long-term survival after resection for intrahepatic cholangiocarcinoma: an east and west experience. JAMA Surg. 2014;149:432–8.
17. Spolverato G, Ejaz A, Kim Y, Sotiropoulos G, Pau A, Alexandrescu S, et al. Tumor size predicts vascular invasion and histologic grade among patients undergoing resection of intrahepatic cholangiocarcinoma. J Gastrointest Surg. 2014;18:1284–91.
18. Yuan D, Garcia-Beccaria M, Heikenwalder M. Intrinsic and environmental factors in intrahepatic cholangiocarcinoma development. Oncoscience. 2017;4(9–10):117–9.
19. Guglielmi A, Ruzzenente A, Campagnaro T, Pachera S, Valdegamberi A, Nicoli P, et al. Intrahepatic cholangiocarcinoma: prognostic factors after surgical resection. World J Surg. 2009;33(6):1247–54.
20. Kang S, Hwang S, Lee Y, Kim K, Ahn C, Moon D, Ha T, Song G, Jung D, Lee S. Prognostic comparison of the 7th and 8th editions of the American Joint Committee on Cancer staging system for intrahepatic cholangiocarcinoma. J Hepatobiliary Pancreat Sci. 2018;25:240–8.
21. Spolverato G, Bagante F, Weiss M, Alexandrescu S, Marques H, Aldrighetti L, et al. Comparative performances of the 7th and the 8th editions of the American Joint Committee on Cancer staging systems for intrahepatic cholangiocarcinoma. J Surg Oncol. 2017;115:696–703.
22. Kim Y, Moris DP, Zhang X-F, Bagante F, Spolverato G, Schmidt G, Dilhoff M, Pawlik TM. Evaluation of the 8th edition American Joint Commission on Cancer (AJCC) staging system for patients with intrahepatic cholangiocarcinoma: a surveillance, epidemiology, and end results (SEER) analysis. J Surg Oncol. 2017;116:643–50.
23. Wang Y, Li J, Xia Y, Gong R, Wang K, Yan Z, et al. Prognostic nomogram for intrahepatic cholangiocarcinoma after partial hepatectomy. J Clin Oncol. 2013;31(9):1188–95.
24. Hepatobiliary Cancers. In: NCCN guidelines version 3.2018. 2018. https://www.nccn.org/professionals/physician_gls/pdf/hepatobiliary.pdf. Accessed 22 Sept 2018.
25. Bridgewater J, Galle PR, Khan SA, Llovet JM, Park J-W, Patel T, Pawlik T, Gores G. Guidelines for the diagnosis and management of intrahepatic cholangiocarcinoma. J Hepatol. 2014;60:1268–89.

26. Luo X, Yuan L, Wang Y, Ge R, Sun Y, Wei G. Survival outcomes and prognostic factors of surgical therapy for all potentially resectable intrahepatic cholangiocarcinoma: a large single-center cohort study. J Gastrointest Surg. 2014;18:562–72.
27. Endo I, Gonen M, Yopp A, Dalal K, Zhou Q, Klimstra D, et al. Intrahepatic cholangiocarcinoma: rising frequency, improved survival, and determinants of outcome after resection. Ann Surg. 2008;248(1):84–96.
28. Squires MH, Cloyd JM, Dillhoff M, Schmidt C, Pawlik TM. Challenges of surgical management of intrahepatic cholangiocarcinoma. Expert Rev Gastroenterol Hepatol. 2018;12(7):671–81.
29. Amini N, Ejaz A, Spolverato G, Maithel S, Kim Y, Pawlik T. Management of lymph nodes during resection of hepatocellular carcinoma and intrahepatic cholangiocarcinoma: a systematic review. J Gastrointest Surg. 2014;18:2136–48.
30. Bagante F, Spolverato G, Weiss M, Alexandrescu S, Marques HP, Aldrighetti L, et al. Assessment of the lymph node status in patients undergoing liver resection for intrahepatic cholangiocarcinoma: the new eighth edition AJCC staging system. J Gastrointest Surg. 2018a;22:52–9.
31. Goere D, Wagholikar GD, Pessaux P, Carrere N, Sibert A, Vilgrain V, et al. Utility of staging laparoscopy in subsets of biliary cancers: laparoscopy is a powerful diagnostic tool in patients with intrahepatic and gallbladder carcinoma. Surg Endosc. 2006;20(5):721–5.
32. D'Angelica M, Fong Y, Weber S, Gonen M, DeMatteo R, Conlon K, Blumgart L, Jarnagin W. The role of staging laparoscopy in hepatobiliary malignancy: prospective analysis of 401 cases. Ann Surg Oncol. 2003;10(2):183–9.
33. Bergquist JR, Puig CA, Shubert CR, Groeschl T, Habermann E, Kendrick M, et al. Carbohydrate antigen 19-9 elevation in anatomically resectable, early-stage pancreatic cancer is independently associated with decreased overall survival and an indication for neoadjuvant therapy: a national cancer database study. J Am Coll Surg. 2016a;223:52–65.
34. Ohtsuka M, Ito H, Kimura F, Shimizu H, Togawa A, Yoshidome H, et al. Results of surgical treatment for intrahepatic cholangiocarcinoma and clinicopathological factors influencing survival. Br J Surg. 2002;89:1525–31.
35. Bergquist JR, Ivanics T, Storlie C, Groeschl R, Tee M, Habermann E, et al. Implications of Ca19-9 elevation for survival, staging, and treatment sequencing in intrahepatic cholangiocarcinoma: a national cohort analysis. J Surg Onc. 2016b;114(4):475–82.
36. Rocha F, Lee H, Katabi N, DeMatteo R, Fong Y, D'Angelica M, Allen P, Klimstra D, Jarnagin W. Intraductal papillary neoplasm of the bile duct: a biliary equivalent to intraductal papillary mucinous neoplasm of the pancreas? Hepatology. 2012;56(4):1352–60.
37. Bagante F, Spolverato G, Weiss M, Alexandrescu S, Marques HP, Aldrighetti L, et al. Impact of morphological status on long-term outcome among patients undergoing liver surgery for intrahepatic cholangiocarcinoma. Ann Surg Oncol. 2017;24:2491–501.
38. Shimada K, Sano T, Sakamoto Y, Esaki M, Kosuge T, Ojima H. Surgical outcomes of the mass-forming plus periductal infiltrating types of intrahepatic cholangiocarcinoma: a comparative study with the typical mass-forming type of intrahepatic cholangiocarcinoma. World J Surg. 2007;31(10):2016–22.
39. Jarnagin WR, Bowne W, Klimstra DS, Ben-Porat L, Roggin K, Cymes K, et al. Papillary phenotype confers improved survival after resection of hilar cholangiocarcinoma. Ann Surg. 2005;241:703–12.
40. Dover LL, Jacob R, Wang TN, Richardson JH, Redden DT, Li P, et al. Improved postoperative survival for intraductal-growth subtype of intrahepatic cholangiocarcinoma. Am Surg. 2016;82:1133–9.
41. Luvira V, Somsap K, Pugkhem A, Eurboonyanun C, Luvira V, Bhudhisawasdi V, et al. Morphological classification of intraductal papillary neoplasm of the bile duct with survival correlation. Asian Pac J Cancer Prev. 2017;18:207–13.
42. Bagante F, Weiss M, Alexandrescu S, Marques HP, Aldrighetti L, Maithel SK, et al. Long-term outcomes of patients with intraductal growth sub-type of intrahepatic cholangiocarcinoma. HPB. 2018b; https://doi.org/10.1016/j.hpb.2018.05.017.

43. Paik K, Jung J, Heo J, Choi S, Choi D, Kim Y. What prognostic factors are important for resected intrahepatic cholangiocarcinoma? J Gastroenterol Hepatol. 2008;23:766–70.
44. Konstadoulakis M, Roayaie S, Gomatos IP, Labow D, Fiel MI, Miller C, Schwartz M. Fifteen-year, single-center experience with the surgical management of intrahepatic cholangiocarcinoma: operative results and long-term outcome. Surgery. 2008;143:366–74.
45. Ribero D, Pinna A, Guglielmi A, Ponti A, Nuzzo G, Guilini S, et al. Surgical approach for long-term survival of patients with intrahepatic cholangiocarcinoma: a multi-institutional analysis of 434 patients. Arch Surg. 2012;147:1107–13.
46. Tamandl D, Herberger B, Gruenberger B, Puhalla H, Klinger M, Gruenberger T. Influence of hepatic resection margin on recurrence and survival in intrahepatic cholangiocarcinoma. Ann Surg Oncol. 2008;15:2787–94.
47. Park H, Yun S, Lee E, Lee S, Han S, Kim S, Park S. Outcomes for patients with recurrent intrahepatic cholangiocarcinoma after surgery. Ann Surg Oncol. 2016;23:4392–400.
48. Valle J, Wasan H, Palmer DH, Cunningham D, Anthoney A, Maraveyas A, et al. Cisplatin plus gemcitabine versus gemcitabine for biliary tract cancer. N Engl J Med. 2010;362:1273–81.
49. Lee J, Park SH, Chang HM, Kim JS, Choi HJ, Lee MA, et al. Gemcitabine and oxaliplatin with or without erlotinib in advanced biliary tract cancer: a multicentre, open-label, randomised, phase 3 study. Lancet Oncol. 2013;(13):181–8.
50. Subbiah IM, Subbiah V, Tsimberidou AM, Naing A, Kaseb AO, Javle M, et al. Targeted therapy of advanced gallbladder cancer and cholangiocarcinoma with aggressive biology: eliciting early response signals from phase 1 trials. Oncotarget. 2013;4:153–62.
51. Jeong S, Cheng Q, Huang L, Wang J, Sha M, Tong Y, et al. Risk stratification system to predict recurrence of intrahepatic cholangiocarcinoma after hepatic resection. BMC Cancer. 2017;17:464–73.
52. Doussot A, Groot-Koerkamp B, Wiggers JK, Chou J, Gonen M, DeMatteo R. Outcomes after resection of intrahepatic cholangiocarcinoma: external validation and comparison of prognostic models. J Am Coll Surg. 2015;221(2):452–61.
53. Raoff M, Dumitra S, Ituarte P, Melstrom L, Warner S, Fong Y, Singh G. Development and validation of a prognostic score for intrahepatic cholangiocarcinoma. JAMA Surg. 2017;152(5) https://doi.org/10.1001/jamasurg.2017.0117.
54. Meng Z, Pan W, Hong H, Chen J, Chen Y. Macroscopic types of intrahepatic cholangiocarcinoma and the eighth edition of AJCC/UICC TNM staging system. Oncotarget. 2017;8(60):101165–74.
55. Compton CC, Byrd DR, Garcia-Aguilar J, Kurtzman SH, Olawaiye A, editors. AJCC cancer staging atlas. A companion to the seventh editions of the AJCC cancer staging manual and handbook. New York: Springer; 2012.

Chapter 4
Imaging

Pegah Khoshpouri, Timothy M. Pawlik, and Ihab R. Kamel

Introduction

Cholangiocarcinoma comprises less than 2% of all malignancies [1]. Even though it is a rare type of cancer, it is the second most common primary malignancy of the liver [2], accounting for 10–15% of all primary liver cancers. Imaging has a fundamental role in the diagnosis, staging, management, and assessment of response to therapy of cholangiocarcinoma. To date, surgery is the only potentially curative treatment for cholangiocarcinoma and imaging plays a significant role in surgical planning.

Most cases of cholangiocarcinoma are extrahepatic (80–90%) [3]. Intrahepatic cholangiocarcinoma can be divided into three subtypes including mass-forming, periductal-infiltrating, and intraductal growing. The most common intrahepatic subtype is the mass-forming cholangiocarcinoma (>85%), which is also called peripheral cholangiocarcinoma. ICC usually has central fibrosis with progressive centripetal enhancement on the delayed phase. The periductal-infiltrating subtype mostly arises at the hilum of the liver, where it is called a Klatskin tumor. The growth of periductal-infiltrating cholangiocarcinoma along the biliary ductal walls results in both dilatation and narrowing of the biliary tree. The intraductal growing subtype conveys a better prognosis due to its slow growth. This subtype often causes focal dilatation of the biliary system likely due to mucin production [4]. These three subtypes of intrahepatic cholangiocarcinoma are differentiated on imaging by different features.

P. Khoshpouri · I. R. Kamel (✉)
Russell H. Morgan Department of Radiology and Radiological Sciences,
Johns Hopkins Hospital, Baltimore, MD, USA
e-mail: pkhoshp1@jhmi.edu; ikamel@jhmi.edu

T. M. Pawlik
Wexner Medical Center, The Ohio State University Wexner Medical Center,
Columbus, OH, USA
e-mail: Tim.Pawlik@osumc.edu

T. M. Pawlik et al. (eds.), *Intrahepatic Cholangiocarcinoma*,
https://doi.org/10.1007/978-3-030-22258-1_4

Imaging Techniques

Ultrasonography

Ultrasonography is often the first diagnostic imaging modality utilized in patients with jaundice or right upper quadrant pain, which can be the initial presentation of cholangiocarcinoma due to proximal biliary dilatation. A curved linear array transducer (2–6 MHz range) is suitable for assessment of the liver parenchyma.

Ultrasonography is also useful intraoperatively to guide surgical planning for several reasons: (1) Ultrasonography provides live images that are free of radiation risk. (2) Intraoperative ultrasonography can clearly demonstrate the intrahepatic vasculature, which is very valuable for surgical procedures, for instance, during partial hepatectomies. (3) Known and occult masses can be detected by intraoperative ultrasonography, which is especially helpful during laparoscopic surgery, when palpation of the mass is not possible [5]. (4) Intraoperative ultrasonography also provides valuable information about intraductal biliary stones before their removal. (5) Intraoperative ultrasonography can guide oncologic treatments such as radiofrequency ablation of liver tumors [6].

Computed Tomography (CT)

Computed tomography using multiphasic contrast enhancement protocol is very useful for assessment of intrahepatic cholangiocarcinoma. Intraductal calculi could be better differentiated from an intraductal mass on the pre-contrast phase imaging, since the intraductal mass could enhance after the administration of the intravenous contrast [7]. The arterial phase (20–25 sec postinjection) is useful to assess the vasculature anatomy in surgical planning. Both the portal venous phase (60 sec postinjection) and delayed phase (150–180 sec after the portal venous phase or 3–10 min after contrast injection) can show progressive/persistent enhancement of the fibrous stroma [8].

Magnetic Resonance Imaging (MRI)

MRI with different sequences provides excellent tissue characterization. Useful sequences for the detection and characterization of cholangiocarcinoma include T1-weighted sequence (including pre and post-contrast, and in and out of phase sequences), T2-weighted sequence, and diffusion-weighted imaging (DWI). Fat suppression is important in reduction of fat signal within the liver parenchyma and in the porta hepatis on T1-weighted imaging. Post-contrast images can be obtained at different predetermined times including the arterial phase (20–25 sec postinjection), portal venous phase (60 sec postinjection), and delayed phase (3 min postinjection). Bolus tracking technique can also be used to accurately time post-contrast images [7, 9].

Hepatobiliary contrast agents including gadobenic acid (MultiHance) and gadoxetate disodium (EOVIST) are lipophilic. Therefore, these agents are useful in functional assessment of hepatocytes when taken up by hepatocytes and then secreted into the biliary system. Both gadobenic acid and gadoxetate disodium are hyperintense on T1-weighted sequence images. Hepatobiliary phase imaging can be obtained approximately 120 min post-administration of MultiHance and 10–20 min after administration of EOVIST. Due to the combined extracellular and rapid hepatobiliary features of EOVIST, cholangiocarcinoma demonstrates some progressive enhancement from arterial phase to delayed phase on post-EOVIST T1-weighted sequence images. However, it still appears hypoenhanced compared with the liver parenchyma on the delayed phase. The best tumor delineation can be appreciated on the delayed phase images due to high uptake of contrast by liver parenchyma [10]. In patients with poor hepatic function, the liver parenchyma and the biliary system will be poorly opacified [11].

Magnetic Resonance Cholangiopancreaticography (MRCP)

MRCP obtained by a heavily T2-weighted signal sequence is very helpful for assessment of cholangiocarcinoma. MRCP shows detailed anatomy of the biliary system, which can help distinguish benign from malignant obstruction. Unlike endoscopic retrograde cholangiopancreaticography (ERCP) that is limited to the assessment of biliary system distal to the area of obstruction, MRCP is a noninvasive imaging modality that can assess the biliary system proximal to the area of obstruction. On MRCP, slow-moving fluids including bile, appear hyperintense, while fast-moving fluids, like blood, and background soft tissue including liver parenchyma and fat appear hypointense. At least 4-hour fasting is recommended for MRCP to distend the gallbladder and decrease gastric secretions and bowel movements [12].

It is well documented that DWI increases sensitivity of MRI for detection of cholangiocarcinoma. DWI is based on the fact that intact cell membrane limits motion of the water molecules. Highly cellular microenvironments, like malignant neoplasms, cause restricted diffusion and low ADC values. Therefore, DWI may help in distinguishing malignant from benign strictures which is critical for periductal-infiltrating subtypes of cholangiocarcinoma. The degree of restriction on DWI-MR has been shown to be an independent preoperative prognostic biomarker for intrahepatic cholangiocarcinoma [13].

Positron Emission Tomography (PET)

Functional imaging of cholangiocarcinoma is feasible by PET. PET can be fused with CT or MRI to add anatomic details to functional assessment. PET is based on increased utilization of glucose by tumor cells. A radiotracer, 18-fluorodeoxyglucose

(18 FDG), is administered intravenously and is transferred into the tumor cells by glucose transporter type 1 (GLUT-1). FDG is then trapped inside the cell after phosphorylation by a hexokinase into FDG-6-phosphate. Overexpression of GLUT-1 and hexokinase by tumor cells causes FDG accumulation inside the cells, which is detected as hot spots on PET. Although not all the neoplasms are FDG avid, all types of intrahepatic cholangiocarcinoma are FDG avid, which makes PET a useful functional imaging modality for assessment of cholangiocarcinoma [3, 14].

Detection of distant metastasis can significantly affect medical and surgical management of patients with cholangiocarcinoma. PET provides sensitivity close to 100% for detection of cholangiocarcinoma metastasis >1 cm, and therefore, can add value to surgical planning [14]. Although PET is less helpful with infiltrative tumors, it can detect focal tumors as small as 1 cm [15]. Of note, the sensitivity of PET is higher in the detection of intrahepatic cholangiocarcinoma (90%) compared to extrahepatic cholangiocarcinoma (60%) [14].

Mass-Forming Cholangiocarcinoma

Ultrasonography

Ultrasonographic manifestation of mass-forming cholangiocarcinoma depends on tumor size. Tumors less than 3 cm are usually isoechoic to hypoechoic, while tumors greater than 3 cm are usually echogenic relative to the surrounding liver parenchyma. A hypoechoic halo is noted in 35% of cases, which corresponds to tumor compression on, and infiltration into, the peripheral liver parenchyma [16, 17] (Fig. 4.1a). Mass-forming cholangiocarcinoma usually has a well-demarcated, yet irregular margin. Capsular retraction is often an additional imaging feature [18].

Computed Tomography

On noncontrast CT, mass-forming cholangiocarcinomas are usually seen as homogeneously hypodense masses with lobular margins [19]. In the arterial and portal venous phase images, heterogeneous peripheral enhancement is seen, with progressive central enhancement in the delayed phases [19, 20] (Fig. 4.1b, c). The amount of delayed enhancement indicates the fibrous tissue content of the tumor. More fibrotic interstitial tissue is usually associated with a worse prognosis. Some data suggest that more than two-thirds enhancement of the tumor on delayed phase images is associated with a poor prognosis [19, 21].

CT can show biliary dilatation distal to the mass [21]. Cholangiocarcinoma rarely invades the vasculature to cause tumor thrombosis; however, narrowing of the hepatic and portal veins can be seen on CT [22]. In case of severe portal stenosis, atrophy of the associated liver segment can occur [23]. Similar to ultrasonography, liver capsular retraction can be appreciated on CT [20] (Fig. 4.1c).

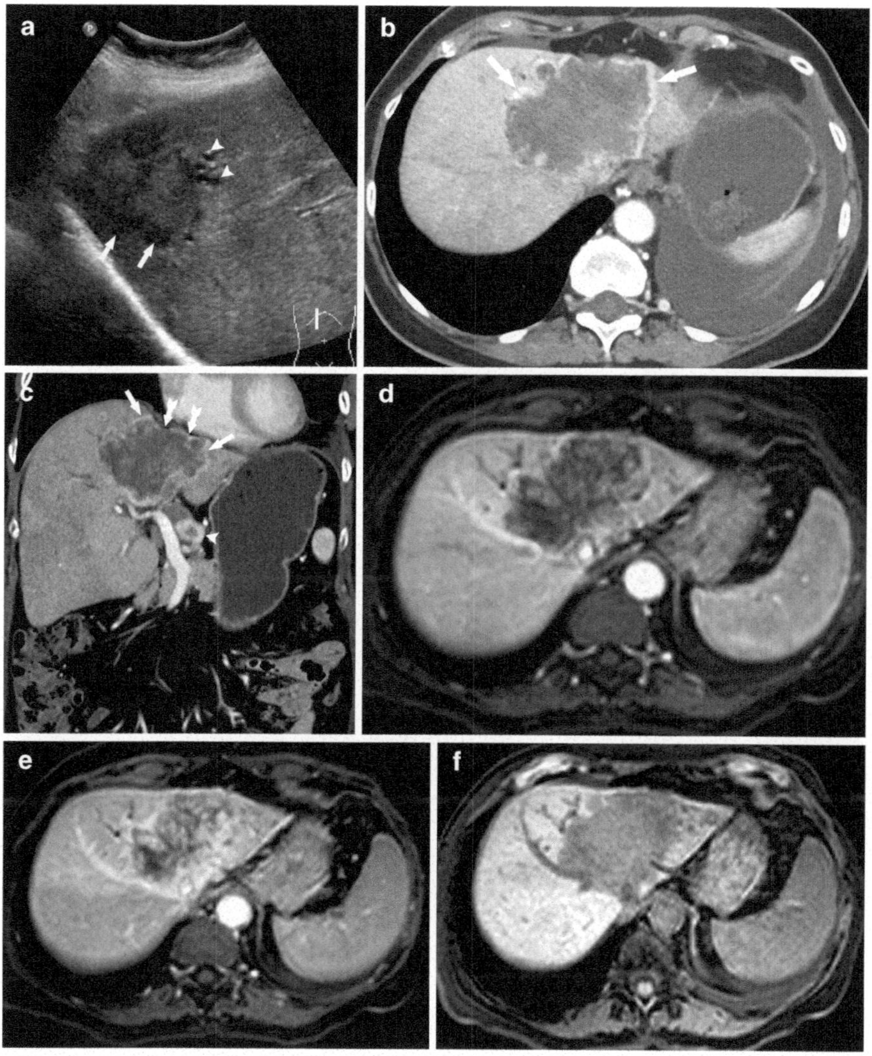

Fig. 4.1 Mass-forming cholangiocarcinoma. Ultrasonography (**a**) shows a heterogeneous echotexture mass with hypoechoic halo (arrows) and dilated bile ducts (arrowheads). Axial (**b**) and coronal (**c**) contrast-enhanced CT in portal venous phase shows a centrally hypoenhancing mass with lobular enhancing margins (arrows). Capsular retraction adjacent to the tumor (notched arrows) and necrotic hilar adenopathy (arrowhead) are also noted on coronal (**c**) view. T1-weighted post-contrast images (**d–f**) demonstrate progressive centripetal enhancement of the mass that correlates with progressive enhancement of the fibrous stroma. T2-weighted sequence (**g**) shows central dark signal suggestive of fibrous stroma (arrow). DWI sequence (**h**) shows peripheral diffusion restriction of the tumor (arrows). PET CT (**i**) demonstrates high FDG uptake in the periphery of the tumor (arrows)

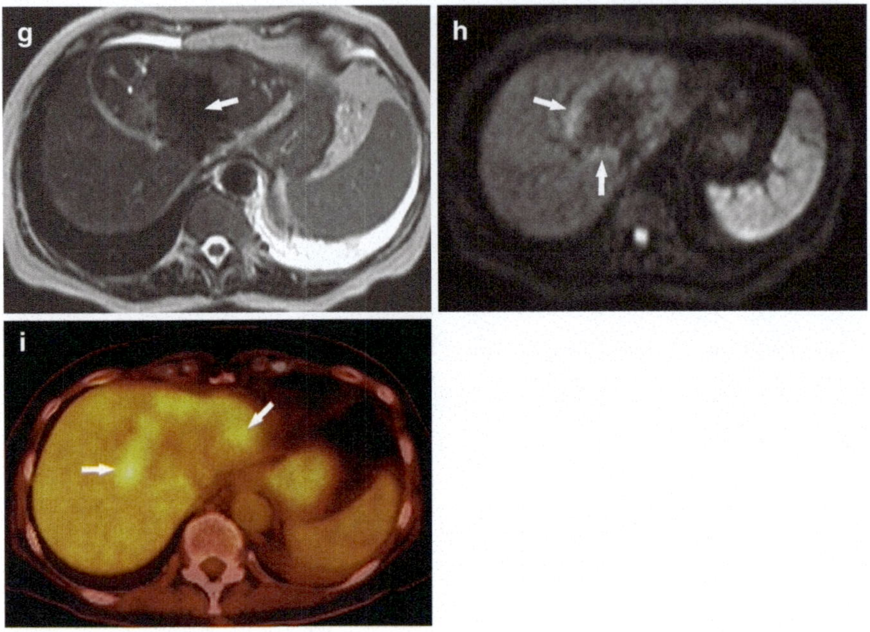

Fig. 4.1 (continued)

Magnetic Resonance Imaging and Magnetic Resonance Cholangiopancreatography

Mass-forming cholangiocarcinoma appears as a homogeneous T1 hypointense and T2 hyperintense mass with an irregular border. Peripheral biliary dilatation can be seen similar to that on CT imaging. Contrast enhancement is also similar to that on CT, with early peripheral and progressive central enhancement on more delayed phase imaging (Fig. 4.1d–f). Slow diffusion of contrast through the tumor is attributable to the fibrous stroma. A central low signal focus on T2-weighted imaging represents severe fibrosis (Fig. 4.1g). Peripheral early enhancement and rapid washout correspond to an area of active growth [17, 24]. The tumor is hypoenhancing on the delayed and hepatobiliary phases using a hepatobiliary contrast agent, due to lack of normal hepatocytes in the tumor.

Cholangiocarcinoma can be differentiated from hepatocellular carcinoma (HCC) based on its enhancement pattern. HCC demonstrates diffuse heterogeneous enhancement on early post-contrast phase imaging and washout of contrast on delayed imaging. In addition, cholangiocarcinoma usually does not invade the hepatic vasculature which is more common in HCC. The presence of cirrhosis favors HCC over cholangiocarcinoma [25, 26]. There can be an overlap in dynamic contrast enhancement pattern of intrahepatic cholangiocarcinoma and HCC in tumors less than 3 cm. DWI may help distinguish these tumors when other sequences are equivocal [13] (Fig. 4.1h).

Positron Emission Tomography

Sensitivity of FDG PET imaging to detect mass-forming intrahepatic cholangiocarcinoma is 85% versus only 18% for infiltrating cholangiocarcinoma [15]. High tracer uptake indicates high metabolism of the lesion that determines the activity of the tumor (Fig. 4.1i).

Periductal-Infiltrating Cholangiocarcinoma

Ultrasonography

Periductal-infiltrating cholangiocarcinoma is characterized by biliary duct narrowing/obliteration or dilatation without a mass-forming tumor [27]. Periductal-infiltrating cholangiocarcinoma can present as thickening of the biliary system with or without a mass-like lesion around dilated or narrowed bile ducts. Findings are usually isoechoic, but echogenicity is not specific and the tumor can be hypoechoic or hyperechoic [24]. Non-visualization of the right and left biliary duct junction is a characteristic ultrasonographic finding for periductal-infiltrating cholangiocarcinoma at the liver hilum, also known as Klatskin tumor [27].

Computed Tomography

CT presentation of periductal-infiltrating cholangiocarcinoma includes biliary dilatation or narrowing with periductal parenchymal thickening. Segmental dilatation of the biliary system indicates more proximal tumor involvement [23, 28]. These tumors are usually hilar and present with biliary dilatation in both liver lobes and contraction of the gallbladder (Fig. 4.2a–c). Peripheral tumors are usually not purely periductal-infiltrating and are often associated with mass-forming cholangiocarcinoma [28]. Normal bile ducts demonstrate water density unless there is intraductal sludge or stone.

Hilar periductal-infiltrating cholangiocarcinoma can be confused with periportal lymphangitic metastasis of an extrahepatic tumor. Unlike periductal-infiltrating cholangiocarcinoma, periportal metastasis usually involves both hepatic lobes and may not cause ductal dilatation [23, 29].

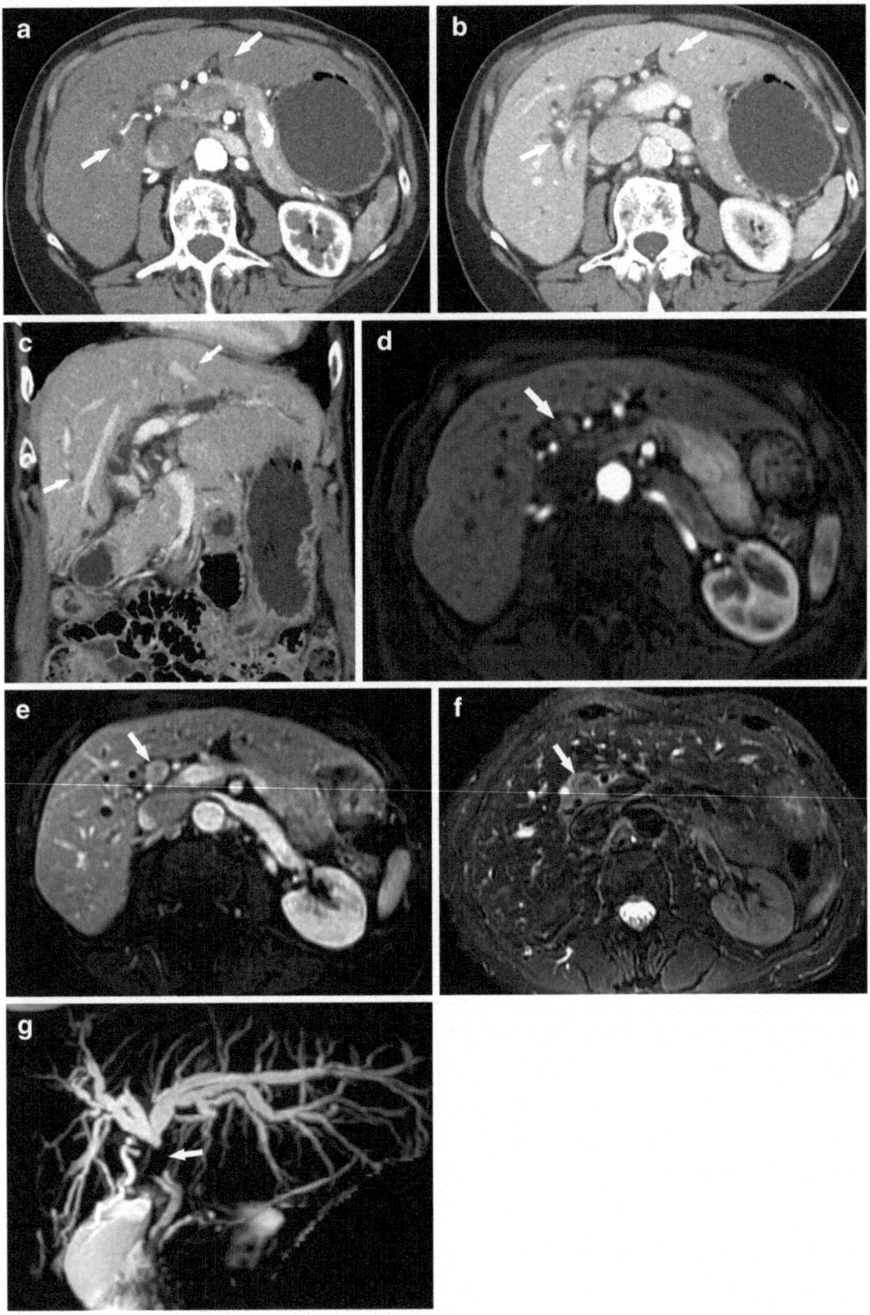

Fig. 4.2 Periductal-infiltrating cholangiocarcinoma (Klatskin tumor). Axial CT in arterial phase (**a**), portal venous phase (**b**), and coronal reconstruction (**c**) demonstrate dilatation of the biliary tree in both liver lobes (arrows). T1-weighted MR images show small heterogeneously enhancing lesion (arrow) adjacent to the hepatic hilum with progressive enhancement during arterial phase (**d**) and portal venous phase (**e**) T2-weighted sequence (**f**) shows centrally hypointense signal (arrow). MRCP (**g**) demonstrates significant dilatation of the biliary system in both liver lobes with abrupt cut-off in the hepatic hilum at the level of tumor (arrow)

Magnetic Resonance Imaging and Magnetic Resonance Cholangiopancreatography

Elongated and branching growth pattern along an irregularly narrowed or dilated bile duct is characteristic of periductal-infiltrating cholangiocarcinoma. This tumor demonstrates periductal thickening and increased enhancement and is T1 hypointense and T2 hyperintense (Fig. 4.2d–f). Benign stricture in its early stages can present similar to periductal-infiltrating cholangiocarcinoma on MRCP. These tumors present as irregular wall thickening of the bile duct, which is suggestive of cholangiocarcinoma when the thickening is greater than 5 mm. There is also upstream dilation of the intrahepatic ducts [5, 23] (Fig. 4.2g). The tumor demonstrates progressive enhancement on delayed phase. Portal vein invasion is also possible, which can be detected on MR (Fig. 4.3).

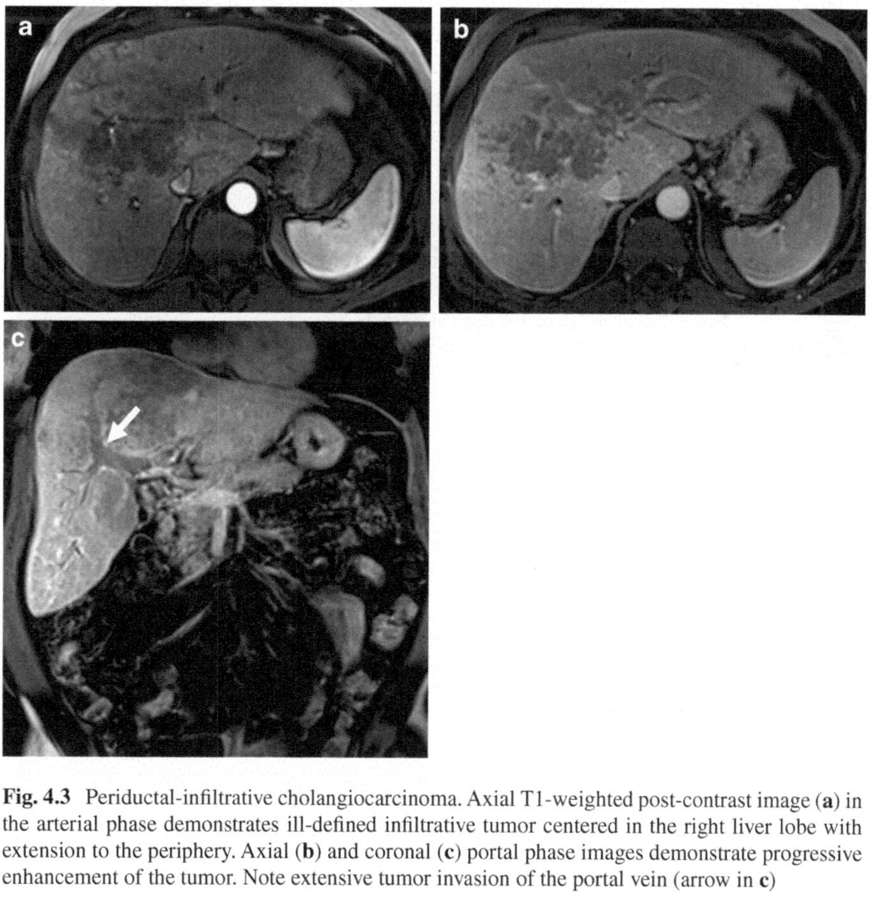

Fig. 4.3 Periductal-infiltrative cholangiocarcinoma. Axial T1-weighted post-contrast image (**a**) in the arterial phase demonstrates ill-defined infiltrative tumor centered in the right liver lobe with extension to the periphery. Axial (**b**) and coronal (**c**) portal phase images demonstrate progressive enhancement of the tumor. Note extensive tumor invasion of the portal vein (arrow in **c**)

Intraductal Cholangiocarcinoma

Ultrasonography

Intraductal growing cholangiocarcinoma usually presents with biliary duct dilatation and sometimes ductal narrowing. Occasionally, a polypoid hyperechoic mass can be seen, which is usually confined to the wall of the biliary system. Anechoic mucin that is produced by the tumor can obscure visualization of the mass [7, 30].

Computed Tomography

Intraductal growing cholangiocarcinoma usually manifests as biliary ectasia on CT. This subtype of cholangiocarcinoma can present as a polypoid intraductal lesion with proximal ductal dilatation, as intraductal cast-like lesion with biliary stricture and proximal duct ectasia, or as diffuse biliary dilatation with or without a polypoid intraductal lesion [17, 30]. Mucin production by tumor can result in biliary dilatation with intraductal material higher in attenuation than simple fluid. Biliary dilatation can be out of proportion to the tumor size [18, 31, 32].

Since these tumors are intraductal, these lesions can be mistaken with intraductal stones. As such, accurate interpretation of images can be challenging when intraductal cholangiocarcinoma and hepatolithiasis coexist. The tumor itself, if visualized, shows enhancement on post-contrast images. Noncontrast images can be helpful, which show high attenuation in intraductal stones. Intraductal cholangiocarcinoma is hypoattenuating on noncontrast CT when large enough (more than 1 cm) to be seen [17, 33]. Hepatolithiasis can cause benign biliary strictures secondary to inflammation, which should be differentiated from malignant biliary stricture caused by cholangiocarcinoma [7, 34]. Imaging features to suggest malignant stricture include asymmetric and irregular long segment narrowing, presence of enhancing ducts and periductal lesion, and lymphadenopathy [23, 35].

Magnetic Resonance Imaging and Magnetic Resonance Cholangiopancreatography

Intraductal growing cholangiocarcinoma lesions are usually hypointense on T1-weighted sequence and hyperintense on T2-weighted sequence. These lesions demonstrate heterogeneous enhancement on the arterial and portal venous phase post-contrast, and nodular, well-defined mass-like progressively enhancing lesions are visible on the more delayed phase. This feature reflects the desmoplastic nature of intraductal cholangiocarcinoma tumors [13]. Proximal biliary duct dilatation can be appreciated on different sequences. High tissue characterization of MRI allows detection of multifocal tumors since these tumors are spreading along the mucosal surface of the biliary tree [30].

Response to Treatment

Surgical resection is still the only well-established treatment option for patients with intrahepatic cholangiocarcinoma [36]. However, less than a third of cases are resectable at the time of diagnosis [37]. Systemic intravenous chemotherapy provides a limited benefit for unresectable cases. Recent studies have suggested an increased survival with intra-arterial therapies including trans-arterial chemoembolization (TACE) [38]. Assessment of treatment response after intra-arterial treatment of unresectable intrahepatic cholangiocarcinoma can be challenging. Traditionally, decrease in size and enhancement of the tumor on axial view have been accepted as indicators of tumor response to therapy by the World Health Organization, the Response Evaluation Criteria in Solid Tumors (RECIST), the modified RECIST (mRECIST), and the European Association for the Study of the Liver [39] (Fig. 4.4).

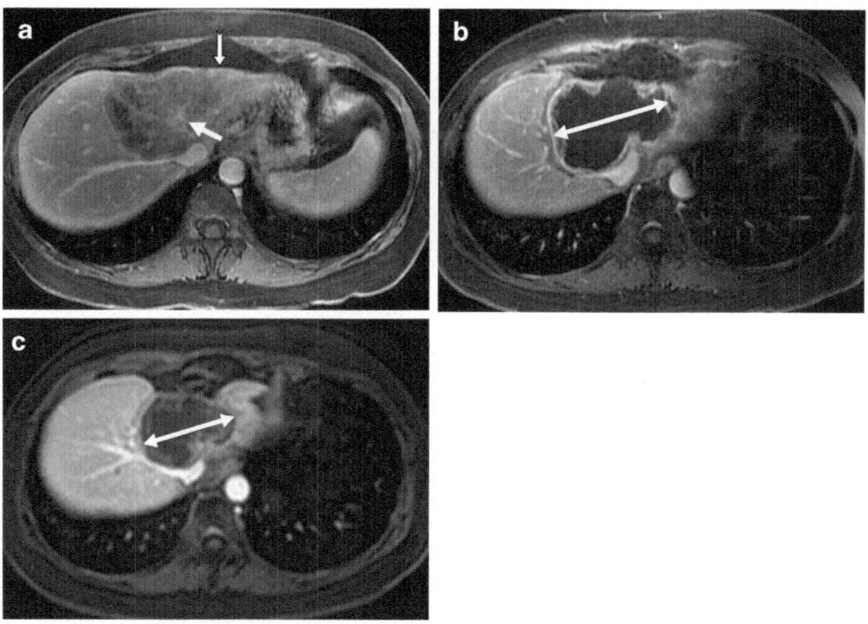

Fig. 4.4 Baseline T1-weighted post-contrast image (**a**) shows a mass-forming intrahepatic cholangiocarcinoma with central enhancement (arrow) and capsular retraction (notched arrow) before treatment. T1-weighted post-contrast images show favorable response to trans-arterial chemoembolization therapy with decrease in tumor enhancement and size (double arrows), 4 months (**b**) and 10 months (**c**) following therapy, respectively

Since cholangiocarcinoma is a hypovascular tumor with irregular peripheral rim enhancement, assessment of enhancement on bidirectional images could be suboptimal. Rather, volumetric enhancement can be measured more reliably [40]. Changes in size of the tumor after treatment may also be delayed, while functional MR techniques can provide information about early cellular changes. Diffusion-weighted imaging, apparent diffusion coefficient (ADC) map, and contrast-enhanced volumetric MR imaging can add value in assessment of tumor response to treatment. In particular, DWI and ADC values can provide information on tumor viability and structure. Specifically, intact cellular membrane in viable tissue restricts motion of water molecules that results in low ADC values. In contrast, increased permeability of cell membrane in necrotic tissue allows free motion of water molecules, which results in higher ADC values. Volumetric ADC, percentage viable tumor volume, and viable tumor burden and changes after treatment are novel MR imaging parameters that provide prognostic information in unresectable intrahepatic cholangiocarcinoma undergoing TACE [39, 41]. In addition, baseline multiparametric MRI assessment including percentage viable tumor volume and volumetric ADC can help predict mortality among patients with intrahepatic cholangiocarcinoma undergoing TACE [42].

Conclusion

Imaging has a significant role in diagnosis, staging, management, and assessment of response to treatment for intrahepatic cholangiocarcinoma. MRI/MRCP and PET can add value to the management of these patients. Recent advances in MR technology have revolutionized assessment of response of unresectable intrahepatic cholangiocarcinoma to more modern treatment options.

References

1. Breitenstein S, Apestegui C, Clavien P. Positron emission tomography (PET) for cholangiocarcinoma. HPB (Oxford). 2008;10(2):120–1.
2. Meza-Junco J, Montano-Loza AJ, Ma M, Wong W, Sawyer MB, Bain VG. Cholangiocarcinoma: has there been any progress? Can J Gastroenterol. 2010;24:52–7.
3. Blechacz B, Gores G. Cholangiocarcinoma. Clin Liver Dis. 2008;12(1):131–50.
4. Poultsides G, Zhu A, Choti M, Pawlik T. Intrahepatic cholangiocarcinoma. Surg Clin North Am. 2010;90(4):817–37.
5. Patel NA, Roh MS. Utility of intraoperative liver ultrasound. Surg Clin N Am. 2004;84:513–24.
6. Zacharoulis D, Asopa V, Navarra G, Nicholls JP, Jensen SL, Habib NA. Hepatectomy using intraoperative ultrasound-guided radiofrequency ablation. Int Surg. 2003;88(2):80–2.
7. Chung YE, Kim M-J, Park YN, Choi J-Y, Pyo JY, Kim YC, et al. Varying appearances of cholangiocarcinoma: radiologic-pathologic correlation. Radiographics. 2009;29(3):683–700.
8. Zhang Y, Uchida M, Abe T, Nishimura H, Hayabuchi N, Nakashima Y. Intrahepatic peripheral cholangiocarcinoma: comparison of dynamic CT and dynamic MRI. J Comput Assist Tomogr. 1999;23(5):670–7.

9. Maetani Y, Itoh K, Watanabe C, Shibata T, Ametani F, Yamabe H, et al. MR imaging of intrahepatic cholangiocarcinoma with pathologic correlation. AJR Am J Roentgenol. 2001;176(6):1499–507.
10. Péporté ARJ, Sommer WH, Nikolaou K, Reiser MF, Zech CJ. Imaging features of intrahepatic cholangiocarcinoma in Gd-EOB-DTPA-enhanced MRI. Eur J Radiol. 2013;82(3):e101–6.
11. Semelka RC. In: Semelka RC, Brown MA, Altun E, editors. Abdominal-Pelvis MRI. 4th ed. Hoboken, NJ: Wiley Blackwell; 2016.
12. Bonekamp S, Corona-Villalobos CP, Halappa VG, Kamel IR. MR (including MR cholangiopancreatography). In: Herman JM, Pawlik TM, Thomas CRJ, editors. Biliary tract and gallbladder cancer. 2nd ed. Berlin, Heidelberg: Springer; 2014. p. 145–58.
13. Fábrega-Foster K, Ghasabeh MA, Pawlik TM, Kamel IR. Multimodality imaging of intrahepatic cholangiocarcinoma. HepatoBiliary Surg Nutr. 2017;6(2):67–78.
14. Petrowsky H, Wildbrett P, Husarik DB, Hany TF, Tam S, Jochum W, et al. Impact of integrated positron emission tomography and computed tomography on staging and management of gallbladder cancer and cholangiocarcinoma. J Hepatol. 2006;45(1):43–50.
15. Anderson CD, Rice MH, Pinson CW, Chapman WC, Chari RS, Delbeke D. Fluorodeoxyglucose PET imaging in the evaluation of gallbladder carcinoma and cholangiocarcinoma. J Gastrointest Surg. 2004;8(1):90–7.
16. Vilgrain V, Van Beers BE, Flejou JF, Belghiti J, Delos M, Gautier AL, et al. Intrahepatic cholangiocarcinoma: MRI and pathologic correlation in 14 patients. J Comput Assist Tomogr. 1997;21(1):59–65.
17. Lim JH, Kim M-H, Kim TK, Lee M-G, Lee SS, Lee JW, et al. Papillary neoplasms of the bile duct that mimic biliary stone disease. Radiographics. 2003;23(2):447–55.
18. Brant WE, Helms CA. Fundamentals of diagnostic radiology. Philadelphia: Lippincott-Williams; 2012. p. 886–7.
19. Sainani NI, Catalano OA, Holalkere N-S, Zhu AX, Hahn PF, Sahani DV. Cholangiocarcinoma: current and novel imaging techniques. Radiographics. 2008;28(5):1263–87.
20. Valls C, Gumà A, Puig I, Sanchez A, Andía E, Serrano T, et al. Intrahepatic peripheral cholangiocarcinoma: CT evaluation. Abdom Imaging. 2000;25(5):490–6.
21. Asayama Y, Yoshimitsu K, Irie H, Tajima T, Nishie A, Hirakawa M, et al. Delayed-phase dynamic CT enhancement as a prognostic factor for mass-forming intrahepatic cholangiocarcinoma. Radiology. 2006;238(1):150–5.
22. Han JK, Choi BI, Kim AY, An SK, Lee JW, Kim TK, et al. Cholangiocarcinoma: pictorial essay of CT and cholangiographic findings. Radiographics. 2002;22(1):173–87.
23. Park HS, Lee JM, Kim SH, Jeong JY, Kim YJ, Lee KH, et al. CT differentiation of cholangiocarcinoma from periductal fibrosis in patients with hepatolithiasis. Am J Roentgenol. 2006;187(2):445–53.
24. Worawattanakul S, Semelka RC, Noone TC, Calvo BF, Kelekis NL, Woosley JT. Cholangiocarcinoma: spectrum of appearances on MR images using current techniques. Magn Reson Imaging. 1998;16(9):993–1003.
25. Shaib YH, Davila JA, McGlynn K, El-Serag HB. Rising incidence of intrahepatic cholangiocarcinoma in the United States: a true increase? J Hepatol. 2004;40(3):472–7.
26. Ito H, Ito K, D'Angelica M, Gonen M, Klimstra D, Allen P, et al. Accurate staging for gallbladder cancer. Ann Surg. 2011;254(2):320–5.
27. Laing F. The gallbladder and bile ducts. In: Rumack C, Wilson S, Charboneau J, editors. Diagnostic ultrasound. St. Louis: Mosby-Year Book; 1998. p. 175–223.
28. Lee JW, Han JK, Kim TK, Kim YH, Choi BI, Han MC, et al. CT features of intraductal intrahepatic cholangiocarcinoma. Am J Roentgenol. 2000;175(3):721–5.
29. Tada H, Morimoto M, Shima T, Hirana H, Nakagawa Y, Shimamoto K, et al. Progressive jaundice due to lymphangiosis carcinomatosa of the liver: CT appearance. J Comput Assist Tomogr. 1996;20(4):650–2.
30. Lim JH, Yi CA, Lim HK, Lee WJ, Lee SJ, Kim SH. Radiological spectrum of intraductal papillary tumors of the bile ducts. Korean J Radiol. 2002;3(1):57–63.

31. Honda H, Onitsuka H, Yasumori K, Hayashi T, Ochiai K, Gibo M, et al. Intrahepatic peripheral cholangiocarcinoma: two-phased dynamic incremental ct and pathologic correlation. J Comput Assist Tomogr. 1993;17(3):397–402.
32. Pavone P, Laghi A, Passariello R. MR cholangiopancreatography in malignant biliary obstruction. Semin Ultrasound CT MR. 1999;20(5):317–23.
33. Neitlich JD, Topazian M, Smith RC, Gupta A, Burrell MI, Rosenfield AT. Detection of choledocholithiasis: comparison of unenhanced helical CT and endoscopic retrograde cholangiopancreatography. Radiology. 1997;203(3):753–7.
34. Kawakatsu M, Vilgrain V, Zins M, Vullierme MP, Belghiti J, Menu Y. Radiologic features of papillary adenoma and papillomatosis of the biliary tract. Abdom Imaging. 1997;22(1):87–90.
35. Bader TR, Beavers KL, Semelka RC. MR imaging features of primary sclerosing cholangitis: patterns of cirrhosis in relationship to clinical severity of disease. Radiology. 2003;226(3):675–85.
36. Weber SM, Ribero D, O'Reilly EM, Kokudo N, Miyazaki M, Pawlik TM. Intrahepatic cholangiocarcinoma: expert consensus statement. HPB. 2015;17(8):669–80.
37. DeOliveira ML, Cunningham SC, Cameron JL, Kamangar F, Winter JM, Lillemoe KD, et al. Cholangiocarcinoma: thirty-one-year experience with 564 patients at a single institution. Ann Surg. 2007;245(5):755–62.
38. Seidensticker R, Seidensticker M, Doegen K, Mohnike K, Schütte K, Stübs P, et al. Extensive use of interventional therapies improves survival in unresectable or recurrent intrahepatic cholangiocarcinoma. Gastroenterol Res Pract. 2016;2016:1–13.
39. Zarghampour M, Fouladi DF, Pandey A, Ghasabeh MA, Pandey P, Varzaneh FN, et al. Utility of volumetric contrast-enhanced and diffusion-weighted MRI in differentiating between common primary hypervascular liver tumors. J Magn Reson Imaging. . [Internet]. 2018 Apr 6; Available from: http://doi.wiley.com/10.1002/jmri.26032.
40. Heye T, Merkle EM, Reiner CS, Davenport MS, Horvath JJ, Feuerlein S, et al. Reproducibility of dynamic contrast-enhanced MR imaging. Part II. Comparison of intra- and interobserver variability with manual region of interest placement versus semiautomatic lesion segmentation and histogram analysis. Radiology. 2013;266(3):812–21.
41. Halappa VG, Bonekamp S, Corona-Villalobos CP, Li Z, Mensa M, Reyes D, et al. Intrahepatic cholangiocarcinoma treated with local-regional therapy: quantitative volumetric apparent diffusion coefficient maps for assessment of tumor response. Radiology. 2012;264(1):285–94.
42. Pandey A, Pandey P, Aliyari Ghasebeh M, Zarghampour M, Khoshpouri P, Ameli S, et al. Baseline volumetric multiparametric MRI: can it be used to predict survival in patients with Unresectable intrahepatic cholangiocarcinoma undergoing transcatheter arterial chemoembolization? Radiology [Internet]. 2018. Available from: https://pubs.rsna.org/doi/10.1148/radiol.2018180450.

Chapter 5
Surgical Treatment

Georgios Antonios Margonis and George A. Poultsides

Introduction

Intrahepatic cholangiocarcinoma (ICC) is the second most common malignancy (after hepatocellular carcinoma) arising from the liver, comprising 10–15% of liver tumors. Importantly, its incidence is increasing worldwide. ICC arises from cholangiocytes in peripheral bile ducts proximal to the second-order bile ducts and can grow in different patterns. Specifically, it can grow as a mass within the liver (i.e., mass-forming subtype), along the bile duct in a longitudinal fashion (i.e., periductal infiltration subtype), or within the bile duct lumen (i.e., intraductal subtype). Irrespective of growth pattern, ICC commonly lacks specific symptoms, such as jaundice (as only a portion of intrahepatic bile ducts are usually obstructed and a sufficient number of liver segments have adequate biliary drainage), and, in turn, is frequently diagnosed incidentally or at an advanced stage. Surgery is the mainstay of treatment and the only modality that can potentially achieve cure in a small subset of patients. Unfortunately, only a minority (20–30%) of patients present with resectable disease at the time of diagnosis. As such, defining and expanding resectability criteria both from technical and oncologic perspectives are critical.

G. A. Margonis
John L. Cameron Division of Pancreatic and Hepatobiliary Surgery, Department of Surgery, The Johns Hopkins Hospital, Baltimore, MD, USA
e-mail: gmargon1@jhu.edu

G. A. Poultsides (✉)
Department of Surgery, Stanford University Hospital, Stanford, CA, USA
e-mail: gpoultsides@stanford.edu

T. M. Pawlik et al. (eds.), *Intrahepatic Cholangiocarcinoma*,
https://doi.org/10.1007/978-3-030-22258-1_5

Resectability and Patient Selection

As with any solid tumor, resectability is defined by technical and oncologic parameters. Regarding the former, technically resectable ICCs are those that can be completely extirpated with preservation of an adequate future liver remnant (FLR), namely two or more continuous segments, with intact hepatic arterial and portal venous inflow, hepatic venous outflow, and biliary drainage. What percentage of liver constitutes an adequate FLR depends on the quality of the liver parenchyma. According to the generic 20/30/40 rule, an FLR of at least 20% is needed in patients with otherwise healthy livers, at least 30% in those pretreated with chemotherapy or with steatosis, and at least 40% in those with early cirrhosis [1]. FLR can be estimated by several ways. The ratio of future liver remnant (FLR) volume to standardized total liver volume has been traditionally used. In cases where the FLR is borderline or less than the abovementioned cut offs, portal vein embolization (PVE) can be used to induce FLR hypertrophy. The degree of hypertrophy and kinetic growth rate have also been found to be protective factors against postoperative liver failure, in addition to FLR volume, for patients undergoing resection of colorectal liver metastasis after PVE [2]. PVE has been studied specifically in biliary tract cancers, and its benefit for patients with advanced biliary cancer who are to undergo extended, complex hepatectomies has been confirmed [3]. Nonetheless, it has been shown that FLR function may precede FLR size. For example, 99mTc-mebrofenin hepatobiliary scintigraphy (HBS), a technique that assesses the function of the FLR instead of its volume, is more predictive of postoperative liver failure compared to traditional CT volumetry [4].

After establishing that a patient with ICC is technically resectable, the surgeon needs to assess the oncologic benefit conferred by the operation. Lymph node metastasis beyond the porta hepatis or distant metastatic disease (including intrahepatic metastases) is a clear contraindication to resection. Regarding the latter, besides cross-sectional imaging including Positron Emission Tomography (PET), diagnostic laparoscopy (DL) can be used to enhance detection of metastatic disease. Prior studies have demonstrated that the use of DL can identify occult metastatic disease in 25–36% [5]. As such, the National Comprehensive Cancer Network (NCCN) guidelines suggest that, if imaging does not reveal any metastatic disease, DL to rule out unresectable disseminated disease should be considered [6]. The Americas Hepato-Pancreato-Biliary Association (AHPBA) expert consensus recommended DL, but only in high-risk patients [7], such as patients with multicentric disease, elevated CA 19-9, questionable vascular invasion, or suspicion for peritoneal disease. Further, they suggested adding laparoscopic intraoperative ultrasound of the liver in high-risk patients to assess for intrahepatic tumors and vascular invasion. In contrast with the liberal policy of NCCN and the more restrictive of AHPBA, The International Liver Cancer Association (ILCA) guidelines did not support routine use of DL because of limited amount of supportive data and suggested further research [8]. Lastly, a recent expert commentary suggested that, in some cases, DL may not be sufficient to safely determine resectability and an open exploration with at least a mini-laparotomy may be required [9].

If a patient is technically resectable and distant metastatic disease has been ruled out, patient selection for surgery may be further refined by evaluating factors associated with poor outcomes, such as microscopically positive surgical margin, nodal status, tumor size, multifocality, and major vascular invasion [10].

Surgical Margin Status

R0 Versus R1 Although an R0 margin is the gold standard in most malignancies, the fact that ICC is commonly diagnosed at an advanced stage (e.g., large tumors, invading adjacent structures) often renders an R0 resection technically challenging. As such, many studies have assessed whether an R1 resection truly impairs long-term outcomes. Some earlier studies (before 2010) failed to demonstrate a survival detriment from R1 resections [11, 12], but may have been underpowered to detect survival differences between R0 and R1. Larger subsequent studies have indicated oncological benefit from R0 resections. For example, in a large cohort of 224 patients with ICC, Yeh et al. compared R0 vs R1 vs R2 and showed that median survival was 26.2 vs 11.4 vs only 5.8 months, respectively [13]. Similarly, a 2016 meta-analysis that collectively analyzed all eligible studies concluded that "patients with negative surgical margin had significantly favorable overall survival and progression-free survival after surgical resection for ICC." [14] Thus, there is a consensus that surgeons should strive for an R0 margin as it is substantially associated with long-term outcomes.

This is reflected in various guidelines. For example, the ILCA guidelines published in 2014 stated that "The goal of surgical resection is to remove all the disease with negative microscopic (R0) margins while preserving an adequate remnant liver volume." [8] Similarly, the AHPBA expert consensus statement from 2015 concluded that "Resectability for ICC is defined by the ability to completely remove the disease with curative intent (R0) while leaving an adequate liver remnant." [7] Lastly, the 2014 NCCN guidelines stated that "Available evidence (although not conclusive) supports the recommendation that hepatic resection with negative margins should be the goal of surgical therapy for patients with potentially resectable disease." [6]

Width of Negative Margin Given the consensus on the necessity of R0 margins, the next question centers around the optimal margin width. Although many studies have compared R0 vs R1, a much smaller number of studies examined margin width. Farges et al. were among the first to suggest an optimal margin width [15]. They demonstrated that among patients with N0 disease, an incremental increase of margin width was associated with improved median survival (≤1 mm: 15 months; 2–4 mm: 36 months; 5–9 mm: 57 months; ≥10 mm: 64 months, $P < 0.001$), and a margin >5 mm independently predicted long-term survival (OR 2.2). Subsequently, in the largest study to date (n = 583), our group suggested that surgeons should strive to achieve at least a 1 cm margin when resecting ICC to optimize long-term

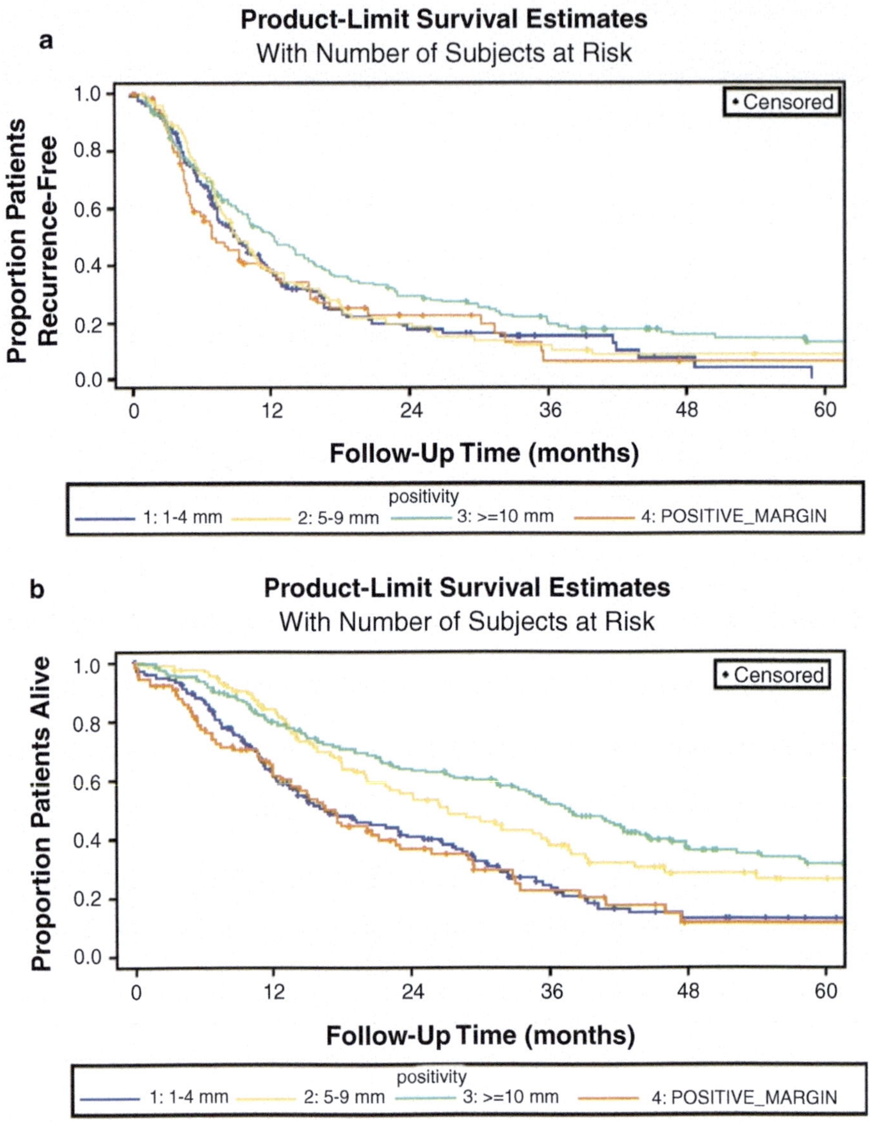

Fig. 5.1 Recurrence-free (**a**) and overall survival (**b**) following hepatic resection in 583 patients with intrahepatic cholangiocarcinoma stratified by margin status and width of negative margin. R1 margin status was associated with an inferior long-term outcome. Moreover, there was an incremental worsening RFS and OS as margin width decreased. (Adapted with permission from SpringerNature: Spolverato et al. [16])

outcomes (Fig. 5.1) [16]. This conclusion was confirmed by a study from Hong Kong that found that the disease-free survival increased from 14.1 to 86 months with a width of more than 1 cm ($P = 0.008$) [17]. Similarly, a meta-analysis performed in 2016 confirmed that 10 mm should be the optimal margin width when overall survival outcome was the main endpoint [18].

In contrast with margin status (R0 vs R1), the most recent guidelines do not make any specific recommendations regarding the optimal margin width. Specifically, neither the NCCN guidelines or the AHPBA expert consensus, nor the ILCA guidelines specify an optimal margin width [6–8]. The lack of specific recommendations may be attributed to the fact that, with the exception to the Farges study, all other studies and the meta-analysis were published after the guidelines were proposed. Given that margin width is the only surgeon-controlled variable, we believe that the aforementioned studies on optimal margin width will form the basis for specific recommendations in the upcoming revision of the consensus guidelines for ICC.

Surgical Margin Versus Extent of Resection Performing an R0 resection and striving for a wide margin may warrant a more extensive hepatectomy. In fact, to achieve an R0 margin, extended hepatectomy and/or resection of the extrahepatic bile duct bifurcation may be necessary in 78% and 29% of ICC cases, respectively [19]. In turn, one could hypothesize that these major resections, and not the margin width per se, may be the reason why survival is improved with wide margins. To our knowledge, only one study explicitly addressed this question. In 2017, Zhang et al. demonstrated that margin width, rather than the extent of resection, was associated with long-term outcomes. As such, if parenchymal-sparing resections can achieve a margin width of ≥5 mm, they should be preferable to major hepatic resections for ICC [20].

Margin Status and Nodal Disease Although there is a consensus that surgical margin status impacts survival, two studies have demonstrated that this is not applicable in the setting of nodal metastases. First, Farges et al. found that although an R1 resection was an independent predictor of poor survival in N0 patients, survival was comparable between R0 and R1 patients in those with N1 disease [15]. In 2014, Luo and colleagues similarly showed that while surgical margin was a strong prognostic factor in N0 patients, in the presence of LN metastasis, patients with R0 resections had similar survival as those with R1 resections. In fact, in the presence of nodal disease, the 5-year OS rates for the two groups were equally unfavorable (0% and 5.3%, $P = 0.266$) [21]. The surgeon should keep this information in mind when treating an ICC patient with N1 disease, as extending the resection to address a potential R1 margin may increase the morbidity of the surgery without an associated improvement in long-term outcome.

Margin Status and Adjuvant Therapy In surgical oncology, adjuvant therapy is used in theory to "sterilize" an R1 margin and eradicate microscopic residual disease. Although prospective data are lacking, there are a few retrospective studies that have explored whether adjuvant therapy may be useful in the R1 setting. For example, a meta-analysis identified patients with an R1 resection as one of the few groups that derived the greatest benefit from adjuvant therapy [22]. However, this meta-analysis included different biliary tract cancers, and ICC was underrepresented. More recently, ICC was the sole focus of a retrospective analysis of National Cancer Database data, which showed that ICC patients with an R1/R2 surgical margin were among the few subsets of patients who derived oncological benefit from adjuvant chemotherapy (19.5 vs. 11.6 months; $P = 0.006$) [23]. Subset analyses, stratified by margin status, of the recently presented BILCAP trial (a multicenter phase III trial randomizing patients to adjuvant capecitabine versus observation after resection of cholangiocarcinoma or gallbladder cancer) and the publication of ongoing trials such as the ACTICCA-1 (a multicenter phase III trial randomizing patients to adjuvant gemcitabine and cisplatin versus observation, after resection of cholangiocarcinoma or gallbladder cancer) will shed further light on the role of adjuvant therapy, but still these trials may be underpowered for ICC specifically (as this is the rarest type of biliary tract cancers) [24, 25].

Although, similar to adjuvant chemotherapy, prospective data on the use of adjuvant radiation are lacking, retrospective studies have suggested that adjuvant radiation therapy may be of value. In fact, given that 60–80% of all recurrences are locoregional, adjuvant radiation may be indicated at least for those with confirmed or suspected locoregional residual disease (e.g., R1 resections, preoperative major vascular involvement, or N1 disease) [26, 27]. Regarding the latter, in a study of patients who underwent R0 resections but had ICC adherent to major blood vessels, median OS was marginally better in the adjuvant intensity modulated radiotherapy (IMRT) group compared to the surgery-only group (21.8 months vs 15 months, $P = 0.049$) [28]. Similarly, another study demonstrated that tumor recurrence was common (60.8%), even after an R0 resection, and suggested that adjuvant RT might prevent locoregional recurrence [27]. Limited data on the use of adjuvant transarterial chemoembolization (TACE), on the other hand, showed no association with improved recurrence-free survival [29]. Lastly, stereotactic body radiation therapy (SBRT) has been used for locally advanced, unresectable ICC, with some proposing extrapolation of these results in the adjuvant setting [30].

Nodal Disease

Portal lymphadenectomy is routinely recommended for ICC to facilitate staging and inform prognosis. There is no doubt that regional lymph node metastasis is one of the strongest negative prognostic factors, as it likely reflects aggressive tumor biology. In fact, its prognostic significance is so strong that when patients are classified by LN status, other prognostic factors lose their significance. Nodal status has a profound impact on AJCC staging. For example, in the 7th edition of AJCC, ICC with regional lymph node metastasis was classified as stage IVA. Subsequently in the 8th edition, regional lymph node metastasis was downstaged from IVA to IIIB. To accurately establish N staging, previous data from our group have suggested that at least three nodes should be removed from the porta hepatis [31]. However, the most recent recommendation of the AJCC staging schema is to dissect at least six lymph nodes.

N staging is not only informative but may guide the selection of neoadjuvant or adjuvant treatment, which in turn may improve outcomes. The issue is that, as discussed in the case of R1, no phase III data exist on outcomes in ICC patients with nodal disease treated with adjuvant treatment. However, three phase III trials (that include other biliary tract cancers and have been recently completed or are underway) have evaluated the use of adjuvant therapy in resected ICC. The PRODIGE 12–ACCORD 18 study was completed recently and did not identify any subset of patients who may benefit from adjuvant GEMOX. In the BILCAP study, a prespecified sensitivity analysis noted a statistically significant difference in overall survival in favor of the capecitabine group, after adjusting for nodal status (along with other risk factors) [32]. Of note, the BILCAP study included a higher number of patients with LN-positive disease compared to PRODIGE 12 (54% vs 37%), which may in part explain the different result. The results of the ACTICCA-1 study are pending. Similar to BILCAP, both a meta-analysis of adjuvant treatment in biliary tract cancer (in which, however, ICC was dramatically underrepresented) and a recent retrospective study exclusively on ICC patients suggested that, among all patients with resected disease, those with nodal disease may derive the greatest benefit from adjuvant treatment (OR: 0.49 and HR: 0.54, respectively) [22, 33]. Lastly, a retrospective analysis of NCDB data demonstrated that, although median OS between adjuvant chemotherapy and surgery alone was comparable (23 versus 20 months), when stratified by lymph node status, chemotherapy was associated with a significant improvement in median OS among N1 patients (19.8 vs. 10.7 months, $P < 0.001$) [23].

As such, LN dissection may help select patients who will benefit from adjuvant therapy. With regard to adjuvant therapy in N1 disease, the guidelines are conservative but consistent. Specifically, the AHPBA expert consensus suggested that "For node-positive ICC, systemic therapy with either gemcitabine or 5-FU, or 5-FU-based radiation should be considered." [7] The NCCN guidelines state that lymph node metastasis, among other factors, is a risk factor that could be considered as a criterion for selecting patients for adjuvant treatment [6]. Similar to the other two guidelines, the ILCA guidelines state that "For those patients undergoing resection–especially those with N1 disease – adjuvant therapy should be strongly considered." [8]

Tumor Size and Multifocal Disease

Some earlier studies suggested that surgical resection for multifocal disease may be futile due to high rates of local failure and poor survival [12]. However, in 2015, our group compared patients with large or multifocal disease, defined as ≥7 cm or ≥2 tumors, vs those with single, solitary tumors and concluded that, although survival is decreased in the former cohort, this group should still be carefully assessed for the possibility of surgical resection [34]. In particular, patients with large or multifocal tumors without any of three additional risk factors (more than three tumors, nodal metastasis, and poor tumor differentiation) had a 5-year OS rate of 28.8%, which was comparable to the 30.5% OS rate of patients with a small, solitary tumor. In a subsequent study from Pittsburgh, Wright et al. defined multifocal disease as two or more tumors and compared intra-arterial treatments (IAT) vs surgery in those patients [35]. Although no tumor size cut off was used as an inclusion criterion, median tumor size of the surgery group was 7.5 cm, which is comparable to the tumor size in our study (all tumors were equal or larger than 7 cm), compared to 10.6 cm for the IAT group. As expected, the surgery and IAT groups were not comparable. Many adverse prognostic factors were more commonly associated with the IAT group: macrovascular invasion (44.1% vs 24.6%, $P = 0.027$), nodal metastases (57.6% vs 28.6%, $P = 0.002$), bilobar disease, (88.1% vs 47.4%, $P < 0.001$), and portal vein thrombosis (22% vs 10.5%, $P = 0.09$). As such, the IAT group was heavily biased towards worse baseline prognosis. Interestingly, despite this, survival was comparable in the two groups (20 months for surgery vs 16 months for IAT, $P = 0.627$). As such, surgery did not appear to confer any significant incremental benefit over IAT to those patients with multifocal ICC. A third study from Kyoto University compared survival in patients with intrahepatic metastasis (IM), vascular invasion (VI), and regional lymph node metastasis (LM). Among the three groups, patients with nodal disease had the worst survival at 12.8 months vs 18.7 for IM and 23.4 for VI. After comparing with similar but non-resected patients, they concluded that surgical resection may be justified for some advanced ICC patients with IM, VI, or LM [36].

Of note, a potential pitfall in interpreting outcomes of studies in patients with multifocal ICC concerns satellite lesions vs intrahepatic metastases. In the aforementioned Pittsburgh study, the authors mentioned that they did not distinguish between those two and both were included as multifocal disease. In our study, there is no specific mention to these two entities. In an editorial, however, it was suggested that, before including them in the same category, it should first be investigated whether these two entities are prognostically different [37]. To this end, a recent study from Italy compared the long-term outcomes of patients with satellite nodules in the same liver segment vs those with multifocal scattered tumors in different liver segments [38]. The former may correspond to nodules that spread from the primary tumor, while the latter may correspond to "true" metastatic disease. Importantly, 5-year overall survival after resection was much lower in the latter group (34.2% vs 9.9%, $P < 0.001$), indicating that "true" metastatic disease may reflect more aggressive tumor biology, compared to nodules that are spread in a close distance from the primary tumor. Perhaps, more importantly, from a practical standpoint, they found that, specifically in patients with "true" metastatic disease, the presence of LN metastases and the inability to achieve an R0 resection portend such poor prognosis that surgical resection should not be considered.

The cited studies on multifocal ICC are not directly comparable as both design (single vs multi-institutional design) and comparison groups (Surgery vs IAT, Surgery in multifocal vs Surgery in unifocal, "true" multifocal vs satellite nodules) differed. Interestingly, although the conclusions drawn about eligibility for surgery of patients with multifocal ICC appear disparate, the results are similar to an extent. Specifically, median OS of the multifocal group was 21.1 months in the study from our group vs 20 months in the Pittsburgh study vs 18.7 months in the Kyoto study vs 25–30 months in the Italian study. As such, the decision to offer surgery in a patient with multifocal ICC should take into consideration the morbidity of the surgery, the number and location of additional tumors (distance from main tumor), the presence of other unfavorable factors (nodal disease, anticipated margin), and the efficacy of alternative treatments.

ILCA guidelines recommend that "Patients demonstrating intrahepatic metastases should not undergo resection; Recommendation B1." [8] This recommendation is in line with that made by the AHPBA expert consensus statement: "Multiple bilobar or multicentric tumours are formal contraindications to resection." [7] In contrast, NCCN guidelines are more liberal and state that "although multifocal liver disease is generally representative of metastatic disease and is a contraindication to resection, in highly selected cases with limited multifocal disease resection can be considered." [6] It is obvious, from the variability of the aforementioned guidelines, that further study is warranted to more accurately define what constitutes "highly selected ICC cases with limited multifocal disease," where surgical resection may be of benefit. Furthermore, future guidelines and studies will need to assess the "optimal threshold" between the two ends of the spectrum of multifocal disease, one being limited satellitosis and the other being "true" intrahepatic metastases.

Major Vascular Invasion

A study from Kyoto University suggested that major vascular invasion into the Portal Vein (PV) or Inferior Vena Cava (IVC) may be the least harmful of all prognostic factors and that surgical resection in this case may be associated with acceptable oncological outcomes [36]. Indeed, Ali et al. from Mayo Clinic found that median OS in those with treated major vascular invasion (n = 14) was not worse than OS in patients without major vascular invasion (32 vs. 49 months, respectively, P = 0.268) [39]. The most recent study by Reames et al. (n = 128) corroborated those findings by reporting comparable median OS between the two patient groups (33.4 vs 40.2, $P > 0.05$) [40]. These two studies also demonstrated that rates of perioperative morbidity and mortality are not increased when major vascular resection is performed. Collectively, PV or IVC invasion should not be considered a contraindication to resection, at least when performed at experienced centers. These studies are in line with the AHPBA consensus statement, which states that "even patients with advanced complex tumors that will require extensive resections and major vascular and biliary reconstruction should be considered as potential candidates for resection" [7].

Long-Term Outcomes Following Surgery

Overall Survival

A systematic review and meta-analysis from 2014 summarized data from a large number of studies and reported on a median and 5-year overall survival of 28 months and 35%, respectively [10]. These data are most probably representative, as they are consistent with the median and 5-year OS reported by the largest 5 studies included in the same review (18–33 months and 21–35%). Unfortunately, it appears that survival has not improved in more contemporary studies. For example, although most cohorts of the studies analyzed in the meta-analysis included patients from the early 90s, Raoof et al. reported a median survival of 35 months for a cohort who underwent surgery for ICC between 2004 and 2013, a value similar to OS rates reported in the meta-analysis of older studies [41]. Of note, markedly better outcomes can be expected in subsets of patients, like those with solitary ICC ≤5 cm. Specifically, these patients can achieve 5-year survival rates up to 71% [42].

Intrahepatic Recurrence and Repeat Hepatectomy

The 5-year recurrence risk following curative-intent resection of ICC is around 70% [43]. Given that around 60% of these recurrences occur in an intrahepatic location, repeat hepatectomy may be considered, at least for a subset of those patients. Some studies report a small fraction of patients with recurrence (9%) being treated with repeat resection, but with only modest outcomes [43]. Although modest, these survival rates were better compared to those for patients treated with intra-arterial therapy or systemic chemotherapy (26.1 months vs. 9.6 months vs. 16.8 months, respectively. $P = 0.01$). In another study, 72 patients underwent repeat R0 resection for liver-only recurrence and had a 5-year OS rate of 41.9% [44]. A survival benefit was noted particularly in those who recurred at least 1 year after the first surgery (3-year recurrence-to-death survival: 46.6% vs 23.0%, $P = 0.022$). Similarly, a study by Zhang et al. demonstrated that patients with early recurrence fared worse than those with late recurrence (median OS: 10 versus 18 months, respectively; $P = 0.029$) [45]. This phenomenon may be attributed to different patterns of recurrence associated with the timing of recurrence. Specifically, patients with early recurrence were more likely to develop extrahepatic disease (44.1% vs 28.3%, $P < 0.001$), whereas those with late recurrence were more likely to have liver-only recurrence (71.7% vs 55.9%, $P < 0.001$). Interestingly, independent factors associated with early intrahepatic recurrence included tumor-related factors such as tumor size, number of lesions, and satellite lesions, whereas only the presence of liver cirrhosis was independently associated with late intrahepatic recurrence. This is an interesting finding, as it suggests that early recurrences are related to the dissemination of the original tumor, while late recurrences may be associated with "de novo" metachronous ICCs, which is similar to what is occasionally observed in HCC. Studies assessing clonality of tumors are needed to confirm this hypothesis.

Long-Term Survivors

Despite the overall moderate prognosis, long-term survival may be feasible for a small subset of patients with ICC. A study from Asia demonstrated that around 8% of ICC patients may be "cured" (survive at least 10 years after their surgery). Low serum tumor marker levels and favorable tumor-related characteristics such as solitary, small N0 tumors were associated with "cure". A Western study defined long-term survivors as those who survived ≥5 years and identified 153 patients (22.5%) as long-term survivors [46]. Interestingly, around 10% of those long-term survivors had negative prognostic factors such as perineural invasion, multifocal disease, nodal disease, and large tumors. As such, the mere presence of these negative factors at the time of surgery did not preclude patients from surviving 5 years post-resection. This seemingly paradoxical observation may be explained by the concept of "conditional survival," which refers to the changing probability of survival over time and has been applied to other malignancies [47]. Specifically, the more time that accrues from the date of surgery, the higher the likelihood that some patients with worse baseline disease will live longer than was expected at the time of surgery.

Neoadjuvant Therapy

No prospective randomized data exist on outcomes in ICC patients treated with preoperative systemic or locoregional treatment. In turn, no formal indications for the use of pre-hepatectomy therapy exist. Nonetheless, based on extrapolation of data from the ABC-02 trial performed among patients with stage 4 biliary tract adenocarcinomas, gemcitabine and cisplatin combination has been employed in the neoadjuvant setting as well (Fig. 5.2). A few retrospective studies have assessed the outcomes of these therapies, which are administered either to eradicate occult metastatic disease or facilitate resection by downstaging initially unresectable ICC. Regarding the former indication, in the largest study to date, Buettner and colleagues compared propensity-score matched patients (matched based on the factors associated with receipt of pre-hepatectomy chemotherapy) who received pre-hepatectomy chemotherapy to patients who had upfront surgery [48]. Although a trend for improved OS and DFS was noted in the pre-hepatectomy chemotherapy group, these differences did not reach statistical significance.

Regarding the latter indication, a few retrospective studies have assessed the role of pre-hepatectomy transarterial therapies and chemotherapy in downstaging locally

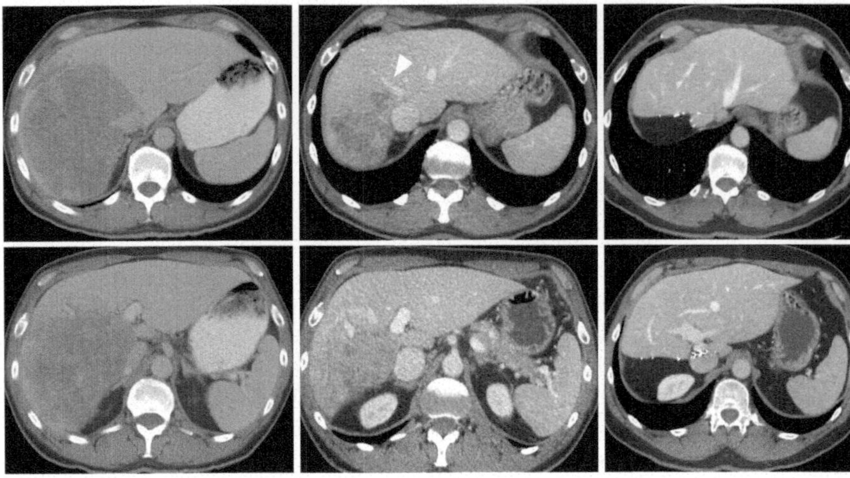

Fig. 5.2 Locally advanced intrahepatic cholangiocarcinoma managed with neoadjuvant chemotherapy and surgical resection: Fifty-one year old man who presented with abdominal pain and weight loss. Computed tomography (CT) at presentation (left column) showed a large liver tumor encasing the retrohepatic IVC and right hepatic vein origin (top left image), in addition to abutting the left portal vein (bottom left image, green arrow). There was no evidence of portal lymphadenopathy or distant metastatic disease. Given the borderline resectable nature of the tumor, 4 months of gemcitabine-cisplatin chemotherapy were administered. CT images (middle column) after neoadjuvant chemotherapy and before resection show significant response in terms of size with persistent vascular abutment (top middle image: white arrow, middle hepatic vein). The patient underwent an extended right hepatectomy and portal lymphadenectomy. No IVC or portal vein resection was required intraoperatively. The tumor was 90% viable, and there was carcinoma within 1 mm of the surgical margin. All 7 portal lymph nodes were negative. The tumor was unifocal. The patient received 2 more months of adjuvant gemcitabine-cisplatin chemotherapy and is alive with no evidence of disease 4 years postoperatively (right column)

advanced, unresectable ICC to allow for curative-intent resection. For example, Rayar et al. reported on ten patients with a single locally advanced ICC (mostly tumors invading major vascular structures) that were deemed unresectable [49]. After receiving a combination of yttrium-90 radioembolization and chemotherapy, eight of the ten patients were successfully downstaged and subsequently underwent a curative-intent resection. Of those eight patients, two died postoperatively and other two recurred (at 19 and 7 months after surgery, respectively). The limited follow-up, the small cohort size, and the lack of a comparison arm do not allow to draw conclusions regarding the oncologic benefit of downstaging. A different approach of downstaging unresectable ICC has been reported by the Memorial Sloan Kettering group [50]. Specifically, 236 patients with locally advanced ICC (tumor confined to the liver) or with metastatic regional lymph nodes (but no evidence of distant extrahepatic disease) were treated with either hepatic artery infusion (HAI) floxuridine (FUDR), systematic chemotherapy, or the combination of the two. Only eight patients (one had received HAI alone, four had received systemic chemotherapy alone, and three had received a combination of the two) had their initially unresectable tumors converted and, in turn, underwent a curative-intent resection. Of those eight patients, two patients died perioperatively and five patients recurred within 1 year. The conversion rate in the study was low and, similar to the Rayar study, definitive conclusions on long-term outcomes following conversion cannot be made. Collectively, systemic chemotherapy and locoregional modalities such as Y^{90} radioembolization and HAI may be selectively employed as a downstaging therapy for patients with initially unresectable ICC without evidence of extrahepatic disease, although only a small minority of patients is likely to ultimately achieve a curative resection [9].

Liver Transplantation

Earlier studies that evaluated outcomes of orthotopic liver transplantation (OLT) in ICC included patients with both hilar and intrahepatic cholangiocarcinoma. Given that these two entities differ significantly, it may be hard to interpret those results. Nonetheless, their outcomes have been so poor for ICC that OLT has been contraindicated for ICC in most transplant centers globally. As such, it may not be surprising that most recent OLT series for ICC include patients who were either transplanted because of decompensated cirrhosis and were found to have a small ICC in the remnant, or were transplanted with an erroneous preoperative diagnosis of HCC and were only proved to be ICC in the explant. Interestingly, post hoc analysis, mainly from UNOS (n = 440), and an international, multi-institutional collaboration (n = 48) have revitalized interest in OLT for ICC [51, 52]. In fact, the latter study identified a group of patients who benefited the most from OLT. Namely, these were patients with "very early" ICC (defined as single tumor ≤2 cm,) who fared much better when compared to those who had "advanced disease" (i.e., single tumor >2 cm or multifocal disease) with 5-year OS of 65% vs 45%, respectively, and recurrence risk at 5 years of 18% vs 61%, respectively. Of note, according to a subsequent study, these favorable outcomes may be limited only to patients with well-differentiated tumors [53]. Although another study from Mayo Clinic reported on a higher recurrence rate of 33.3% for early ICC, notably, they grouped hepatocellular carcinoma-cholangiocarcinoma cases together with ICC, thus rendering the three studies incomparable [54]. Prospective studies and matched comparisons with resected "very early" ICC (well differentiated, solitary and <2 cm) are needed to investigate whether OLT has a role in ICC patients, although these small solitary tumors may also be adequately managed with thermal ablation, SBRT, or other locoregional modalities in patients with cirrhosis. At this time, OLT for ICC patients should only be considered in this cohort of very early stage, select tumors, ideally on a clinical trial protocol.

Conclusion and Future Directions

Although surgical resection is associated with moderate survival, it remains the best option for many patients with ICC, and in fact, some of them may survive long enough to be considered cured. Margin negative resection and adequate regional lymphadenectomy remain the mainstay of appropriate surgical therapy. Advances in surgical techniques, systemic chemotherapy, and locoregional therapies will increase the "pool" of technically resectable patients. In parallel, as our understanding of this disease will evolve to further comprehend the prognostic significance of margin status, tumor size, multifocality, and vascular invasion, we will have a more balanced approach between "what can be technically removed" and "whether resection will provide a long-term benefit". At present, this notion is limited by the lack of studies about the interplay between traditional clinicopathologic factors and tumor biology. In the future, along with progress made in systemic therapy (including targeted and immunologic therapies), biomarkers may aid in answering questions such as when to operate on patients with large, multifocal disease, when to offer neoadjuvant therapy (and what type), and what the optimal margin width should be. Similar approaches have been suggested for other liver malignancies [55].

References

1. Adams RB, Aloia TA, Loyer E, Pawlik TM, Taouli B, Vauthey JN, et al. Selection for hepatic resection of colorectal liver metastases: expert consensus statement. HPB (Oxford). 2013;15:91–103. https://doi.org/10.1111/j.1477-2574.2012.00557.x.
2. Shindoh J, Truty MJ, Aloia TA, Curley SA, Zimmitti G, Huang SY, et al. Kinetic growth rate after portal vein embolization predicts posthepatectomy outcomes: toward zero liver-related mortality in patients with colorectal liver metastases and small future liver remnant. J Am Coll Surg. 2013;216:201–9. https://doi.org/10.1016/j.jamcollsurg.2012.10.018.
3. Nagino M, Kamiya J, Nishio H, Ebata T, Arai T, Nimura Y. Two hundred forty consecutive portal vein embolizations before extended hepatectomy for biliary cancer: surgical outcome and long-term follow-up. Ann Surg. 2006;243:364–72. https://doi.org/10.1097/01.sla.0000201482.11876.14.
4. de Graaf W, van Lienden KP, Dinant S, Roelofs JJ, Busch OR, Gouma DJ, et al. Assessment of future remnant liver function using hepatobiliary scintigraphy in patients undergoing major liver resection. J Gastrointest Surg. 2010;14:369–78. https://doi.org/10.1007/s11605-009-1085-2.
5. Goere D, Wagholikar GD, Pessaux P, Carrere N, Sibert A, Vilgrain V, et al. Utility of staging laparoscopy in subsets of biliary cancers: laparoscopy is a powerful diagnostic tool in patients with intrahepatic and gallbladder carcinoma. Surg Endosc. 2006;20:721–5. https://doi.org/10.1007/s00464-005-0583-x.
6. Benson AB 3rd, D'Angelica MI, Abrams TA, Are C, Bloomston PM, Chang DT, et al. Hepatobiliary cancers, version 2.2014. J Natl Compr Cancer Netw. 2014;12:1152–82.
7. Weber SM, Ribero D, O'Reilly EM, Kokudo N, Miyazaki M, Pawlik TM. Intrahepatic cholangiocarcinoma: expert consensus statement. HPB (Oxford). 2015;17:669–80. https://doi.org/10.1111/hpb.12441.
8. Bridgewater J, Galle PR, Khan SA, Llovet JM, Park JW, Patel T, et al. Guidelines for the diagnosis and management of intrahepatic cholangiocarcinoma. J Hepatol. 2014;60:1268–89. https://doi.org/10.1016/j.jhep.2014.01.021.

9. Squires MH, Cloyd JM, Dillhoff M, Schmidt C, Pawlik TM. Challenges of surgical management of intrahepatic cholangiocarcinoma. Expert Rev Gastroenterol Hepatol. 2018;12:671–81. https://doi.org/10.1080/17474124.2018.1489229.
10. Mavros MN, Economopoulos KP, Alexiou VG, Pawlik TM. Treatment and prognosis for patients with intrahepatic cholangiocarcinoma: systematic review and meta-analysis. JAMA Surg. 2014;149:565–74. https://doi.org/10.1001/jamasurg.2013.5137.
11. Tamandl D, Herberger B, Gruenberger B, Puhalla H, Klinger M, Gruenberger T. Influence of hepatic resection margin on recurrence and survival in intrahepatic cholangiocarcinoma. Ann Surg Oncol. 2008;15:2787–94. https://doi.org/10.1245/s10434-008-0081-1.
12. Endo I, Gonen M, Yopp AC, Dalal KM, Zhou Q, Klimstra D, et al. Intrahepatic cholangiocarcinoma: rising frequency, improved survival, and determinants of outcome after resection. Ann Surg. 2008;248:84–96. https://doi.org/10.1097/SLA.0b013e318176c4d3.
13. Yeh CN, Hsieh FJ, Chiang KC, Chen JS, Yeh TS, Jan YY, et al. Clinical effect of a positive surgical margin after hepatectomy on survival of patients with intrahepatic cholangiocarcinoma. Drug Des Devel Ther. 2015;9:163–74. https://doi.org/10.2147/DDDT.S74940.
14. Li MX, Bi XY, Li ZY, Huang Z, Han Y, Zhao JJ, et al. Impaction of surgical margin status on the survival outcome after surgical resection of intrahepatic cholangiocarcinoma: a systematic review and meta-analysis. J Surg Res. 2016;203:163–73. https://doi.org/10.1016/j.jss.2016.02.012.
15. Farges O, Fuks D, Boleslawski E, Le Treut YP, Castaing D, Laurent A, et al. Influence of surgical margins on outcome in patients with intrahepatic cholangiocarcinoma: a multicenter study by the AFC-IHCC-2009 study group. Ann Surg. 2011;254:824–9;. ; discussion 830. https://doi.org/10.1097/SLA.0b013e318236c21d.
16. Spolverato G, Yakoob MY, Kim Y, Alexandrescu S, Marques HP, Lamelas J, et al. The impact of surgical margin status on long-term outcome after resection for intrahepatic cholangiocarcinoma. Ann Surg Oncol. 2015;22:4020–8. https://doi.org/10.1245/s10434-015-4472-9.
17. Ma KW, Cheung TT, She WH, Chok KS, Chan AC, Ng IO, et al. The effect of wide resection margin in patients with intrahepatic cholangiocarcinoma: a single-center experience. Medicine (Baltimore). 2016;95:e4133. https://doi.org/10.1097/MD.0000000000004133.
18. Tang H, Lu W, Li B, Meng X, Dong J. Influence of surgical margins on overall survival after resection of intrahepatic cholangiocarcinoma: a meta-analysis. Medicine (Baltimore). 2016;95:e4621. https://doi.org/10.1097/MD.0000000000004621.
19. Sotiropoulos GC, Bockhorn M, Sgourakis G, Brokalaki EI, Molmenti EP, Neuhauser M, et al. R0 liver resections for primary malignant liver tumors in the noncirrhotic liver: a diagnosis-related analysis. Dig Dis Sci. 2009;54:887–94. https://doi.org/10.1007/s10620-008-0408-6.
20. Zhang XF, Bagante F, Chakedis J, Moris D, Beal EW, Weiss M, et al. Perioperative and long-term outcome for intrahepatic cholangiocarcinoma: impact of major versus minor hepatectomy. J Gastrointest Surg. 2017;21:1841–50. https://doi.org/10.1007/s11605-017-3499-6.
21. Luo X, Yuan L, Wang Y, Ge R, Sun Y, Wei G. Survival outcomes and prognostic factors of surgical therapy for all potentially resectable intrahepatic cholangiocarcinoma: a large single-center cohort study. J Gastrointest Surg. 2014;18:562–72. https://doi.org/10.1007/s11605-013-2447-3.
22. Horgan AM, Amir E, Walter T, Knox JJ. Adjuvant therapy in the treatment of biliary tract cancer: a systematic review and meta-analysis. J Clin Oncol. 2012;30:1934–40. https://doi.org/10.1200/JCO.2011.40.5381.
23. Miura JT, Johnston FM, Tsai S, George B, Thomas J, Eastwood D, et al. Chemotherapy for surgically resected intrahepatic cholangiocarcinoma. Ann Surg Oncol. 2015;22:3716–23. https://doi.org/10.1245/s10434-015-4501-8.
24. Edeline J, Bonnetain F, Phelip JM, Watelet J, Hammel P, Joly J-P, et al. Gemox versus surveillance following surgery of localized biliary tract cancer: results of the PRODIGE 12-ACCORD 18 (UNICANCER GI) phase III trial. American Society of Clinical Oncology; 2017.
25. Primrose JN, Fox R, Palmer DH, Prasad R, Mirza D, Anthoney DA, et al. Adjuvant capecitabine for biliary tract cancer: the BILCAP randomized study. J Clin Oncol. 2017;35:4006. https://doi.org/10.1200/JCO.2017.35.15_suppl.4006.

26. Song S, Kim K, Chie EK, Kim S, Park HJ, Yi NJ, et al. Locoregional recurrence after curative intent resection for intrahepatic cholangiocarcinoma: implications for adjuvant radiotherapy. Clin Transl Oncol. 2015;17:825–9. https://doi.org/10.1007/s12094-015-1312-0.
27. Gil E, Joh JW, Park HC, Yu JI, Jung SH, Kim JM. Predictors and patterns of recurrence after curative liver resection in intrahepatic cholangiocarcinoma, for application of postoperative radiotherapy: a retrospective study. World J Surg Oncol. 2015;13:227. https://doi.org/10.1186/s12957-015-0637-z.
28. Jia AY, Wu JX, Zhao YT, Li YX, Wang Z, Rong WQ, et al. Intensity-modulated radiotherapy following null-margin resection is associated with improved survival in the treatment of intrahepatic cholangiocarcinoma. J Gastrointest Oncol. 2015;6:126–33. https://doi.org/10.3978/j.issn.2078-6891.2014.102.
29. Shen WF, Zhong W, Liu Q, Sui CJ, Huang YQ, Yang JM. Adjuvant transcatheter arterial chemoembolization for intrahepatic cholangiocarcinoma after curative surgery: retrospective control study. World J Surg. 2011;35:2083–91. https://doi.org/10.1007/s00268-011-1171-y.
30. Shen ZT, Zhou H, Li AM, Li B, Shen JS, Zhu XX. Clinical outcomes and prognostic factors of stereotactic body radiation therapy for intrahepatic cholangiocarcinoma. Oncotarget. 2017;8:93541–50. https://doi.org/10.18632/oncotarget.19972.
31. Kim Y, Spolverato G, Amini N, Margonis GA, Gupta R, Ejaz A, et al. Surgical management of intrahepatic cholangiocarcinoma: defining an optimal prognostic lymph node stratification Schema. Ann Surg Oncol. 2015;22:2772–8. https://doi.org/10.1245/s10434-015-4419-1.
32. Siebenhuner AR, Seifert H, Bachmann H, Seifert B, Winder T, Feilchenfeldt J, et al. Adjuvant treatment of resectable biliary tract cancer with cisplatin plus gemcitabine: a prospective single center phase II study. BMC Cancer. 2018;18:72. https://doi.org/10.1186/s12885-017-3967-0.
33. Sur MD, In H, Sharpe SM, Baker MS, Weichselbaum RR, Talamonti MS, et al. Defining the benefit of adjuvant therapy following resection for intrahepatic cholangiocarcinoma. Ann Surg Oncol. 2015;22:2209–17. https://doi.org/10.1245/s10434-014-4275-4.
34. Spolverato G, Kim Y, Alexandrescu S, Popescu I, Marques HP, Aldrighetti L, et al. Is hepatic resection for large or multifocal intrahepatic cholangiocarcinoma justified? Results from a multi-institutional collaboration. Ann Surg Oncol. 2015;22:2218–25. https://doi.org/10.1245/s10434-014-4223-3.
35. Wright GP, Perkins S, Jones H, Zureikat AH, Marsh JW, Holtzman MP, et al. Surgical resection does not improve survival in multifocal intrahepatic cholangiocarcinoma: a comparison of surgical resection with intra-arterial therapies. Ann Surg Oncol. 2018;25:83–90. https://doi.org/10.1245/s10434-017-6110-1.
36. Yoh T, Hatano E, Yamanaka K, Nishio T, Seo S, Taura K, et al. Is surgical resection justified for advanced intrahepatic cholangiocarcinoma? Liver Cancer. 2016;5:280–9. https://doi.org/10.1159/000449339.
37. Abou-Alfa GK, Geschwind JF, Choti M, d'Angelica MI. Consensus conference on intrahepatic cholangiocarcinoma. HPB (Oxford). 2015;17:661–3. https://doi.org/10.1111/hpb.12438.
38. Conci S, Ruzzenente A, Vigano L, Ercolani G, Fontana A, Bagante F, et al. Patterns of distribution of hepatic nodules (single, satellites or multifocal) in intrahepatic cholangiocarcinoma: prognostic impact after surgery. Ann Surg Oncol. 2018; https://doi.org/10.1245/s10434-018-6669-1.
39. Ali SM, Clark CJ, Zaydfudim VM, Que FG, Nagorney DM. Role of major vascular resection in patients with intrahepatic cholangiocarcinoma. Ann Surg Oncol. 2013;20:2023–8. https://doi.org/10.1245/s10434-012-2808-2.
40. Reames BN, Ejaz A, Koerkamp BG, Alexandrescu S, Marques HP, Aldrighetti L, et al. Impact of major vascular resection on outcomes and survival in patients with intrahepatic cholangiocarcinoma: a multi-institutional analysis. J Surg Oncol. 2017;116:133–9. https://doi.org/10.1002/jso.24633.
41. Raoof M, Dumitra S, Ituarte PHG, Melstrom L, Warner SG, Fong Y, et al. Development and validation of a prognostic score for intrahepatic cholangiocarcinoma. JAMA Surg. 2017;152:e170117. https://doi.org/10.1001/jamasurg.2017.0117.

42. Tarchi P, Tabrizian P, Prigoff J, Schwartz M. Outcomes of resection for solitary </=5 cm intrahepatic cholangiocarcinoma. Surgery. 2018;163:698–702. https://doi.org/10.1016/j.surg.2017.09.058.
43. Spolverato G, Kim Y, Alexandrescu S, Marques HP, Lamelas J, Aldrighetti L, et al. Management and outcomes of patients with recurrent intrahepatic cholangiocarcinoma following previous curative-intent surgical resection. Ann Surg Oncol. 2016;23:235–43. https://doi.org/10.1245/s10434-015-4642-9.
44. Si A, Li J, Xing X, Lei Z, Xia Y, Yan Z, et al. Effectiveness of repeat hepatic resection for patients with recurrent intrahepatic cholangiocarcinoma: factors associated with long-term outcomes. Surgery. 2017;161:897–908. https://doi.org/10.1016/j.surg.2016.10.024.
45. Zhang XF, Beal EW, Bagante F, Chakedis J, Weiss M, Popescu I, et al. Early versus late recurrence of intrahepatic cholangiocarcinoma after resection with curative intent. Br J Surg. 2018;105:848–56. https://doi.org/10.1002/bjs.10676.
46. Bagante F, Spolverato G, Weiss M, Alexandrescu S, Marques HP, Aldrighetti L, et al. Defining long-term survivors following resection of intrahepatic cholangiocarcinoma. J Gastrointest Surg. 2017;21:1888–97. https://doi.org/10.1007/s11605-017-3550-7.
47. Margonis GA, Buettner S, Andreatos N, Wagner D, Sasaki K, Barbon C, et al. Prognostic factors change over time after hepatectomy for colorectal liver metastases: a multi-institutional, international analysis of 1099 patients. Ann Surg. 2018; https://doi.org/10.1097/SLA.0000000000002664.
48. Buettner S, Koerkamp BG, Ejaz A, Buisman FE, Kim Y, Margonis GA, et al. The effect of preoperative chemotherapy treatment in surgically treated intrahepatic cholangiocarcinoma patients-a multi-institutional analysis. J Surg Oncol. 2017;115:312–8. https://doi.org/10.1002/jso.24524.
49. Rayar M, Sulpice L, Edeline J, Garin E, Levi Sandri GB, Meunier B, et al. Intra-arterial yttrium-90 radioembolization combined with systemic chemotherapy is a promising method for downstaging unresectable huge intrahepatic cholangiocarcinoma to surgical treatment. Ann Surg Oncol. 2015;22:3102–8. https://doi.org/10.1245/s10434-014-4365-3.
50. Konstantinidis IT, Groot Koerkamp B, Do RK, Gonen M, Fong Y, Allen PJ, et al. Unresectable intrahepatic cholangiocarcinoma: systemic plus hepatic arterial infusion chemotherapy is associated with longer survival in comparison with systemic chemotherapy alone. Cancer. 2016;122:758–65. https://doi.org/10.1002/cncr.29824.
51. Vilchez V, Shah MB, Daily MF, Pena L, Tzeng CW, Davenport D, et al. Long-term outcome of patients undergoing liver transplantation for mixed hepatocellular carcinoma and cholangiocarcinoma: an analysis of the UNOS database. HPB (Oxford). 2016;18:29–34. https://doi.org/10.1016/j.hpb.2015.10.001.
52. Sapisochin G, Facciuto M, Rubbia-Brandt L, Marti J, Mehta N, Yao FY, et al. Liver transplantation for "very early" intrahepatic cholangiocarcinoma: international retrospective study supporting a prospective assessment. Hepatology. 2016;64:1178–88. https://doi.org/10.1002/hep.28744.
53. Takahashi K, Obeid J, Burmeister CS, Bruno DA, Kazimi MM, Yoshida A, et al. Intrahepatic cholangiocarcinoma in the liver explant after liver transplantation: histological differentiation and prognosis. Ann Transplant. 2016;21:208–15.
54. Lee DD, Croome KP, Musto KR, Melendez J, Tranesh G, Nakhleh R, et al. Liver transplantation for intrahepatic cholangiocarcinoma. Liver Transpl. 2018;24:634–44. https://doi.org/10.1002/lt.25052.
55. Margonis GA, Sasaki K, Andreatos N, Kim Y, Merath K, Wagner D, et al. KRAS mutation status dictates optimal surgical margin width in patients undergoing resection of colorectal liver metastases. Ann Surg Oncol. 2017;24:264–71. https://doi.org/10.1245/s10434-016-5609-1.

Chapter 6
Management of the Nodal Basin

Alfredo Guglielmi, Fabio Bagante, Andrea Ruzzenente, Tommaso Campagnaro, Simone Conci, and Calogero Iacono

Introduction

Lymph node status is the most important characteristic associated with the prognosis of patients with intrahepatic cholangiocarcinoma (ICC) [1]. While patients without lymph node metastasis can reach a long-term survival after curative-intent surgery, patients with metastatic disease involving lymph nodes are seldom considered amenable for surgery, and when surgically treated, present a poor prognosis after hepatectomy [2]. The importance of lymph node status has also been emphasized by the American Joint Committee on Cancer (AJCC) in the staging of patients with ICC. The 7th edition AJCC staging manual introduced, for the first time, a TNM staging system specific for ICC [3]. While the AJCC 7th edition was based on an analysis of data extracted from a large population-based database, the Surveillance, Epidemiology, and End Results (SEER) program, which included 598 patients who underwent surgery for ICC, it did not adequately stage the tumor and lymph node status [4]. In fact, several studies have reported only a poor to moderate ability to predict the patient's prognosis based on the criteria proposed by the AJCC 7th edition for the lymph-node staging [4, 5]. For these reasons, the new 8th edition of the AJCC staging system has introduced some modifications including a reclassification of the tumor (T) category and for the lymph-node staging [6]. Even though these advantages seem to recognize the importance of an accurate evaluation of the lymph node status, the role and extension of lymphadenectomy for ICC are still debated.

A. Guglielmi · F. Bagante · A. Ruzzenente · T. Campagnaro · S. Conci · C. Iacono (✉)
Department of Surgery, University of Verona, Verona, Italy
e-mail: alfredo.guglielmi@univr.it; andrea.ruzzenente@univr.it; tommaso.campagnaro@ospedaleuniverona.it; calogero.iacono@univr.it

T. M. Pawlik et al. (eds.), *Intrahepatic Cholangiocarcinoma*,
https://doi.org/10.1007/978-3-030-22258-1_6

Anatomy of the Lymph Node Drainage

Similar with the other organs in the human body, the lymphatic vessels and lymph nodes for the liver and the bile duct go with the blood vessels supplying and draining the organ. In particular, the lymph node drainage for the liver includes a superficial and a deep pathway [7]. The superficial lymphatic pathway is found beneath the Glisson's capsule of the liver and can be classified into three major groups. The first group includes the most common lymph node sites of metastasis through the hepatoduodenal and gastro-hepatic ligament pathway (Fig. 6.1a). The second group includes the diaphragmatic lymphatic plexus as the liver is directly in contact with the diaphragm with the liver bare area and indirectly through the coronary and triangular ligaments. The third group is along the falciform ligament to the deep superior epigastric node in the anterior abdominal wall and along the deep superior epigastric artery below the xiphoid cartilage. Moreover, the deep lymphatic drainage follows the portal veins, drains into the lymph nodes at the hilum of the liver, the hepatic lymph nodes, then to the nodes in the hepatoduodenal ligament (Fig. 6.1b). Two major lymph node chains can be identified in the hepatoduodenal ligament: the hepatic artery chain and the posterior periportal chain. The hepatic artery chain follows the common hepatic artery to the node at the celiac axis and then into the cisterna chyli. The posterior periportal chain, located posterior to the portal vein in the hepatoduodenal ligament, drains into the retro-pancreatic nodes and the aortocaval node into the cisterna chyli and the thoracic duct. A more detailed classification of the lymph node basin has been provided by the Japanese Society of Hepato-Biliary-Pancreatic Surgery (JSHBPS), which defined the regional lymph nodes of cholangiocarcinoma as the nodes in the hepatoduodenal ligament (#12), the nodes along the left gastric artery (#7), the nodes along the common hepatic artery (#8), the nodes along the celiac artery (#9), the nodes in the right cardial

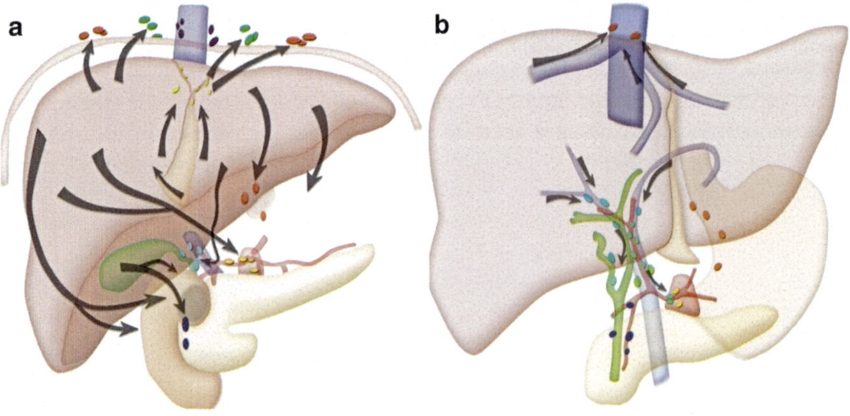

Fig. 6.1 (**a**) Superficial and (**b**) deep pathways of lymphatic drainage for the liver. (From Harisinghani [7])

Table 6.1 Classification of the lymph node basin provided by the Japanese Society of Hepato-Biliary-Pancreatic Surgery (JSHBPS) [8]

No.	Definition
1	Right paracardial LNs
2	Left paracardial LNs
3	LNs along the lesser curvature of the stomach
4	LNs along the greater curvature of the stomach
5	Supra-pyloric LNs
6	Infra-pyloric LNs
7	LNs along the trunk of left gastric artery
8	LNs along the common hepatic artery
9	LNs around the celiac artery
10	LNs at the splenic hilum
11	LNs along the splenic artery including LNs on the distal part of posterior surface of the pancreas end to the left border of the portal vein or superior mesenteric vein
12	LNs in the hepatoduodenal ligament
13	LNs on the posterior surface of the head of the pancreas
14	LNs at the root of the superior mesenteric artery
15	LNs along the middle colic vessels
16	LNs around the abdominal aorta

region (#1), the nodes along the lesser curvature of the stomach (#3), and on the posterior surface of the head of the pancreas (#13) [8]. Furthermore, JSHBPS defined distant lymph node basins as the inter-aortocaval lymph nodes (#16) (Table 6.1).

Recommendation and Staging of Lymph Node Status

The European Society for Medical Oncology (ESMO) recommended in the Clinical Practice Guidelines for Biliary Cancer, published in 2016, a routine lymphadenectomy at the level of the hepatoduodenal ligament during surgery given that the presence of lymph node metastasis is a well-documented prognostic parameter [9, 10]. Conversely, in the National Comprehensive Cancer Network (NCCN) guidelines for ICC, a portal lymphadenectomy is considered only "reasonable," while in the 2014 European Association for the Study of the Liver (EASL) guidelines for ICC, only removal of clinically suspicious nodal disease is defined as "mandatory" and lymphadenectomy be "strongly considered" at the time of surgery [11, 12].

Moreover, different staging systems for ICC have been proposed by the National Cancer Center of Japan (NCCJ) staging system (Okabayashi), the Liver Cancer Study Group of Japan (LCSGJ), and the American Joint Committee on Cancer (AJCC), but the characterization of the lymph node involvement is similar among them [13, 14]. In detail, regional lymph node metastases are defined as N1 disease and include involvement of hilar (hepatoduodenal), periduodenal, and peripancreatic nodes. As reported in the first edition of the LCSGJ guidelines in 1997, regional lymph node dissection of groups 1 and 2 lymph node basins should be performed depending on whether the ICC tumor is located on the right (group 1: #12; group 2: #7, #8, #9, and # 13) or left side (group 1: #12, #1, and #3; group 2: #7, #8, #9, and # 13) of the liver [15, 16]. While first proposed by the LCSGJ, this recommendation has been removed in the last version of the Japanese guidelines given the insufficient data supporting a classification of the lymph nodes basins draining the liver [17]. Recently, the 8th edition of the AJCC TNM staging system has modified the criteria for lymph node staging, adding a minimum number of six lymph nodes harvested for an adequate staging [6].

Lymphadenectomy

Even though the lymph-node status has been identified as the most important factor associated with patient's prognosis, routine lymphadenectomy is not always performed [15, 18–20]. In particular, national and international guidelines recommend removal of clinically suspicious lymph nodes, but the role and extension of routine lymphadenectomy is poorly defined [9, 11, 21, 22]. Moreover, while in the Japanese centers lymphadenectomy is always performed as a fundamental step in the surgical treatment of ICC, lymphadenectomy is not routinely performed at many Western centers [23]. In a recent analysis of 561 patients who underwent curative-intent surgery for ICC at 12 major international hepatobiliary centers in Europe, Asia, Australia, and USA, only 48% ($n = 272$) of patients underwent a concomitant lymphadenectomy and, among these patients, the incidence of metastatic lymph-node (N1 patients) was 45.2% ($n = 123$) [20]. In this study, although other risk factors, such as tumor morphology and number of lesions, contributed to patients' survival, lymph-node status was the strongest independent predictor of disease-specific survival (DSS). Moreover, the authors reported that the DSS of Nx patients varied over the time after surgery. While DSS was worse among Nx patients compared to N0 patients within the first 18 months after surgery, among patients who survived to 18 months after surgery, DSS of Nx patients was comparable to DSS of N0 patients. The authors suggest that the heterogeneous outcomes of Nx patients confirmed the hypothesis that Nx patients are a combination of N0 and (under-staged) N1 patients. Recently, Zangh and colleagues have investigated the trend in lymph-nodal evaluation during the last 13 years using the information of 1496 patients who underwent curative-intent resection for ICC included in the SEER database [24]. The authors reported that, at the time of surgery, a lymphadenectomy was performed only in 52% of patients and that only 11% of patients had six or more than six lymph nodes evaluated [24]. Moreover, while the incidence of lymphadenectomy did not change over time (2000–2004: 50% vs. 2005–2009: 52% vs. 2010–2013: 54%; $p = 0.636$), the proportion of patients who had six or more than six lymph nodes evaluated increased during the study period (2000–2004: 7% vs. 2005–2009: 11% vs. 2009–2013: 14%; $p = 0.003$) [24].

Radiological Assessment of Node Status

The data on the incidence of lymphadenectomy confirm that it is underutilized as a routine practice on patients undergoing surgery for ICC. Some surgeons have pointed out that one of the possible reasons for this trend is that the preoperative imaging might provide enough information to stage patients' lymph node status, allowing a selective use of lymphadenectomy for ICC [25]. To this side, several papers have reported that preoperative imaging might not be reliable to assess nodal status and direct selective lymphadenectomy only in "high-risk" patients, describing only a sensitivity of 40–50% and a specificity of 77–92% to detect nodal metastases with preoperative CT or MRI [21, 26]. Moreover, Bagante et al. compared the concordance between pathological and radiological evaluation of lymph node status among ICC patients who underwent preoperative EUS (2%), CT (49%), MRI (39%), and PET (10%) [5]. Among 317 patients who had data on both radiological and pathological nodal evaluation, the incidence of negative lymph node was 66% among patients initially deemed radiologically negative lymph nodes compared with 42% among patients who were preoperatively staged as suspicious lymph node status. In contrast, the incidence of negative lymph nodes was 35% among patients deemed radiologically metastatic lymph nodes. The incidence of metastatic lymph nodes increased from 34%, among patients who were radiologically negative to 58% and 65% among patients who were radiologically suspicious or radiologically metastatic, respectively ($p < 0.001$). The area under the receiver operating characteristic (ROC) curve comparing radiological and pathological nodal evaluation was only 0.63 [5]. Based on these data, radiological lymph node assessment does not adequately stage the nodal basin and should not replace the pathological evaluation of the lymph node staging.

Number of Lymph Node Harvested

Even though the newly released AJCC 8th edition recommends the recovery of at least six lymph nodes for complete pathologic staging, consistent data supporting this cut-off are still lacking [6]. To validate this indication, a recent analysis of 1154 patients undergoing hepatectomy for ICC between 1990 and 2015 at one of 14 major hepatobiliary centers sought to define outcomes and risk of death among patients who were- "adequately" (≥6 lymph nodes harvested) versus "inadequately" staged (<6 lymph nodes harvested) according to the eighth edition of the AJCC staging manual [5].

The authors reported that, at the time of hepatectomy, lymph nodes were harvested in only 45% of patients with a median number of harvested lymph node of 4 (inter-quartile range, 2–8). Among the 315 patients with negative lymph nodes, 21% of patients had only one harvested lymph node, 42% 2–5 harvested lymph nodes, and 37% ≥6 harvested lymph nodes. While the 5-year OS of patients with negative lymph nodes was 44% compared with 15% for patients with metastatic lymph nodes, patients with negative lymph node and ≥6 harvested lymph nodes had a 5-year OS of 55% compared with 39% for patients with negative lymph nodes and <6 harvested lymph nodes [5].

Extension of Lymphadenectomy

The extension of lymphadenectomy for ICC is not clear based on available data. The majority of recommendations come from retrospective analyses that include heterogeneous groups of patients with bile duct cancers resulting in a low grade of evidence supporting the decision-making process on the extension of lymphadenectomy. There is a general consensus defining the regional lymph node stations as the nodes in the hepatoduodenal ligament (#12), along the left gastric artery (#7), the common hepatic artery (#8), the celiac artery (#9), the nodes in the right cardial region (#1), along the lesser curvature of the stomach (#3), and on the posterior surface of the head of the pancreas (#13). Para-aortic lymph node metastasis has traditionally been defined as distant metastasis [27]. Although the number of metastatic lymph nodes is prognostic, some suggest that the location of the metastatic disease might be associated with the prognosis of patients with bile duct cancers. Several studies have identified the importance of negative para-aortic lymph nodes for a curative resection of ICC [28–31]. Moreover, a recent meta-analysis including ten retrospective studies has reported that an extended lymphadenectomy including regional and para-arotic lymph nodes did not provide a survival benefit for patients with bile duct cancers. This study suggests that radical resection with extended lymphadenectomy should be abandoned when a positive para-aortic lymph node was confirmed pathologically during exploration [32]. Regional lymphadenectomy should include regional lymph node basins as #12, #7, #8, #9, and #13 and might be extended to the stations (#1 and #3) for ICC of the left side of the liver (Fig. 6.2).

Lymphadenectomy in Patients with ICC and Cirrhosis

Lymphadenectomy has been shown to alter short-term outcomes of patients with cirrhosis undergoing surgery for other abdominal malignancies. There is little data regarding the possible implication of lymphadenectomy in ICC patients with cirrhosis. This topic is of particular importance because chronic liver disease and cirrhosis are well-known risk factors of developing ICC and these patients might be at increased risk of morbidity [33]. In recent analysis of the impact of lymphadenectomy on peri-operative outcomes of ICC patients with cirrhosis, the frequency of cirrhotic patients was 10% and lymphadenectomy was associated with an increased risk of complications among these patients compared with non-cirrhotics [34]. The authors reported that patients who had cirrhosis were less likely to undergo a major

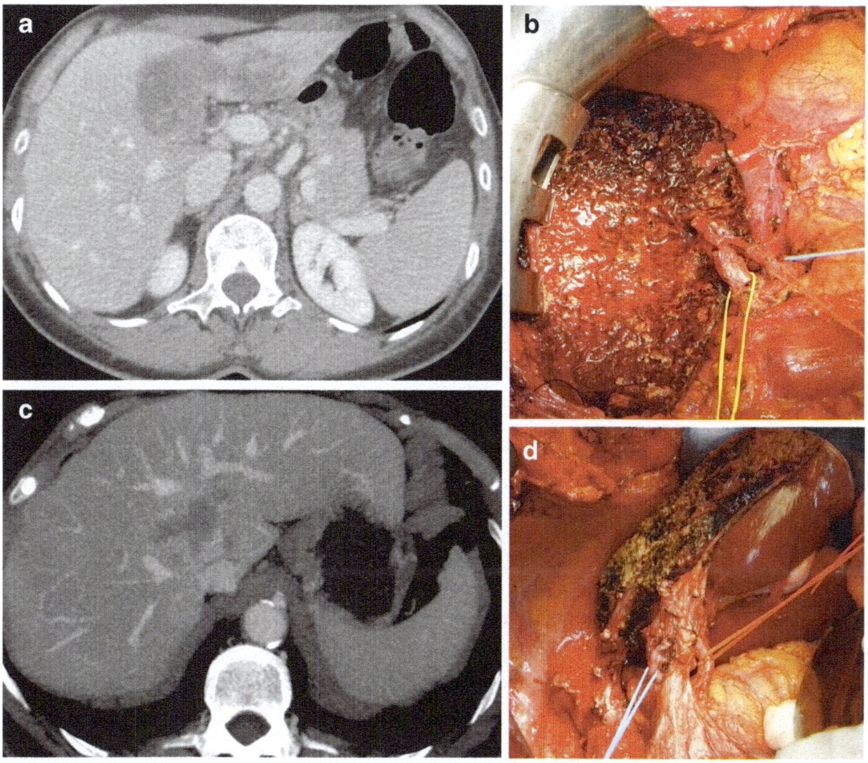

Fig. 6.2 (**a**) CT showing intrahepatic cholangiocarcinoma involving left lobe and anterior segments of the right liver. (**b**) Left trisectionectomy with standard lymphadenectomy (basins #12, #7, #8, #9, and #13) and isolation of the portal vein (blue loop), hepatic artery (red loop), and bile duct (yellow loop). (**c**) CT showing intrahepatic cholangiocarcinoma involving segment 8 and caudate lobe. (**d**) Right hepatectomy extended to caudate lobe standard lymphadenectomy (basins #12, #7, #8, #9, and #13) and isolation of the portal vein (blue loop) and hepatic artery (red loop)

hepatectomy and were about one third less likely to undergo lymphadenectomy at the time of surgery, even though the incidence of metastatic lymph node was comparable among cirrhotic and non-cirrhotic patients when lymph-node evaluation was performed [34]. As such, the AJCC 8th edition recommendation to perform a lymphadenectomy to harvest at least 6 lymph nodes should be considered in light of higher risk of complication when operating on patients with ICC and cirrhosis [34].

What Is the Best Method to Assess Lymph Node Status?

In the recent literature, different approaches have been proposed to estimate the prognostic impact of lymph node status on the prognosis of patients with ICC similar to perihilar cholangiocarcinoma [28]. While the AJCC N-stage system considers only the presence of lymph node metastasis, Kim et al. using the SEER database investigated the impact of the lymph node ratio(LNR) and the logarithm of the ratio of the number of metastatic lymph nodes and the number of negative lymph nodes (LODDS) [35]. The incidence of patients with 1, 2, 3, or ≥4 metastatic lymph nodes was 60%, 18%, 9%, and 13% among patients with positive lymph nodes, respectively. When modeled as a continuous variable, number of metastatic lymph nodes was associated with disease-free survival with a HR 1.26 per each added lymph node metastasis [35]. Moreover, both LODDS and LNR were better predictors of disease-specific survival than the AJCC N staging. In particular, LNR performed well among patients who had >3 lymph nodes harvested, while LODDS was better in predicting the disease specific survival of patients with ≤3 lymph nodes examined [35].

Conclusion

While there is a lack of evidence on the optimal lymph node staging for ICC, several retrospective studies have reported the benefit of lymphadenectomy, confirming the AJCC recommendation to harvest at least six lymph nodes. According to the Liver Cancer Study Group of Japan (LCSGJ) recommendation, lymphadenectomy for ICC should include basin #12 (hepatoduodenal ligament), #7 (left gastric artery), #8 (common hepatic artery), #9 (celiac artery), and # 13 (posterior surface of the head of the pancreas) and might be extended to basin #1 (right cardiac nodes) and #3 (lesser curvature of the stomach) for ICC of the left side of the liver [15, 17]. Furthermore, rather than a simple binary classification (negative vs. positive lymph node status), number of positive nodes and combined scores as lymph node ratio (LNR) and log of odds (LODDS) can improve the prognostic stratification of patients undergoing curative-intent surgery for ICC. Based on the data in the literature and on our center experience, lymph node dissection is a fundamental part of the surgical treatment of ICC.

References

1. Guglielmi A, Ruzzenente A, Campagnaro T, et al. Patterns and prognostic significance of lymph node dissection for surgical treatment of perihilar and intrahepatic cholangiocarcinoma. J Gastrointest Surg. 2013;17:1917–28.
2. Rahnemai-Azar AA, Weisbrod AB, Dillhoff M, et al. Intrahepatic cholangiocarcinoma: current management and emerging therapies. Expert Rev Gastroenterol Hepatol. 2017;11:439–49.
3. Edge SB. American Joint Committee on Cancer: "AJCC cancer staging manual". New York: Springer; 2010.
4. Kim Y, Moris DP, Zhang XF, et al. Evaluation of the 8th edition American Joint Commission on Cancer (AJCC) staging system for patients with intrahepatic cholangiocarcinoma: a surveillance, epidemiology, and end results (SEER) analysis. J Surg Oncol. 2017;116:643–50.

5. Bagante F, Spolverato G, Weiss M, et al. Assessment of the lymph node status in patients undergoing liver resection for intrahepatic cholangiocarcinoma: the new eighth edition AJCC staging system. J Gastrointest Surg. 2018;22:52–9.
6. Amin MB. American Joint Committee on Cancer, American Cancer Society: "AJCC cancer staging manual". Chicago: American Joint Committee on Cancer, Springer; 2017.
7. Harisinghani MG. Atlas of lymph node anatomy. New York: Springer; 2013.
8. Miyazaki M, Ohtsuka M, Miyakawa S, et al. Classification of biliary tract cancers established by the Japanese Society of Hepato-Biliary-Pancreatic Surgery: 3(rd) English edition. J Hepatobiliary Pancreat Sci. 2015;22:181–96.
9. de Jong MC, Nathan H, Sotiropoulos GC, et al. Intrahepatic cholangiocarcinoma: an international multi-institutional analysis of prognostic factors and lymph node assessment. J Clin Oncol. 2011;29:3140–5.
10. Valle JW, Borbath I, Khan SA, et al. Biliary cancer: ESMO clinical practice guidelines for diagnosis, treatment and follow-up. Ann Oncol. 2016;27:v28–37.
11. Bridgewater J, Galle PR, Khan SA, et al. Guidelines for the diagnosis and management of intrahepatic cholangiocarcinoma. J Hepatol. 2014;60:1268–89.
12. Benson AB 3rd, D'Angelica MI, Abbott DE, et al. NCCN guidelines insights: hepatobiliary cancers, version 1.2017. J Natl Compr Cancer Netw. 2017;15:563–73.
13. Nathan H, Pawlik TM. Staging of intrahepatic cholangiocarcinoma. Curr Opin Gastroenterol. 2010;26:269–73.
14. Ronnekleiv-Kelly SM, Pawlik TM. Staging of intrahepatic cholangiocarcinoma. Hepatobiliary Surg Nutr. 2017;6:35–43.
15. Shimada M, Yamashita Y, Aishima S, et al. Value of lymph node dissection during resection of intrahepatic cholangiocarcinoma. Br J Surg. 2001;88:1463–6.
16. The Liver Cancer Study Group of Japan: "Classification of Primary Liver Cancer". Tokyo: Kanehara; 1997.
17. The Liver Cancer Study Group of Japan: "General rules for the clinical and pathological study of primary liver cancer". Tokyo: Kanehara; 2003.
18. Vitale A, Moustafa M, Spolverato G, et al. Defining the possible therapeutic benefit of lymphadenectomy among patients undergoing hepatic resection for intrahepatic cholangiocarcinoma. J Surg Oncol. 2016;113:685–91.
19. Nuzzo G, Giuliante F, Ardito F, et al. Improvement in perioperative and long-term outcome after surgical treatment of hilar cholangiocarcinoma: results of an Italian multicenter analysis of 440 patients. Arch Surg. 2012;147:26–34.
20. Bagante F, Gani F, Spolverato G, et al. Intrahepatic cholangiocarcinoma: prognosis of patients who did not undergo lymphadenectomy. J Am Coll Surg. 2015;221:1031–1040.e1031–1034.
21. Morine Y, Shimada M. The value of systematic lymph node dissection for intrahepatic cholangiocarcinoma from the viewpoint of liver lymphatics. J Gastroenterol. 2015;50:913–27.
22. Shimada K, Sano T, Nara S, et al. Therapeutic value of lymph node dissection during hepatectomy in patients with intrahepatic cholangiocellular carcinoma with negative lymph node involvement. Surgery. 2009;145:411–6.
23. Kim DH, Choi DW, Choi SH, et al. Is there a role for systematic hepatic pedicle lymphadenectomy in intrahepatic cholangiocarcinoma? A review of 17 years of experience in a tertiary institution. Surgery. 2015;157:666–75.
24. Zhang XF, Chen Q, Kimbrough CW, et al. Lymphadenectomy for intrahepatic cholangiocarcinoma: has nodal evaluation been increasingly adopted by surgeons over time? A national database analysis. J Gastrointest Surg. 2018;22:668–75.
25. Zhang XF, Chakedis J, Bagante F, et al. Trends in use of lymphadenectomy in surgery with curative intent for intrahepatic cholangiocarcinoma. Br J Surg. 2018;105:857–66.
26. Seo S, Hatano E, Higashi T, et al. Fluorine-18 fluorodeoxyglucose positron emission tomography predicts lymph node metastasis, P-glycoprotein expression, and recurrence after resection in mass-forming intrahepatic cholangiocarcinoma. Surgery. 2008;143:769–77.

27. Sano T, Shimizu Y, Senda Y, et al. Assessing resectability in cholangiocarcinoma. Hepat Oncol. 2014;1:39–51.
28. Nakayama T, Tsuchikawa T, Shichinohe T, et al. Pathological confirmation of para-aortic lymph node status as a potential criterion for the selection of intrahepatic cholangiocarcinoma patients for radical resection with regional lymph node dissection. World J Surg. 2014;38:1763–8.
29. Aoba T, Ebata T, Yokoyama Y, et al. Assessment of nodal status for perihilar cholangiocarcinoma: location, number, or ratio of involved nodes. Ann Surg. 2013;257:718–25.
30. Conci S, Ruzzenente A, Sandri M, et al. What is the most accurate lymph node staging method for perihilar cholangiocarcinoma? Comparison of UICC/AJCC pN stage, number of metastatic lymph nodes, lymph node ratio, and log odds of metastatic lymph nodes. Eur J Surg Oncol. 2017;43:743–50.
31. Kitagawa Y, Nagino M, Kamiya J, et al. Lymph node metastasis from hilar cholangiocarcinoma: audit of 110 patients who underwent regional and paraaortic node dissection. Ann Surg. 2001;233:385–92.
32. Gu J, Xia L, Xu B, et al. Clinical prognostic significance of regional and extended lymphadenectomy for biliary cancer with para-aortic lymph node metastasis: a systematic review and meta-analysis. Dig Liver Dis. 2016;48:717–25.
33. Shin HR, Oh JK, Masuyer E, et al. Epidemiology of cholangiocarcinoma: an update focusing on risk factors. Cancer Sci. 2010;101:579–85.
34. Bagante F, Spolverato G, Weiss M, et al. Surgical management of intrahepatic cholangiocarcinoma in patients with cirrhosis: impact of lymphadenectomy on peri-operative outcomes. World J Surg. 2018;42:2551–60.
35. Kim Y, Spolverato G, Amini N, et al. Surgical management of intrahepatic cholangiocarcinoma: defining an optimal prognostic lymph node stratification schema. Ann Surg Oncol. 2015;22:2772–8.

Chapter 7
Pathologic Assessment

Benjamin J. Swanson

Introduction

The diagnosis of intrahepatic cholangiocarcinoma (ICC) is usually made by needle biopsy of a liver mass. The vast majority of ICCs are adenocarcinomas, with the most common growth pattern being acinar or tubular growth. Other less common types include mucinous, clear cell, and adenosquamous carcinoma. Precursor lesions include biliary intraepithelial neoplasia and intraductal papillary neoplasms of bile ducts. The differential diagnosis of ICC is large and includes many tumors metastatic to the liver. The most common tumors to metastasize to the liver include colorectal, breast, lung, pancreas and upper gastrointestinal tract. In addition, hepatocellular carcinoma (HCC) enters the differential diagnosis whenever the tumor is poorly differentiated. Immunohistochemistry is very helpful to distinguish ICC from several metastatic tumors and hepatocellular carcinoma. Brush cytology can also be used to diagnose suspicious intrahepatic strictures, with fluorescent in-situ hybridization analysis employed for challenging cases. Specimens resected for ICC should be evaluated for their gross growth pattern, precursor lesions, and other pathologic risk factors. Ancillary testing includes DNA mismatch repair immunohistochemistry and next generation DNA sequencing. In this chapter, we provide a comprehensive review of the histopathologic assessment of ICC.

B. J. Swanson (✉)
Department of Pathology and Microbiology, University of Nebraska Medical Center, Omaha, NE, USA
e-mail: bjswanso@unmc.edu

T. M. Pawlik et al. (eds.), *Intrahepatic Cholangiocarcinoma*,
https://doi.org/10.1007/978-3-030-22258-1_7

Biopsy Interpretation of Intrahepatic Cholangiocarcinoma

The vast majority of intrahepatic cholangiocarcinomas (ICC) are adenocarcinomas. Like adenocarcinomas throughout the gastrointestinal and biliary system, they are composed of malignant glands [1]. The precursor for ICC is thought to be a progenitor/stem cell of biliary epithelium. Thus, the cells of ICC are cuboidal cells that lack mucin, recapitulating their progenitor. The most common growth pattern is gland forming, also known as tubular or acinar (Fig. 7.1a). The tumors can also grow in trabecular (ribbon-like) and micropapillary (glands with projections and tufts that lack fibrovascular cores) patterns. Tumors are conventionally graded as well-differentiated (>95% of the tumor composed of glands), moderately differentiated (50–95% gland formation), and poorly differentiated (<50% gland formation).

The typical immunohistochemical staining pattern for ICC is that they are positive for CK7, variably positive for CK20, and variably positive for CDX2 [2]. The tumors are also positive for CK19, and broad spectrum keratins such as AE1/AE3 and CAM5.2. Usually, the tumors are negative for TTF-1, GATA3, estrogen receptor, and progesterone receptor.

When greater than 50% of the glands show mucinous morphology (malignant glands floating in mucin), the diagnosis of mucinous adenocarcinoma is made (Fig. 7.1b). This is a very rare tumor that may have a worse prognosis compared to conventional ICC [3]. A minor (<50%) mucinous component can also be seen in conventional (acinar) cholangiocarcinoma. Some studies have suggested that the immunochemistry profile for these tumors is CK7 positive, CK20 negative, CDX2 negative. This variant of ICC must be distinguished from metastatic mucinous adenocarcinoma, especially from the colon. Metastatic mucinous adenocarcinoma from the colon is usually CK7 negative, CK20 positive, and CDX2 positive by immunohistochemistry.

Signet ring cell morphology is defined by discohesive cells with an eccentrically placed nucleus and a mucin vacuole[4]. Tumors with greater than 50% signet rings (signet ring cell carcinoma) are incredibly rare. Signet ring cells are more commonly a minor component (<50%) of a mucinous adenocarcinoma (Fig. 7.1e).

Clear cell ICC is diagnosed when the tumor is predominately (>50%) composed of optically clear cells (by H&E) with well-defined cell borders (Fig. 7.1c) [5]. The tumors may be interspersed with a more conventional adenocarcinoma. HCC with clear cell features and metastasis from other anatomic sites (especially the kidney) must be excluded by performing immunohistochemistry (clear cell carcinoma from the kidney is PAX8 positive, CK7 negative, CK20 negative).

When a primary tumor of the liver demonstrates both glandular and squamous differentiation, a diagnosis of adenosquamous carcinoma is made. The squamous component is recognized by keratinization (Fig. 7.1d) and intercellular bridges between polygonal cells [6], whereas the glandular component may also contain mucin. At least one meta-review of prior case studies of adenosquamous carcinoma suggests this may have a worse prognosis compared to conventional ICC [7].

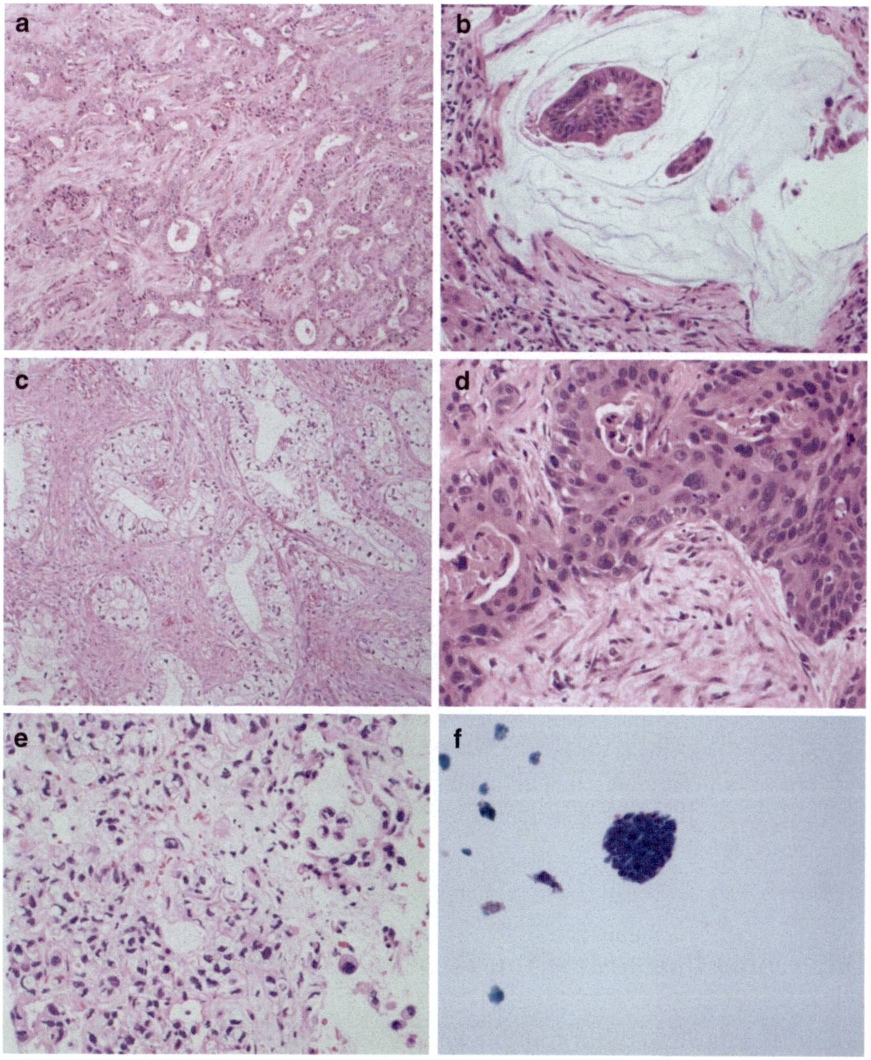

Fig. 7.1 (**a**) Typical acinar growth pattern of cholangiocarcinoma with gland formation. (**b**) Mucinous adenocarcinoma with abundant extracellular mucin and cells floating in mucin. (**c**) Clear cell adenocarcinoma with optically clear cytoplasm and well-defined cell borders. (**d**) Squamous differentiation within an adenosquamous carcinoma demonstrating focal keratinization. (**e**) Signet ring cell morphology with multiple discohesive cells, eccentric nuclei, and mucin vacuoles. (**f**) Brush cytology of cholangiocarcinoma with a disorganized group of cells showing hyperchromasia

Lymphoepithelial-like cholangiocarcinoma is a rare variant of ICC that in some studies is related to Epstein-Barr virus (EBV) [8]. Similar to other EBV-related carcinomas elsewhere in the body, the tumor grows as syncytial sheets of undifferentiated malignant cells. Also present is an intense inflammatory reaction composed of lymphocytes and plasma cells that intermingle with the undifferentiated malignant cells. The tumor will mark with keratin markers (AE1/AE3, CAM5.2, etc.) and may show nuclear reactivity for EBV by in-situ hybridization (EBER).

Brush Cytology for Intrahepatic Cholangiocarcinoma

Cytologic and brush examination of ICC shows findings similar to other pancreaticobiliary adenocarcinomas such as extrahepatic cholangiocarcinoma and pancreatic ductal adenocarcinoma. Low power examination of smear slides demonstrates a hypercellular background. High power microscopic examination shows disorganized groups of cells. The individual cells show nuclear pleomorphism, irregular nuclear membranes, loss of nuclear polarity, and conspicuous nucleoli (Fig. 7.1f). Brush cytology of suspicious intrahepatic bile duct strictures has excellent specificity for diagnosing carcinoma, however, the sensitivity may be less than 40% [9]. When tissue is present in the cell block, immunohistochemistry can be performed to exclude metastatic tumors.

Fluorescent in-situ hybridization (FISH) testing can be performed on brush cytologic specimens of intrahepatic lesions to help diagnose ICC. Some studies have suggested that FISH analysis of regions 1q21 (*MCL1*), 7p12 (*EGFR*), 8q24 (*MYC*), and 9p21 (*CDKN2A*) which detect chromosomal gain and losses of the above regions are sensitive and specific in the diagnosis of pancreaticobiliary adenocarcinomas [10]. These FISH probe sets are not widely available in all anatomic pathology practices. Therefore, in our practice, we utilize FISH analysis in clinical scenarios where the clinical suspicion for ICC is high but the brush cytology diagnosis is not definitive.

Differential Diagnosis of Intrahepatic Cholangiocarcinoma

It may be difficult to distinguish benign and malignant biliary tract tumors. Bile duct adenomas are benign proliferations of bile ductules that can sometimes enter into the differential diagnosis with ICC, especially during frozen section analysis. The benign biology of bile duct adenomas is reflected in their histologic appearance. They are composed of bland, uniform glands which lack nuclear pleomorphism and mitotic figures (Fig. 7.2a). They have a smooth/rounded interface with the surrounding hepatic architecture and do not invade adjacent tissue. Bile duct adenomas are usually small and are rarely greater in size than 2 cm. They are usually located in the subcapsule of the liver [11]. By comparison, ICC shows greater variation in nuclear size and contour as well as conspicuous mitotic figures. Furthermore, ICCs are usually quite large and not subcapsular. ICCs have infiltrative borders with the adjacent tissue.

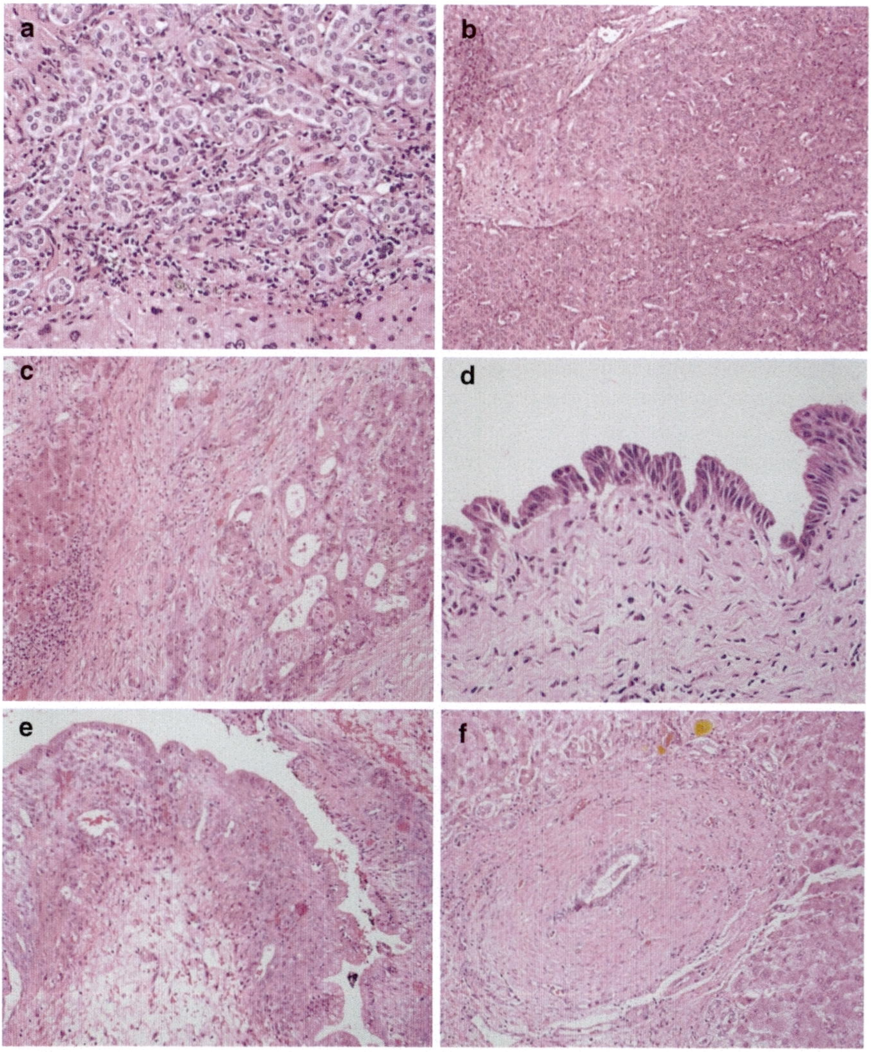

Fig. 7.2 (**a**) Bile duct adenoma with bland cell morphology and a smooth interface with surrounding hepatocytes. (**b**) Hepatocellular component of combined hepatocellular-cholangiocarcinoma with oncocytic neoplastic hepatocytes. (**c**) Cholangiocarcinoma component of combined hepatocellular-cholangiocarcinoma with gland formation. (**d**) Biliary intraepithelial neoplasia-3 shows severe dysplasia with loss of nuclear polarity. (**e**) Mucinous cystic neoplasm is composed of mucinous epithelium with ovarian-type stroma. (**f**) Periductal ("onion-skin") fibrosis of primary sclerosing cholangitis

Whenever the diagnosis of adenocarcinoma within the liver is entertained, metastatic tumors must be excluded. The incidence of adenocarcinomas metastatic to the liver is greater than the incidence of primary liver tumors. Moreover, by H&E morphology, ICC and metastatic adenocarcinomas can be indistinguishable. Thus, the distinction of metastasis from ICC is a very common problem in anatomic pathology that can sometimes be difficult. Immunohistochemistry is employed to aid in the distinction. The most common tumors to metastasize to the liver include colorectal, breast, lung, pancreas, and upper gastrointestinal tract (gastric and esophageal) [1]. Many tumors can reliably be distinguished from ICC, though pancreatic and upper gastrointestinal tumors are more challenging.

The classic morphologic feature of colorectal adenocarcinomas is luminal necrosis of the glands, referred to as "dirty" necrosis, although this histologic feature is not always present. Conversely, ICCs do not have "dirty" necrosis within central lumens. By immunohistochemistry, colorectal adenocarcinomas are usually CK20 positive, CK7 negative, CDX2 positive, and SATB2 positive [12].

Both lobular and ductal adenocarcinomas of the breast can spread to the liver. Ductal adenocarcinomas of the breast most closely morphologically resemble ICC and must be excluded in women. The typical immunochemical profile of ductal breast adenocarcinoma is CK7 positive, CK20 negative, CDX2 negative, GATA3 positive, gross cystic disease fluid protein 15 (GCDFP-15) positive, and mammaglobin positive [13]. Furthermore, depending on the subtype of breast cancer, there may be a variable expression of estrogen receptor, progesterone receptor, and HER2/Neu [14].

Non-small cell carcinomas of the lung include squamous cell carcinoma, adenocarcinoma, and large cell neuroendocrine carcinoma. Adenocarcinomas of the lung can closely resemble ICC. The typical immunoprofile of lung adenocarcinoma is CK7 positive, CK20 positive, CDX2 negative, TTF-1 positive, and Napsin A positive [15].

Pancreatic adenocarcinomas which metastasize to the liver usually closely mimic ICC by both morphology and immunohistochemistry. Unfortunately, there are not reliable pathologic features that can confidently separate these entities [16]. Thus, pathologic reports use the term pancreatobiliary to convey this ambiguity. Clinical correlation is often needed to distinguish the two.

Upper gastrointestinal cancers (esophageal and gastric adenocarcinomas) can similarly be impossible to distinguish from ICC by pathologic examination. Their immunohistochemical profile closely resembles ICC: CK7 positive, CK20 variable, CDX2 variable [17]. Furthermore, the H&E morphology of upper gastrointestinal tract tumors is similar to ICC. Therefore, surgical pathology reports usually include upper gastrointestinal tract tumors in the differential diagnosis.

HCC enters into the differential diagnosis of ICC when the tumor is poorly differentiated. Histologic features, which favor ICC, include mucin production as well as background liver that is non-cirrhotic. By comparison, H&E features which favor poorly differentiated hepatocellular carcinoma include bile production and background liver that is cirrhotic. Immunohistochemical markers for adenocarcinoma (MOC-31, aka Ep-CAM) and hepatocellular lesions (Hepatocyte antibody (HepPar-1, Arginase) can be of great use in this distinction. ICCs are MOC31 positive, HepPar-1negative, Arginase negative, whereas Hepatocellular carcinomas are MOC31 negative, HepPar-1 positive, Arginase positive [18].

Combined Hepatocellular-Cholangiocarcinoma is a WHO-defined tumor that contains histologic elements of both hepatocellular carcinoma and cholangiocarcinoma [19]. The current definition does not require a minimum amount of each component. This tumor is thought to arise from a common progenitor cell (stem cell) that gives rise to both the hepatocellular carcinoma component and cholangiocarcinoma component. This tumor is associated with risk factors similar to HCC (cirrhosis, viral hepatitis C infection, viral hepatitis B infection). Histologically, the hepatocellular component is identified by bile production as well as oncocytic neoplastic hepatocytes (Fig. 7.2b) that may show any degree of differentiation. The hepatocellular component can also be identified by immunohistochemistry with positive staining for HepPar-1 and Arginase. The cholangiocarcinoma component is histologically identified by gland formation and mucin production (Fig. 7.2c). Positivity for CK19 can help define the portions of the tumor that are cholangiocarcinoma. Given the theorized stem cell origin of this tumor, subtypes with stem cell features have been recognized by the WHO: typical, cholangiocellular, and intermediate-cell subtypes. Immunostains which are positive in the stem cell subtypes include CD56 and c-kit. The clinical significance of identifying the stem cell subtypes in combined hepatocellular-cholangiocarcinoma is unclear.

The distinction of ICC from combined hepatocellular-cholangiocarcinoma can be very challenging on needle biopsy due to sampling limitations. Whenever a tumor is biopsied in a patient with cirrhosis or history of viral hepatitis B/C infection, combined hepatocellular-cholangiocarcinoma should be considered in the differential diagnosis. However, this tumor may only be definitively diagnosed after surgical resection.

Pathologic Interpretation of Surgical Resections of Intrahepatic Cholangiocarcinoma

Surgical resections for ICC should be evaluated according to the College of American Pathologists checklist for tumors of intrahepatic bile ducts (https://documents.cap.org/protocols/cp-intrahepatic-bileducts-17protocol-4000.pdf).

The growth pattern of ICC should be discerned by both gross pathologic examination as well as H&E findings. The major growth patterns for ICC include mass-forming, periductal infiltrating, and a mixed mass-forming/periductal infiltrating. The growth pattern may help predict the prognosis for the patient [20, 21].

As its name applies, the mass-forming growth pattern of ICC presents as a large nodule that is often singular. This is the most common gross subtype of ICC. The periductal-infiltrating subtype of ICC grows in a tree-like fashion along portal tracts. Therefore, it is multifocal and may be more difficult to appreciate grossly. Sometimes, a tumor may show mixed features of both mass-forming and periductal-infiltrating growth patterns.

Precursor Lesions and Predisposing Conditions for Intrahepatic Cholangiocarcinoma

Resected ICC should be pathologically evaluated for both precursor lesions and pathologic risk factors. Precursor lesions include biliary dysplasia, intraductal papillary neoplasm of bile ducts, and mucinous cystic neoplasms. Risk factors include primary sclerosing cholangitis, hepatolithiasis (biliary stones should be mentioned in pathology reports), liver flukes, and viral hepatitis B and C infection.

Flat dysplasia of bile ducts is thought to be a precursor for intrahepatic cholangiocarcinoma. The terminology has been proposed [22, 23] that these lesions are described as biliary intraepithelial neoplasia (BilIN) similar to pancreatic intraepithelial neoplasia (PanIN). Histologically, BilIN shows nuclear and architectural features similar to cholangiocarcinoma; however, they lack invasion of the basement membrane. A three-tiered system from low-grade dysplasia (BilIN-1) to high-grade dysplasia/carcinoma in-situ (BilIN-3) has been proposed. The cells of BilIN-1 demonstrate mild to moderate nuclear changes (hyperchromasia, irregular nuclear membranes) with maintenance of nuclear polarity. In contrast, BilIN-3 is more similar to cholangiocarcinoma with severe nuclear atypia and frank loss of nuclear polarity (Fig. 7.2d). BilIN-2 is reserved for lesions between BilIN-1 and BilIN-3. The presence of dysplasia/BilIN should be noted at any biliary margin of a surgical resection specimen.

Intraductal papillary neoplasms of bile ducts (IPNB) are another potential precursor lesion to ICC. Their nomenclature, growth pattern, and risk of progression to invasive carcinoma are similar to intraductal papillary neoplasms (IPMNs) of the pancreas [24]. IPNB can occur in both intrahepatic and extrahepatic anatomic locations [25]. Due to their papillary and intraluminal growth pattern, IPNB will dilate an intrahepatic bile duct to form a grossly visible cystic mass. IPNB sometimes produce mucin, which may be evident grossly. Histologic subtypes of IPNB include pancreatobiliary, gastric, intestinal, and oncocytic. These neoplasms may show a mixture of each histologic subtype that can be recognized by H&E examination. Pancreatobiliary IPNB histologically demonstrates cuboidal type epithelium with papillary growth that lacks goblet cells. When invasive adenocarcinoma arises from a pancreatobiliary IPNB, it is most likely to have an acinar growth pattern. Intestinal IPNB histologically resembles colonic epithelium with innumerable goblet cells and mucin production. Invasive mucinous cholangiocarcinoma is more likely to occur with the intestinal subtype of IPNB. The gastric IPNB subtype demonstrates columnar epithelium with mucin that is histologically similar to gastric foveolar epithelium. Oncocytic IPNB has bright eosinophilic cytoplasm with a complex arborizing papillary growth pattern. The degree of dysplasia should be documented similar to IPMN of the pancreas with a two-tiered system of low- and high-grade dysplasia [26].

Mucinous cystic neoplasms of the liver (also known as biliary cystadenoma) can very rarely give rise to ICC [27]. The cyst wall lining of biliary cystadenoma is mucinous epithelium with characteristic ovarian-type stroma (Fig. 7.2e). The ovarian-type stroma can be identified by immunohistochemical stains for CD10, estrogen receptor, progesterone receptor, and inhibin.

Primary sclerosing cholangitis is a cholestatic disorder of the liver that affects bile ducts anywhere in the biliary system. The etiology of the disease is not well understood; however, it is thought that the disease may be autoimmune-related since there is a strong correlation with inflammatory bowel disease, especially ulcerative colitis. Pathologically, PSC shows damage of both intra- and extrahepatic bile ducts [28]. Within the liver, the bile ducts show intraepithelial inflammation composed predominately of lymphocytes. In addition, the bile ducts will show periductal fibrosis, also known as "onion-skin" fibrosis (Fig. 7.2f). As the inflammation and fibrosis progress in PSC, the bile ducts will undergo senescence and atrophy. A secondary biliary ductal proliferation around the portal tracts also occurs as the liver progresses toward cirrhosis. Similar to other cholestatic diseases which cause cirrhosis, the pattern of cirrhosis in PSC is described as "jig-saw" rather than the more common nodular pattern seen with viral hepatitis.

Molecular Assessment of Intrahepatic Cholangiocarcinoma

With the widespread use of next generation sequencing panels, clinically relevant mutations have been identified in ICC. Common mutations in ICC include *TP53*, *CDKN2A/B*, *KRAS*, and *ARID1A* [30]. Mutations that more frequently occur in ICC that may have a targeted inhibitor include *IDH1*, *IDH2*, *FGFR1*, *FGFR2*, *EPHA1*, and *BAP1* [31]. However, this field will likely significantly change with the advent of larger next generation sequencing panels as well as further research into the molecular underpinnings of this cancer.

Defective DNA mismatch repair can be caused by either Lynch syndrome or may occur sporadically. Defective mismatch repair can be pathologically assessed by immunohistochemistry for DNA mismatch repair proteins (MLH1, MSH2, MSH6, and PMS2) or by polymerase chain reaction (PCR) testing of mononucleotide microsatellite instability (MSI). When tumors are mismatch repair deficient or have high-levels of microsatellite instability, they are much more likely to respond to immune checkpoint inhibitors. Unfortunately, only approximately 1% of ICC show defective mismatch repair [29].

Conclusion

The diagnosis of intrahepatic cholangiocarcinoma can be challenging given its similar histopathologic appearance to other primary and metastatic liver cancers. While morphologic and immunohistochemical assessment serves as the basis for diagnosing and staging ICC, the importance of molecular testing continues to increase as potentially targetable mutations are identified.

References

1. Bosman FT, Carneiro F, Hruban RH, Theise ND. WHO classification of tumors of the digestive system. 4th ed. Lyon: IARC; 2010.
2. Chiu C-T, Chiang J-M, Yeh T-S, Tseng J-H, Chen T-C, Jan Y-Y, et al. Clinicopathological analysis of colorectal cancer liver metastasis and intrahepatic cholangiocarcinoma: are they just apples and oranges? Dig Liver Dis. 2008;40(9):749–54.
3. Chi Z, Bhalla A, Saeed O, Cheng L, Curless K, Wang HL, et al. Mucinous intrahepatic cholangiocarcinoma: a distinct variant. Hum Pathol. 2018;78:131–7.
4. Nakanuma Y, Sato Y, Harada K, Sasaki M, Xu J, Ikeda H. Pathological classification of intrahepatic cholangiocarcinoma based on a new concept. World J Hepatol. 2010;2(12):419–27.
5. Haas S, Gütgemann I, Wolff M, Fischer H-P. Intrahepatic clear cell cholangiocarcinoma: immunohistochemical aspects in a very rare type of cholangiocarcinoma. Am J Surg Pathol. 2007;31(6):902–6.
6. Nakajima T, Kondo Y, Miyazaki M, Okui K. A histopathologic study of 102 cases of intrahepatic cholangiocarcinoma: histologic classification and modes of spreading. Hum Pathol. 1988;19(10):1228–34.
7. Kobayashi M, Okabayashi T, Okamoto K, Namikawa T, Araki K. A clinicopathologic study of primary adenosquamous carcinoma of the liver. J Clin Gastroenterol. 2005;39(6):544–8.
8. Jeng YM, Chen CL, Hsu HC. Lymphoepithelioma-like cholangiocarcinoma: an Epstein-Barr virus-associated tumor. Am J Surg Pathol. 2001;25(4):516–20.
9. Renshaw AA, Madge R, Jiroutek M, Granter SR. Bile duct brushing cytology: statistical analysis of proposed diagnostic criteria. Am J Clin Pathol. 1998;110(5):635–40.
10. Barr Fritcher EG, Voss JS, Brankley SM, Campion MB, Jenkins SM, Keeney ME, et al. An optimized set of fluorescence in situ hybridization probes for detection of Pancreatobiliary tract cancer in cytology brush samples. Gastroenterology. 2015;149(7):1813–1824.e1.
11. Allaire GS, Rabin L, Ishak KG, Sesterhenn IA. Bile duct adenoma. A study of 152 cases. Am J Surg Pathol. 1988;12(9):708–15.
12. Li Z, Rock JB, Roth R, Lehman A, Marsh WL, Suarez A, et al. Dual stain with SATB2 and CK20/villin is useful to distinguish colorectal carcinomas from other tumors. Am J Clin Pathol. 2018;149(3):241–6.
13. Kawaguchi KR, Lu F-I, Kaplan R, Liu Y-F, Chadwick P, Chen Z, et al. In search of the ideal immunopanel to distinguish metastatic mammary carcinoma from primary lung carcinoma: a tissue microarray study of 207 cases. Appl Immunohistochem Mol Morphol AIMM. 2014;22(4):266–74.
14. Nash JW, Morrison C, Frankel WL. The utility of estrogen receptor and progesterone receptor immunohistochemistry in the distinction of metastatic breast carcinoma from other tumors in the liver. Arch Pathol Lab Med. 2003;127(12):1591–5.
15. Turner BM, Cagle PT, Sainz IM, Fukuoka J, Shen SS, Jagirdar J. Napsin A, a new marker for lung adenocarcinoma, is complementary and more sensitive and specific than thyroid transcription factor 1 in the differential diagnosis of primary pulmonary carcinoma: evaluation of 1674 cases by tissue microarray. Arch Pathol Lab Med. 2012;136(2):163–71.
16. Chu PG, Schwarz RE, Lau SK, Yen Y, Weiss LM. Immunohistochemical staining in the diagnosis of pancreatobiliary and ampulla of Vater adenocarcinoma: application of CDX2, CK17, MUC1, and MUC2. Am J Surg Pathol. 2005;29(3):359–67.
17. Lau SK, Prakash S, Geller SA, Alsabeh R. Comparative immunohistochemical profile of hepatocellular carcinoma, cholangiocarcinoma, and metastatic adenocarcinoma. Hum Pathol. 2002;33(12):1175–81.
18. Radwan NA, Ahmed NS. The diagnostic value of arginase-1 immunostaining in differentiating hepatocellular carcinoma from metastatic carcinoma and cholangiocarcinoma as compared to HepPar-1. Diagn Pathol. 2012;7:149.

19. Akiba J, Nakashima O, Hattori S, Tanikawa K, Takenaka M, Nakayama M, et al. Clinicopathologic analysis of combined hepatocellular-cholangiocarcinoma according to the latest WHO classification. Am J Surg Pathol. 2013;37(4):496–505.
20. Hirohashi K, Uenishi T, Kubo S, Yamamoto T, Tanaka H, Shuto T, et al. Macroscopic types of intrahepatic cholangiocarcinoma: clinicopathologic features and surgical outcomes. Hepato-Gastroenterology. 2002;49(44):326–9.
21. Uno M, Shimada K, Yamamoto Y, Nara S, Esaki M, Sakamoto Y, et al. Periductal infiltrating type of intrahepatic cholangiocarcinoma: a rare macroscopic type without any apparent mass. Surg Today. 2012;42(12):1189–94.
22. Zen Y, Aishima S, Ajioka Y, Haratake J, Kage M, Kondo F, et al. Proposal of histological criteria for intraepithelial atypical/proliferative biliary epithelial lesions of the bile duct in hepatolithiasis with respect to cholangiocarcinoma: preliminary report based on interobserver agreement. Pathol Int. 2005;55(4):180–8.
23. Zen Y, Adsay NV, Bardadin K, Colombari R, Ferrell L, Haga H, et al. Biliary intraepithelial neoplasia: an international interobserver agreement study and proposal for diagnostic criteria. Mod Pathol Off J U S Can Acad Pathol Inc. 2007;20(6):701–9.
24. Zen Y, Fujii T, Itatsu K, Nakamura K, Minato H, Kasashima S, et al. Biliary papillary tumors share pathological features with intraductal papillary mucinous neoplasm of the pancreas. Hepatol Baltim Md. 2006;44(5):1333–43.
25. Ohtsuka M, Kimura F, Shimizu H, Yoshidome H, Kato A, Yoshitomi H, et al. Similarities and differences between intraductal papillary tumors of the bile duct with and without macroscopically visible mucin secretion. Am J Surg Pathol. 2011;35(4):512–21.
26. Adsay V, Mino-Kenudson M, Furukawa T, Basturk O, Zamboni G, Marchegiani G, et al. Pathologic evaluation and reporting of Intraductal papillary mucinous neoplasms of the pancreas and other Tumoral intraepithelial neoplasms of Pancreatobiliary tract: recommendations of Verona consensus meeting. Ann Surg. 2016;263(1):162–77.
27. Quigley B, Reid MD, Pehlivanoglu B, Squires MH, Maithel S, Xue Y, et al. Hepatobiliary mucinous cystic neoplasms with ovarian-type stroma (so-called "hepatobiliary cystadenoma/cystadenocarcinoma"): clinicopathologic analysis of 36 cases illustrates rarity of carcinomatous change. Am J Surg Pathol. 2018;42(1):95–102.
28. Nakanishi Y, Saxena R. Pathophysiology and diseases of the proximal pathways of the biliary system. Arch Pathol Lab Med. 2015;139(7):858–66.
29. Goeppert B, Roessler S, Renner M, Singer S, Mehrabi A, Vogel MN, et al. Mismatch repair deficiency is a rare but putative therapeutically relevant finding in non-liver fluke-associated cholangiocarcinoma. Br J Cancer. 2019;120(1):109–14.
30. Javle M, Bekaii-Saab T, Jain A, Wang Y, Kelley RK, Wang K, et al. Biliary cancer: utility of next-generation sequencing for clinical management. Cancer. 2016;122(24):3838–47.
31. Nakamura H, Arai Y, Totoki Y, Shirota T, Elzawahry A, Kato M, et al. Genomic spectra of biliary tract cancer. Nat Genet. 2015;47(9):1003–10.

Chapter 8
Systemic Therapy

Ning Jin and Laith Abushahin

Introduction

Intrahepatic cholangiocarcinoma (ICC) represents the second most common primary liver cancer and its incidence is rising [1]. Patients with ICC have an extremely poor prognosis, with a median survival of less than 1 year [2–5]. Only 10–15% of patients with cholangiocarcinoma are amenable to surgery [6]. Furthermore, among those who undergo surgery, the majority will have disease recurrence [7], with the risk of recurrence being linked to nodal metastasis, tumor size, multicentricity, and vascular invasion [8]. Adjuvant chemotherapy is, therefore, an important treatment approach that aims to enhance the curative potential of resection of localized ICC. Alternatively, for patients with locally advanced or metastatic ICC, systemic chemotherapy with gemcitabine- or fluoropyrimidine-based combinations in the first-line and second-line settings, respectively, may offer improvements in quality of life and prolong the overall survival [9]. This chapter reviews the current approaches for both adjuvant and definitive chemotherapy for ICC and discusses novel combinations of chemotherapy with biological agents and targeted agents used for the treatment of ICC.

N. Jin (✉)
Department of Oncology, The Ohio State University Wexner Medical Center, Columbus, OH, USA
e-mail: Ning.Jin2@osumc.edu

L. Abushahin
Department of Oncology, The Ohio State University Wexner Medical Center, Columbus, OH, USA

Division of Medical Oncology, Department of Internal Medicine, Columbus, OH, USA
e-mail: Laith.Abushahin@osumc.edu

T. M. Pawlik et al. (eds.), *Intrahepatic Cholangiocarcinoma*,
https://doi.org/10.1007/978-3-030-22258-1_8

Adjuvant Chemotherapy

The optimal adjuvant chemotherapy for resected ICC remains controversial for several reasons. First, given its relative rarity, most studies have included ICC with other biliary tract cancers (BTC) despite their unique biological and clinical features. Second, as is the case with many uncommon cancers, the majority of cases have been reported through retrospective series. Third, prospective trials have been limited by significant heterogeneity in their risk for recurrence due to underlying negative prognostic factors (e.g., margin status and lymph node status).

In one of the earliest reported series of patients with ICC undergoing hepatic resection, Ercolani et al. reported on 72 patients of which 25 received gemcitabine-based adjuvant chemotherapy [10]. Although the 5-year overall survival was higher among patients who received chemotherapy (65 vs. 40 months ($p < 0.05$)), the favorable prognostic effect of adjuvant chemotherapy could not be maintained on multivariate analysis. Two National Cancer Database (NCDB) studies have also attempted to address this question [11, 12]. In the first study, 638 patients with ICC who underwent surgical resection between 1998 and 2006 were identified. Among them, 12% were treated with adjuvant chemotherapy and 23% with adjuvant chemoradiation. On multivariate analysis, there was a statistically significant survival benefit associated with both chemotherapy and chemoradiation. After adjusting for other prognostic factors, the improvement in survival with adjuvant therapy was restricted to patients with positive lymph nodes and/or resection margins [11]. In the second NCDB publication, 985 patients who underwent resection between 1998 and 2011 and who received adjuvant chemotherapy were compared to a propensity-matched cohort of patients who did not receive adjuvant chemotherapy. Similar to the earlier study, a benefit with adjuvant chemotherapy was observed among patients with nodal metastases and positive margins [12]. Of interest, 53% of patients who received chemotherapy did not have an R0 resection indicating a large proportion of patients with a positive margin on the cohort.

Several prospective trials have been performed to evaluate the role of adjuvant chemotherapy for ICC, though most have included other BTCs as well. Takada et al. randomized 436 patients with pancreatobiliary cancers, including 118 with BTCs, to either postoperative chemotherapy with 5-fluorouracil (5-FU) and mitomycin C (MMC) or surgery alone [13, 14]. The chemotherapy group received MMC (6 mg/m^2 intravenous (IV)) at the time of surgery and 5-FU (310 mg/m^2 IV) in 2 courses of treatment for 5 consecutive days during postoperative Weeks 1 and 3, followed by 5-FU (100 mg/m^2 rally) daily from postoperative Week 5 until disease recurrence. While there were no apparent differences in 5-year survival or 5-year disease-free rate, only 118 patients were categorized as bile duct cancers without further classification as intrahepatic or extrahepatic cholangiocarcinoma.

While it did not specifically include ICC, the European Study Group for Pancreatic Cancer (ESPAC)-3 was a landmark randomized controlled trial (RCT) that evaluated the role of adjuvant chemotherapy in periampullary pancreatobiliary cancers. Of 428 randomized patients, 96 had distal cholangiocarcinomas. Two-thirds of the patients were randomized to either 5-FU or gemcitabine-based adjuvant chemotherapy, while one-third underwent observation [15]. In the 5-FU arm, 143 patients received 20 mg/m^2 of folinic acid via intravenous bolus injection followed by 425 mg/m^2 of 5-FU via intravenous bolus injection administered 1 to 5 days every 28 days for 6 months. In the gemcitabine arm, 141 patients planned to receive 1000 mg/m^2 of IV infusion of gemcitabine once a week for 3 of every 4 weeks for 6 months. Although adjuvant chemotherapy was associated with significantly higher survival among all patients in the trial after adjusting for prognostic factors and performing multiple regression analyses, the value of adjuvant chemotherapy in cholangiocarcinoma was questionable as the median overall survival was numerically higher in the observation group compared to the chemotherapy groups (27.2 months vs. 18.3 months in the 5-FU group and 19.5 months in the gemcitabine group).

In a recent large RCT, the BILCAP study enrolled 447 patients with BTCs of which 19% were ICC. Patients were randomized 1:1 to capecitabine (1250 mg/m^2 days 1–14, every 21 days, for 8 cycles) or observation. This was the first randomized trial to show the benefit of adjuvant therapy that was statistically significant for the "per-protocol" cohort. Although the results of BILCAP were more in favor of adjuvant therapy compared to the prior two randomized trials, several questions remained to be answered including the specific effect on ICC compared to the rest of biliary and periampullary cancers included in the trial [16].

Perhaps the most disappointing findings came from the PRODIGE 12 trial. This was a phase III multicenter RCT evaluating adjuvant gemcitabine and oxaliplatin (GEMOX) versus observation alone in resected biliary cancers. The study randomized 196 patients of which 45% had ICC. Patients were randomized, within 3 months of R0 or R1 resection of a localized intrahepatic, perihilar, extrahepatic cholangiocarcinoma or gallbladder cancer to receive either surveillance or 12 cycles of gemcitabine 1000 mg/m^2 and oxaliplatin 85 mg /m^2 every 2 weeks. The trial results were negative, with no difference in relapse-free survival between study arms. In addition, subgroup analysis by tumor type did not demonstrate any favorable trends [17]. Several factors could have contributed to the lack of proven benefit of therapy in the trial. Inclusion of cases with a lower risk of recurrence may have affected the results as only one-third had node-positive disease and one-half the patients had multifocal tumor. In addition, only 33% of patients in the GEMOX arm received all six cycles of planned treatment. The results of another ongoing large randomized trial of adjuvant chemotherapy with gemcitabine and cisplatin compared to standard of care after curative intent resection of biliary tract cancer (ACTICCA-1) are eagerly awaited (NCT02170090).

While the role for adjuvant systemic chemotherapy continues to be debatable, interest in identifying a suitable adjuvant strategy remains high, given the poor prognosis and high risk of recurrence after surgery. In the meantime, on the basis of the BILCAP trial, adjuvant capecitabine has been established as the standard of care for most resected BTCs including ICC. Nevertheless, all patients with resected ICC are encouraged to enroll in clinical trials to aid our understanding of the optimal adjuvant approach. Smarter trial designs with increased selectivity to ICC with exploration of biologically optimized interventions are necessary. As stated earlier, the recurrence pattern of ICC is different from other biliary cancers as it is primarily in the form of intrahepatic or intraperitoneal recurrence [11]. This could open the way for more anatomic focally directed interventions such as hepatic artery-based therapies.

First-Line Palliative Chemotherapy

For patients with locally advanced or metastatic ICC, systemic chemotherapy remains the mainstay of treatment. In particular, palliative chemotherapy for active symptom control is vital to the management of the disease from the time of initial diagnosis. Compared with best supportive care, palliative chemotherapy offers improvements in quality of life and prolongs the survival for patients with BTCs, including ICC [9]. The data for systemic therapy is limited due to the lack of large prospective randomized clinical trials with head-to-head comparisons. Gemcitabine- and fluoropyrimidine-based (5-FU or capecitabine) chemotherapies are the most frequently studied combinations in phase II trials, with the exception of the combination of gemcitabine and cisplatin, which remains the standard care for the first-line treatment of advanced cholangiocarcinoma. In this next section, we will review chemotherapy regimens including single-agent gemcitabine, 5-FU/capecitabine, and gemcitabine-, fluoropyrimidine-based combinations in the first-line and second-line settings.

The nucleoside analog gemcitabine, as either a single agent or in combination with other chemotherapies, has been extensively studied in patients with BTCs. Data from phase II trials demonstrate that gemcitabine is generally well tolerated with response rates ranging from 0% to 30% [18–21]. In one prospective phase II trial [20], 23 chemotherapy-naïve patients with locally advanced or metastatic biliary tract adenocarcinomas were enrolled and treated with gemcitabine 1000 mg/m^2 on days 1 and 8, every 21 days. Six patients (26.1%) had partial response, while eight patients (34.8%) had stable disease. The overall response rate was 26.1% (95% CI, 22.08–30.12), the median time to disease progression was 8.1 months (95% CI, 3.33–12.87), and the median overall survival was 13.1 months (95% CI, 1.64–24.56). Toxicities were generally mild and included grade 3–4 neutropenia and thrombocytopenia. Treatment was well tolerated and dose omissions or reductions were rare. Overall, results suggest that gemcitabine monotherapy can be a valid first-line treatment method for those with an Eastern Cooperative Oncology Group (ECOG) performance status of 2.

Single-agent 5-FU is a nucleoside metabolic inhibitor that has also been assessed in the first-line. Earlier studies used 5-FU IV bolus; however, the objective response rates were low, and median survival was typically less than 6months [22]. In later trials, continuous infusional 5-FU or leucovorin-modulated 5-FU were studied and showed higher response rates (ranging from 21.4% to 32.1%), although whether this translates into better survival is still unclear [23–27]. In the same class of drugs, capecitabine used as a single agent was also evaluated in patients with cholangiocarcinoma ($n = 18$) and gallbladder cancer ($n = 8$), given as 1000 mg/m^2 twice daily for 14 days, every 21 days. The median survival was 8.1 months (95% CI, 7.4–8.9 months) for patients with cholangiocarcinoma vs. 9.9 months (95% CI, 4.4–15.4 months) for patients with gallbladder cancer [28]. Several phase II studies combining gemcitabine with capecitabine showed response rates of 25–31%, and median survival of 12.7–14 months [29–31].

Multiple phase II studies have also evaluated the combination of gemcitabine with platinum-based compounds, either cisplatin or oxaliplatin in patients with advanced BTCs, showing response rates of 21–36%, and median survival rates of 8.4–15 months [32–35]. A pooled analysis of all published clinical trials from 1985 to 2006 concluded that the addition of oxaliplatin or cisplatin to gemcitabine increases response rate (complete response + partial response), tumor control rate (complete response + partial response + stable disease) and shows a trend towards improved progression-free survival compared with fluoropyrimidine-based regimens, such as 5-FU [36]. However, whether gemcitabine-based combination regimens are superior to fluoropyrimidine-based regimens for advanced BTC is not clear, as the difference in survival times are small and not significant.

In general, gemcitabine-based therapies are used for patients with good performance status, whereas leucovorin-modulated 5-FU based therapies are reasonable options especially for patients with borderline performance status or hyperbilirubinemia in the first-line setting.

Gemcitabine with Cisplatin

The combination of gemcitabine and cisplatin compared with gemcitabine alone was addressed in phase III ABC-02 RCT for patients with locally advanced or metastatic cholangiocarcinoma, gallbladder cancer, or ampullary cancer. Results of this study demonstrated improvements in both progression-free and overall survival in patients who received gemcitabine plus cisplatin, compared to gemcitabine alone. Patients received either cisplatin (25 mg/m^2 on days 1 and 8) followed by gemcitabine (1000 mg/m^2 on days 1 and 8) every 3 weeks for eight cycles or gemcitabine alone (1000 mg/m^2 on days 1, 8 and 15) every 4 weeks for six cycles. Median progression-free survival was 8.0 months vs. 5.0 months (HR, 0.63; 95% CI, 0.51–0.77; $P < 0.001$), and median overall survival was 11.7 months vs. 8.1 months (HR, 0.64; 95% CI, 0.52–0.80; $P < 0.001$). Adverse events were similar in the two groups, with the exception of neutropenia being more frequent in the combination group [37]. This study established the gemcitabine/cisplatin combination as the standard of care in this disease. Notably, this study was supported by a randomized phase II BT22 study of Japanese patients with BTCs, which found median progression-free survival of 5.8 months and overall survival of 11.2 months for gemcitabine/cisplatin, compared with 3.7 and 7.7 months for progression-free and overall survival for gemcitabine alone [38]. A meta-analysis of these two studies showed that the benefit of gemcitabine/cisplatin is most significant among patients with good performance status (ECOG performance status 0–1) and results in improved progression-free and overall survival for intra- and extrahepatic cholangiocarcinoma and gallbladder cancer. However, patients with a performance status of 2 may derive the least benefit from the combination [39].

Gemcitabine with Oxaliplatin (GEMOX)

GEMOX has been evaluated in several studies, and this regimen has been well tolerated [33, 35, 40, 41]. A phase II study of GEMOX examined a cohort of 56 patients with advanced or metastatic BTC, who were treated with gemcitabine (1000 mg/m^2 on day 1) and oxaliplatin(100 mg/m^2 on day 2) every 2 weeks. The patients were divided into two groups: Group A patients (n = 33) had the performance status 0–2, bilirubin <2.5× normal without prior chemotherapy; Group B patients (n = 23) had performance status >2 and/or bilirubin >2.5× normal and/or prior chemotherapy. In Group A, the response rate was 36% and median overall survival duration was 15.4 months, whereas in Group B patients with performance status >2 and prior chemotherapy, the response rate was 22% and median survival was 7.6 months. However, the tolerability of GEMOX in Group B did not differ significantly from that in Group A patients, indicating that this combination is safe in patients who have a poor prognosis or have received prior chemotherapy [33]. Therefore, in patients with a concern about cisplatin toxicity (renal or hearing impairment), oxaliplatin may be substituted for cisplatin in the first-line setting [42].

Gemcitabine with Carboplatin

A phase II study examined a total of 48 patients with advanced BTCs (35 cholangiocarcinoma, 12 gallbladder and 1 ampullary cancer) in the first-line setting, who were treated with a maximum of nine cycles of gemcitabine 1000 mg/m^2 IV on days 1, 8 with carboplatin dosed at an area-under-the-curve (AUC) of 5 on day 1, every 3 weeks. A median of four cycles was administered. The overall response rate for evaluable patients was 31.1%. Median progression-free survival and overall survival were 7.8 months and 10.6 months, respectively. The most common grade 3–4 toxicities include neutropenia and thrombocytopenia [43]. Although severe nonhematological toxicities were uncommon, hematological toxicities associated with gemcitabine and carboplatin, as administered in this protocol, appeared higher compared with the toxicities reported using weekly cisplatin and gemcitabine in the ABC-02 study (Grade 3–4 anemia 12% vs. 6.3%; grade 3–4 thrombocytopenia 20% vs. 8.2% and grade 3–4 neutropenia 37% vs. 22.6%).

Gemcitabine with Capecitabine

In one prospective phase II study, 45 patients were enrolled (53% with cholangiocarcinoma, 47% with gallbladder cancer) and treated with gemcitabine(1000 mg/m^2 on days 1 and 8) and capecitabine (650 mg/m^2 twice daily for 14 days) every 21 days. The overall objective response rate was 31%, with an additional 42% of patients with stable disease. The median progression-free and overall survivals were 7 and 14 months, respectively [29]. This chemotherapy combination was generally well tolerated. In another prospective phase II study, 44 patients who met at least one of the symptoms including impaired Karnofsky performance score of 60 to 80, analgesic consumption ≥10 mg of morphine equivalents per day, or pain score ≥20 mm/100 mm were enrolled (cholangiocarcinoma, $n = 36$; gallbladder cancers, $n = 8$), and were treated with gemcitabine/capecitabine. The objective response rate was 25%, the median time to progression and overall survival were 7.2 months and 13.2 months, respectively. Improved quality of life was observed in patients with a clinical benefit response [30].

5-FU with Oxaliplatin (FOLFOX)

A retrospective cohort study has been conducted to compare the efficacy of FOLFOX vs. gemcitabine as the first-line option in patients with advanced BTC. Twenty-two patients were treated with FOLFOX-4 consisting of oxaliplatin (85 mg/m^2, day 1), leucovorin (200 mg/m^2/day) followed by a 5-FU bolus (400 mg/m^2/day) and 22-hour infusion of 5-FU (600 mg/m^2/day) for two consecutive days, every 2 weeks. Eighteen patients received gemcitabine, 1250 mg/m^2 on days 1 and 8, every 3 weeks. In the FOLFOX-4 group, the overall response rate was 13.6% (95% CI, 4.7–33.3) and there was a 54.5% (95% CI, 34.7–73.1) disease control rate (complete response + partial response + stable disease). Median overall survival was 14.1 months (95% CI, 9.1–18.8) and median progression-free survival was 5.44 months (95% CI, 3.2–6.3). In the gemcitabine group, there was no objective response, whereas 27.7% (95% CI, 12.5–50.9) obtained disease control. Median overall survival was 8.3 months (95% CI, 4.7–12.9) and median progression-free survival was 3.9 months (95% CI, 2.2–5.4). Toxicity, mainly hematological, was acceptable for both treatments [21] (Table 8.1).

Second-Line Palliative Chemotherapy

There is no established second-line systemic therapy following progression after first-line treatment. In fact, only 15–25% of patients are fit enough to receive second-line treatment [44]. In general, for patients who retain adequate performance

Table 8.1 Summary of first-line palliative chemotherapy studies and outcomes in patients with intrahepatocellular cholangiocarcinoma

Treatment	Response rate	Overall survival (median)
Single agents		
Gemcitabine [18–21, 38]	0–30%	5.2–17.3 months
5-FU [23–26]	21.4–32.1%	4.7–10 months
Capecitabine[28]	6%	8.1 months
Combination treatments		
Gemcitabine + cisplatin [32, 34, 36–39]	19.5–33.3%	9.7–11.2 months
Gemcitabine + oxaliplatin (GEMOX) [33, 35, 40]	22–41%	7.6–15.4 months
Gemcitabine + carboplatin [43]	31.1%	10.6 months
Gemcitabine + capecitabine[29–31]	25–31%	12.7–14 months
5-FU + oxaliplatin (FOLFOX) [21]	13.6%	14.1 months

Note: 5-FU when given as continuous infusion or leucovorin-modulated 5-FU

status but progressed on gemcitabine with platinum regimen, FOLFOX, capecitabine with oxaliplatin (CAPOX), 5-FU with irinotecan (FOLFIRI), or capecitabine with irinotecan (XELIRI) can be considered.

In a Phase II study of second-line therapy, 37 patients with advanced BTC who were refractory to gemcitabine/cisplatin chemotherapy were treated with FOLFOX for two consecutive days, every 2 weeks: oxaliplatin (85 mg/m^2, day 1), leucovorin (200 mg/m^2/day) followed by a 5-FU bolus (400 mg/m^2/day) and 22-hour infusion of 5-FU (600 mg/m^2/day). The primary endpoint, the median time to progression, was 3.1 months (95% CI, 2.3–3.6), while the objective response rate was 21.6% (8 with partial response), and disease control rate was 62.2% (15 with stable disease) [45]. Another randomized phase II study evaluated the efficacy and safety of second-line capecitabine and irinotecan vs. irinotecan monotherapy in advanced biliary tract cancer who progressed on gemcitabine and cisplatin. Sixty-four patients were randomized to either irinotecan 180 mg/m^2 on day 1 plus capecitabine 1000 mg/m^2 twice daily on days 1–10 of a 14-day cycle or single-agent irinotecan 180 mg/m^2 on day 1 of a 14-day cycle. Of the 60 patients included in the analysis, the median progression-free survival was 3.7 vs. 2.4 months and median overall survival was 10.1 vs. 7.3 months for capecitabine/irinotecan and irinotecan only arms, respectively. The most common grade 3 or 4 toxicities were leucopoenia and neutropenia [46].

A systematic review of second-line systemic chemotherapies that included 23 studies and 761 patients with advanced BTC, showed that the median overall survival was 7.2 months (95% CI, 6.2–8.2) and the median progression-free survival was 3.2 months (95% CI, 2.7–3.7). No recommendation could be made in regard to the most appropriate second-line regimen. These results underscore the unmet need for prospective RCTs in this setting [47].

Chemotherapies in Combination with Biologic Agents

With the advent of whole-exome and next generation sequencing, multiple molecular aberrations have been identified that contribute to the multistep carcinogenesis in ICC [48–53]. Well established genomic alterations include EGFR (epithelial growth factor receptor) overexpression (11–27%), VEGF (vascular endothelial growth factor) overexpression (54%), KRAS (Kirsten rat sarcoma viral oncogene homolog) mutation (9–24%), and TP53 (tumor protein p53) mutation (3–36%). Results of EGFR inhibitors or VEGF inhibitors in combination with standard chemotherapy have, in general, been disappointing [54–58]. Most of the studies were not biomarker-driven, which may undermine the potential benefit of targeted therapy in distinct patient populations.

Gemcitabine with EGFR Inhibitors

The EGFR family includes HER1/EGFR (human EGFR related 1/EGFR), HER2, HER3, and HER4. EGFR is frequently implicated in the carcinogenesis of cholangiocarcinoma. The majority of EGFR overexpression in BTC is due to DNA copy number gains while activating mutations in EGFR gene are rare events [48, 59]. In a multicenter phase II trial, 44 patients with unresectable cholangiocarcinoma naïve to chemotherapy were enrolled and treated with the EGFR inhibitor cetuximab (400 mg/m^2 at week 1, then 250 mg/m^2 weekly) and gemcitabine (1000 mg/m^2 on days 1, 8 and 15), every 4 weeks. Six-month progression-free survival was 47%, and median overall survival was 13.5 months (95% CI, 9.8–31.8 months). Nine patients (20.4%) had partial response, and the disease control rate was 79.5%. KRAS mutations were found in 7 of 27 patients and had no influence on progression-free survival. Skin toxic effect ≥grade 2 was associated with increased progression-free survival ($P = 0.05$). Grade 3 or 4 treatment-related toxic effects were hematological (52.2%), skin rash (13.6%), and fatigue (11.4%) [60]. Despite these results, randomized studies have failed to demonstrate a survival benefit by combining EGFR inhibitors with gemcitabine/oxaliplatin in advanced cholangiocarcinoma [54–56].

GEMOX with VEGF Inhibitors

VEGF overexpression has been observed in 54% of ICCs [51]. In a retrospective study, the combination therapy of bevacizumab with GEMOX was compared to GEMOX therapy alone in the first-line setting in metastatic BTC. Thirty-two patients were treated with gemcitabine 1000 mg/m^2 followed by 100 mg/m^{2}oxaliplatin, plus bevacizumab 5 mg/kg on day 1, every 2 weeks (GEMOX-bevacizumab, group A). Twenty-five patients were treated with the GEMOX regimen only (group B). The treatment was repeated every 2 weeks until disease progression or unacceptable toxicity. The combination therapy of bevacizumab with GEMOX was associated with a better progression-free survival, compared to that of GEMOX therapy (6.48 months vs. 3.72 months, $p = 0.049$). However, the median overall survival was 11.31 months and 10.34 months in Group A and B ($p = 0.64$), failing to demonstrate a survival benefit of adding bevacizumab to the chemotherapy backbone. Specific grades 3–4 bevacizumab-related adverse events included hypertension (6%), cardiac ischemia (3%), proteinuria (6%), perforation (6%), thrombosis (3%), and bleeding events (3%) [57].

Bevacizumab with Erlotinib

In a multicenter phase II study, patients ($n = 53$) with advanced cholangiocarcinoma ($n = 43$) or gallbladder cancer ($n = 10$) were treated with bevacizumab 5 mg/kg intravenously on days 1, 15 and erlotinib 150 mg by mouth daily on days 1 through 28, in a 28-day cycle. Of 49 evaluable patients, six patients (12%; 95% CI, 6% to 27%) had a confirmed partial response and 25 patients (51%) had documented stable disease. Rash was the most common grade 3 toxicity. Four patients had grade 4 toxicities, including cerebral ischemia and thrombosis. Median overall survival was 9.9 months, and time to progression was 4.4 months. In conclusion, the biologic-only combination of bevacizumab and erlotinib has a demonstrable activity in advanced biliary tract cancers with few grade 3 or 4 adverse events [61].

Novel Targeting Agents

A combination of whole-exome and transcriptome sequencing has been performed to characterize a total of 260 cases of BTC, including 145 cases of ICC, 86 cases of extrahepatic cholangiocarcinoma, and 29 cases of gallbladder cancer. Recurrent mutations in IDH1/2 (isocitrate dehydrogenase 1/2) and BAP1 (BRCA-1 associated protein 1), FGFR2 (fibroblast growth factor receptor 2) fusion are predominantly found in the intrahepatic subtype, whereas ARID1B (AT-rich interactive domain-containing protein 1B) mutation, PRKACA (cAMP-dependent protein kinase catalytic subunit alpha), and PRKACB fusion preferentially occur in extrahepatic subtype [62], indicating that there might be distinctive molecular features among different subtypes of cholangiocarcinoma.

FGFR2 Fusion Inhibitors

FGFR2 mitigates cell differentiation, proliferation, and apoptosis [63]. There is marked variability in the frequency of FGFR2 fusions across studies, ranging from 6% to 50% in ICCs. However, FGFR alterations are rarely found in extrahepatic cholangiocarcinomas [62, 64–66]. FGFR2 fusions are associated with improved survival [49]. In a phase II study, BGJ398, a pan-FGFR tyrosine kinase inhibitor, was evaluated in 61 patients with advanced or metastatic cholangiocarcinoma containing FGFR2 fusions or other FGFR alterations whose disease had progressed on prior therapies. The overall response rate was 14.8%, disease control rate was 75.4%, and estimated median progression-free survival was 5.8 months (95% CI, 4.3 to 7.6 months). Grade 3 or 4 treatment-related adverse events occurred in 25 patients (41%) and included hyperphosphatemia (16.4%), stomatitis (6.6%), and palmar-plantar erythrodysesthesia (4.9%). This study showed meaningful clinical activity against chemotherapy-refractory cholangiocarcinoma containing FGFR2 fusions [67]. There are other FGFR inhibitors that are under investigation (NCT02272998, NCT01752920, NCT03278106).

IDH1/2 Inhibitors

AG-120 is an oral IDH1 inhibitor that is approved for adult patients with relapsed or refractory acute myeloid leukemia (AML) with IDH1 mutations. In a phase I clinical trial in mutated IDH1 advanced solid tumors, 73 patients with cholangiocarcinoma were treated with AG-120 at doses ranging from 100 mg twice daily to 1200 mg once daily. AG-120 demonstrated a favorable safety profile and clinical activity in this study [68]. Among the 72 evaluable patients, 6% ($n = 4$) had a confirmed partial response and 56% ($n = 40$) had stable disease. Progression-free survival rate at 6 months was 40%. Currently, a phase III, multicenter, double-blind study (ClarIDHy) to evaluate the efficacy of AG-120 for patients with mutated IDH1 cholangiocarcinoma is ongoing (NCT02989857).

Conclusion

ICC is a rare but aggressive cancer, with very low 5-year survival rates. While many different chemotherapy regimens have been evaluated in cholangiocarcinoma, only a few studies have shown promising results. For adjuvant chemotherapy, physicians need to discuss treatment options in a multidisciplinary setting and offer the best care to patients using a shared decision-making process. Regarding definitive chemotherapy options for patients with locally advanced and metastatic setting, the appropriate chemotherapies should be considered based on the patient's performance status and liver function. Patient participation in prospective clinical trials is the preferred option for patients with ICC. Ongoing clinical trials will be discussed in greater detail in a later chapter.

References

1. Patel T. Worldwide trends in mortality from biliary tract malignancies. BMC Cancer. 2002;2:10.
2. Yeo CJ, Pitt HA, Cameron JL. Cholangiocarcinoma. Surg Clin North Am. 1990;70(6):1429–47.
3. Bengmark S, Ekberg H, Evander A, Klofver-Stahl B, Tranberg KG. Major liver resection for hilar cholangiocarcinoma. Ann Surg. 1988;207(2):120–5.
4. Nagorney DM, Donohue JH, Farnell MB, Schleck CD, Ilstrup DM. Outcomes after curative resections of cholangiocarcinoma. Arch Surg. 1993;128(8):871–7; discussion 7–9.
5. Kraybill WG, Lee H, Picus J, Ramachandran G, Lopez MJ, Kucik N, et al. Multidisciplinary treatment of biliary tract cancers. J Surg Oncol. 1994;55(4):239–45.
6. Nathan H, Pawlik TM, Wolfgang CL, Choti MA, Cameron JL, Schulick RD. Trends in survival after surgery for cholangiocarcinoma: a 30-year population-based SEER database analysis. J Gastrointest Surg. 2007;11(11):1488–96; discussion 96–7.
7. Spolverato G, Vitale A, Cucchetti A, Popescu I, Marques HP, Aldrighetti L, et al. Can hepatic resection provide a long-term cure for patients with intrahepatic cholangiocarcinoma? Cancer. 2015;121(22):3998–4006.
8. Yamamoto M, Takasaki K, Otsubo T, Katsuragawa H, Katagiri S. Recurrence after surgical resection of intrahepatic cholangiocarcinoma. J Hepato-Biliary-Pancreat Surg. 2001;8(2):154–7.
9. Glimelius B, Hoffman K, Sjoden PO, Jacobsson G, Sellstrom H, Enander LK, et al. Chemotherapy improves survival and quality of life in advanced pancreatic and biliary cancer. Ann Oncol. 1996;7(6):593–600.
10. Ercolani G, Vetrone G, Grazi GL, Aramaki O, Cescon M, Ravaioli M, et al. Intrahepatic cholangiocarcinoma: primary liver resection and aggressive multimodal treatment of recurrence significantly prolong survival. Ann Surg. 2010;252(1):107–14.
11. Sur MD, In H, Sharpe SM, Baker MS, Weichselbaum RR, Talamonti MS, et al. Defining the benefit of adjuvant therapy following resection for intrahepatic cholangiocarcinoma. Ann Surg Oncol. 2015;22(7):2209–17.
12. Miura JT, Johnston FM, Tsai S, George B, Thomas J, Eastwood D, et al. Chemotherapy for surgically resected intrahepatic cholangiocarcinoma. Ann Surg Oncol. 2015;22(11):3716–23.
13. Okamoto M, Yamagata Z, Takeda Y, Yoda Y, Kobayashi K, Fujino MA. The relationship between gallbladder disease and smoking and drinking habits in middle-aged Japanese. J Gastroenterol. 2002;37(6):455–62.
14. Takada T, Amano H, Yasuda H, Nimura Y, Matsushiro T, Kato H, et al. Is postoperative adjuvant chemotherapy useful for gallbladder carcinoma? A phase III multicenter prospective randomized controlled trial in patients with resected pancreaticobiliary carcinoma. Cancer. 2002;95(8):1685–95.
15. Neoptolemos JP, Moore MJ, Cox TF, Valle JW, Palmer DH, McDonald AC, et al. Effect of adjuvant chemotherapy with fluorouracil plus folinic acid or gemcitabine vs observation on survival in patients with resected periampullary adenocarcinoma: the ESPAC-3 periampullary cancer randomized trial. JAMA. 2012;308(2):147–56.
16. Primrose JN, Fox R, Palmer DH, Prasad R, Mirza D, Anthoney DA, et al. Adjuvant capecitabine for biliary tract cancer: the BILCAP randomized study. J Clin Oncol. 2017;35(15_suppl):4006.
17. Edeline J, Bonnetain F, Phelip JM, Watelet J, Hammel P, Joly J-P, et al. Gemox versus surveillance following surgery of localized biliary tract cancer: results of the PRODIGE 12-ACCORD 18 (UNICANCER GI) phase III trial. J Clin Oncol. 2017;35(4_suppl):225.
18. Kubicka S, Rudolph KL, Tietze MK, Lorenz M, Manns M. Phase II study of systemic gemcitabine chemotherapy for advanced unresectable hepatobiliary carcinomas. Hepato-Gastroenterology. 2001;48(39):783–9.
19. Penz M, Kornek GV, Raderer M, Ulrich-Pur H, Fiebiger W, Lenauer A, et al. Phase II trial of two-weekly gemcitabine in patients with advanced biliary tract cancer. Ann Oncol. 2001;12(2):183–6.

20. Park JS, Oh SY, Kim SH, Kwon HC, Kim JS, Jin-Kim H, et al. Single-agent gemcitabine in the treatment of advanced biliary tract cancers: a phase II study. Jpn J Clin Oncol. 2005;35(2):68–73.
21. Novarino AM, Satolli MA, Chiappino I, Giacobino A, Napoletano R, Ceccarelli M, et al. FOLFOX-4 regimen or single-agent gemcitabine as first-line chemotherapy in advanced biliary tract cancer. Am J Clin Oncol. 2013;36(5):466–71.
22. Takada T, Kato H, Matsushiro T, Nimura Y, Nagakawa T, Nakayama T. Comparison of 5-fluorouracil, doxorubicin and mitomycin C with 5-fluorouracil alone in the treatment of pancreatic-biliary carcinomas. Oncology. 1994;51(5):396–400.
23. Ducreux M, Rougier P, Fandi A, Clavero-Fabri MC, Villing AL, Fassone F, et al. Effective treatment of advanced biliary tract carcinoma using 5-fluorouracil continuous infusion with cisplatin. Ann Oncol. 1998;9(6):653–6.
24. Sanz-Altamira PM, Ferrante K, Jenkins RL, Lewis WD, Huberman MS, Stuart KE. A phase II trial of 5-fluorouracil, leucovorin, and carboplatin in patients with unresectable biliary tree carcinoma. Cancer. 1998;82(12):2321–5.
25. Choi CW, Choi IK, Seo JH, Kim BS, Kim JS, Kim CD, et al. Effects of 5-fluorouracil and leucovorin in the treatment of pancreatic-biliary tract adenocarcinomas. Am J Clin Oncol. 2000;23(4):425–8.
26. Chen JS, Jan YY, Lin YC, Wang HM, Chang WC, Liau CT. Weekly 24 h infusion of high-dose 5-fluorouracil and leucovorin in patients with biliary tract carcinomas. Anti-Cancer Drugs. 1998;9(5):393–7.
27. Malik IA, Aziz Z. Prospective evaluation of efficacy and toxicity of 5-fu and folinic acid (Mayo Clinic regimen) in patients with advanced cancer of the gallbladder. Am J Clin Oncol. 2003;26(2):124–6.
28. Patt YZ, Hassan MM, Aguayo A, Nooka AK, Lozano RD, Curley SA, et al. Oral capecitabine for the treatment of hepatocellular carcinoma, cholangiocarcinoma, and gallbladder carcinoma. Cancer. 2004;101(3):578–86.
29. Knox JJ, Hedley D, Oza A, Feld R, Siu LL, Chen E, et al. Combining gemcitabine and capecitabine in patients with advanced biliary cancer: a phase II trial. J Clin Oncol. 2005;23(10):2332–8.
30. Koeberle D, Saletti P, Borner M, Gerber D, Dietrich D, Caspar CB, et al. Patient-reported outcomes of patients with advanced biliary tract cancers receiving gemcitabine plus capecitabine: a multicenter, phase II trial of the Swiss Group for Clinical Cancer Research. J Clin Oncol. 2008;26(22):3702–8.
31. Riechelmann RP, Townsley CA, Chin SN, Pond GR, Knox JJ. Expanded phase II trial of gemcitabine and capecitabine for advanced biliary cancer. Cancer. 2007;110(6):1307–12.
32. Meyerhardt JA, Zhu AX, Stuart K, Ryan DP, Blaszkowsky L, Lehman N, et al. Phase-II study of gemcitabine and cisplatin in patients with metastatic biliary and gallbladder cancer. Dig Dis Sci. 2008;53(2):564–70.
33. Andre T, Tournigand C, Rosmorduc O, Provent S, Maindrault-Goebel F, Avenin D, et al. Gemcitabine combined with oxaliplatin (GEMOX) in advanced biliary tract adenocarcinoma: a GERCOR study. Ann Oncol. 2004;15(9):1339–43.
34. Kim ST, Park JO, Lee J, Lee KT, Lee JK, Choi SH, et al. A phase II study of gemcitabine and cisplatin in advanced biliary tract cancer. Cancer. 2006;106(6):1339–46.
35. Harder J, Riecken B, Kummer O, Lohrmann C, Otto F, Usadel H, et al. Outpatient chemotherapy with gemcitabine and oxaliplatin in patients with biliary tract cancer. Br J Cancer. 2006;95(7):848–52.
36. Eckel F, Schmid RM. Chemotherapy in advanced biliary tract carcinoma: a pooled analysis of clinical trials. Br J Cancer. 2007;96(6):896–902.
37. Valle J, Wasan H, Palmer DH, Cunningham D, Anthoney A, Maraveyas A, et al. Cisplatin plus gemcitabine versus gemcitabine for biliary tract cancer. N Engl J Med. 2010;362(14):1273–81.
38. Okusaka T, Nakachi K, Fukutomi A, Mizuno N, Ohkawa S, Funakoshi A, et al. Gemcitabine alone or in combination with cisplatin in patients with biliary tract cancer: a comparative multicentre study in Japan. Br J Cancer. 2010;103(4):469–74.

39. Valle JW, Furuse J, Jitlal M, Beare S, Mizuno N, Wasan H, et al. Cisplatin and gemcitabine for advanced biliary tract cancer: a meta-analysis of two randomized trials. Ann Oncol. 2014;25(2):391–8.
40. Manzione L, Romano R, Germano D. Chemotherapy with gemcitabine and oxaliplatin in patients with advanced biliary tract cancer: a single-institution experience. Oncology. 2007;73(5–6):311–5.
41. Andre T, Reyes-Vidal JM, Fartoux L, Ross P, Leslie M, Rosmorduc O, et al. Gemcitabine and oxaliplatin in advanced biliary tract carcinoma: a phase II study. Br J Cancer. 2008;99(6):862–7.
42. Valle JW, Borbath I, Khan SA, Huguet F, Gruenberger T, Arnold D, et al. Biliary cancer: ESMO clinical practice guidelines for diagnosis, treatment, and follow-up. Ann Oncol. 2016;27(suppl 5):v28–37.
43. Williams KJ, Picus J, Trinkhaus K, Fournier CC, Suresh R, James JS, et al. Gemcitabine with carboplatin for advanced biliary tract cancers: a phase II single-institution study. HPB (Oxford). 2010;12(6):418–26.
44. Bridgewater J, Palmer D, Cunningham D, Iveson T, Gillmore R, Waters J, et al. Outcome of second-line chemotherapy for biliary tract cancer. Eur J Cancer. 2013;49(6):1511.
45. He S, Shen J, Sun X, Liu L, Dong J. A phase II FOLFOX-4 regimen as second-line treatment in advanced biliary tract cancer refractory to gemcitabine/cisplatin. J Chemother. 2014;26(4):243–7.
46. Zheng Y, Tu X, Zhao P, Jiang W, Liu L, Tong Z, et al. A randomized phase II study of second-line XELIRI regimen versus irinotecan monotherapy in advanced biliary tract cancer patients progressed on gemcitabine and cisplatin. Br J Cancer. 2018;119(3):291–5.
47. Lamarca A, Hubner RA, David Ryder W, Valle JW. Second-line chemotherapy in advanced biliary cancer: a systematic review. Ann Oncol. 2014;25(12):2328–38.
48. Andersen JB. Molecular pathogenesis of intrahepatic cholangiocarcinoma. J Hepatobiliary Pancreat Sci. 2015;22(2):101–13.
49. Churi CR, Shroff R, Wang Y, Rashid A, Kang HC, Weatherly J, et al. Mutation profiling in cholangiocarcinoma: prognostic and therapeutic implications. PLoS One. 2014;9(12):e115383.
50. Ross JS, Wang K, Gay L, Al-Rohil R, Rand JV, Jones DM, et al. New routes to targeted therapy of intrahepatic cholangiocarcinomas revealed by next-generation sequencing. Oncologist. 2014;19(3):235–42.
51. Yoshikawa D, Ojima H, Iwasaki M, Hiraoka N, Kosuge T, Kasai S, et al. Clinicopathological and prognostic significance of EGFR, VEGF, and HER2 expression in cholangiocarcinoma. Br J Cancer. 2008;98(2):418–25.
52. Nakazawa K, Dobashi Y, Suzuki S, Fujii H, Takeda Y, Ooi A. Amplification and overexpression of c-erbB-2, epidermal growth factor receptor, and c-met in biliary tract cancers. J Pathol. 2005;206(3):356–65.
53. Zhu AX, Borger DR, Kim Y, Cosgrove D, Ejaz A, Alexandrescu S, et al. Genomic profiling of intrahepatic cholangiocarcinoma: refining prognosis and identifying therapeutic targets. Ann Surg Oncol. 2014;21(12):3827–34.
54. Lee J, Park SH, Chang HM, Kim JS, Choi HJ, Lee MA, et al. Gemcitabine and oxaliplatin with or without erlotinib in advanced biliary-tract cancer: a multicentre, open-label, randomized, phase 3 study. Lancet Oncol. 2012;13(2):181–8.
55. Malka D, Cervera P, Foulon S, Trarbach T, de la Fouchardiere C, Boucher E, et al. Gemcitabine and oxaliplatin with or without cetuximab in advanced biliary-tract cancer (BINGO): a randomized, open-label, non-comparative phase 2 trial. Lancet Oncol. 2014;15(8):819–28.
56. Chen JS, Hsu C, Chiang NJ, Tsai CS, Tsou HH, Huang SF, et al. A KRAS mutation status-stratified randomized phase II trial of gemcitabine and oxaliplatin alone or in combination with cetuximab in advanced biliary tract cancer. Ann Oncol. 2015;26(5):943–9.
57. Brechon M, Dior M, Dreanic J, Brieau B, Guillaumot MA, Brezault C, et al. Addition of antiangiogenic therapy, bevacizumab, to gemcitabine plus oxaliplatin improves survival in advanced biliary tract cancers. Investig New Drugs. 2018;36(1):156–62.

58. Valle JW, Wasan H, Lopes A, Backen AC, Palmer DH, Morris K, et al. Cediranib or placebo in combination with cisplatin and gemcitabine chemotherapy for patients with advanced biliary tract cancer (ABC-03): a randomized phase 2 trial. Lancet Oncol. 2015;16(8):967–78.
59. Sirica AE. Role of ErbB family receptor tyrosine kinases in intrahepatic cholangiocarcinoma. World J Gastroenterol. 2008;14(46):7033–58.
60. Borbath I, Ceratti A, Verslype C, Demols A, Delaunoit T, Laurent S, et al. Combination of gemcitabine and cetuximab in patients with advanced cholangiocarcinoma: a phase II study of the Belgian Group of Digestive Oncology. Ann Oncol. 2013;24(11):2824–9.
61. Lubner SJ, Mahoney MR, Kolesar JL, Loconte NK, Kim GP, Pitot HC, et al. Report of a multicenter phase II trial testing a combination of biweekly bevacizumab and daily erlotinib in patients with unresectable biliary cancer: a phase II consortium study. J Clin Oncol. 2010;28(21):3491–7.
62. Nakamura H, Arai Y, Totoki Y, Shirota T, Elzawahry A, Kato M, et al. Genomic spectra of biliary tract cancer. Nat Genet. 2015;47(9):1003–10.
63. Tiong KH, Mah LY, Leong CO. Functional roles of fibroblast growth factor receptors (FGFRs) signaling in human cancers. Apoptosis. 2013;18(12):1447–68.
64. Arai Y, Totoki Y, Hosoda F, Shirota T, Hama N, Nakamura H, et al. Fibroblast growth factor receptor 2 tyrosine kinase fusions define a unique molecular subtype of cholangiocarcinoma. Hepatology. 2014;59(4):1427–34.
65. Borad MJ, Champion MD, Egan JB, Liang WS, Fonseca R, Bryce AH, et al. Integrated genomic characterization reveals novel, therapeutically relevant drug targets in FGFR and EGFR pathways in sporadic intrahepatic cholangiocarcinoma. PLoS Genet. 2014;10(2):e1004135.
66. Wu YM, Su F, Kalyana-Sundaram S, Khazanov N, Ateeq B, Cao X, et al. Identification of targetable FGFR gene fusions in diverse cancers. Cancer Discov. 2013;3(6):636–47.
67. Javle M, Lowery M, Shroff RT, Weiss KH, Springfeld C, Borad MJ, et al. Phase II study of BGJ398 in patients with FGFR-altered advanced cholangiocarcinoma. J Clin Oncol. 2018;36(3):276–82.
68. Lowery MA, Bou-Alfa GK, Burris HA, et al. Phase I study of AG-120, an IDH1 mutant enzyme inhibitor: Results from the cholangiocarcinoma dose escalation and expansion cohorts. American Society of Clinical Oncology Annual Meeting. 2017; Abstract 4015.

Chapter 9
Percutaneous Ablation

Guojun Qian, Jinglei Zhang, and Feng Shen

Introduction

Intrahepatic cholangiocarcinoma (ICC) is a primary adenocarcinoma originating from the intrahepatic biliary tree and is the second most common primary liver cancer after hepatocellular carcinoma (HCC) [1]. The incidence of ICC is increasing worldwide according to the recent reports and its development is known to be associated with certain predisposing genetic and environmental factors [2]. Because ICC is often diagnosed at an advanced stage and exhibits aggressive tumor biology, the long-term survival outcomes of patients with ICC remain poor [3]. Among possible treatments for patients with ICC, surgical resection is the only established treatment that may provide long-term survival in well-selected patients, especially when the tumor is completely resected with a negative surgical margin [4, 5]. However, the majority of patients are not candidates for curative-intent surgery due to advanced disease at the time of diagnosis [6]. In addition, tumor recurrence and metastasis are still common even among patients who are able to undergo radical resection.

Image-guided percutaneous ablation is a minimally invasive therapy, which can result in local destruction of multiple types of liver malignancies [7–9]. Although ablative techniques have been well established in the treatment of HCC and isolated liver metastases, demonstrating efficacy even in large liver tumors via stereotactic placement of multiple radiofrequency probes [10], only limited data are currently available on the use of ablation in ICC. In addition, for recurrent ICC after initial

G. Qian · J. Zhang
Department of Ultrasound Interventional Therapy, Eastern Hepatobiliary Surgery Hospital, Naval Medical University, Shanghai, China

F. Shen (✉)
Department of Hepatic Surgery, Eastern Hepatobiliary Surgery Hospital, Naval Medical University, Shanghai, China

T. M. Pawlik et al. (eds.), *Intrahepatic Cholangiocarcinoma*,
https://doi.org/10.1007/978-3-030-22258-1_9

curative resection, the use of repeat hepatectomy is usually limited by poor liver remnant function or multifocal recurrent diseases. In addition to systemic chemotherapy, these patients may be treated with locoregional therapies such as external beam radiation (XRT), radiofrequency ablation (RFA), microwave ablation (MWA), and radioactive implants (RIs) [11, 12].

This chapter reviews the technique, mechanism of action, indications, and outcomes of percutaneous ablation for ICC, highlighting the currently available evidence.

Indications for Percutaneous Ablation for ICC

There is limited research for which to base guidelines on the indications for percutaneous ablation in ICC. In clinical practice, patients with ICC who are not suitable for resection or who have developed relapse after resection are often considered for percutaneous thermal ablation. However, it is not uncommon for patients with ICC to undergo ablation based on a presumptive diagnosis of HCC, for which the use of curative-intent ablation is more established. Since the accurate histopathological evaluation of ablated tumors is usually not possible, this limitation must be considered when evaluating research on ablation for ICC. Percutaneous thermal ablation is commonly used in HCC patients who have a tumor within the Milan criteria, either as a curative-intent treatment or as a bridge to transplantation [13]. However, some authors have reported that the indications for percutaneous ablation should be less stringent: less than 5 nodules, each <5 cm in size, Child-Pugh class A or B liver function, prothrombin time <17 seconds, platelet count >45 cells $\times 10^9$/L, and no evidence of macrovascular invasion and/or extrahepatic distant metastases [14]. However, treatment guidelines for the use of percutaneous thermal ablation in ICC are not comprehensive and immature. Zhang et al. reported that ablation should be considered based on the following criteria: histopathologically proven ICC, primary or recurrent tumor after surgery, maximum tumor size <5 cm, tumor number <3. Whether additional indications beyond this standard are also suitable for ablation is unknown [15].

Therapeutic Mechanism of and Equipment for RFA and WMA

Both RFA and MWA result in cytotoxic destruction of cancer cells via direct thermal injury. The ablation procedures involve placing needles (electrodes/antennas) directly into the targeted tumors. It aims to increase the temperature between 60 and 100 °C in the tumor tissues, which can lead to coagulation necrosis of the tumor while avoiding charring and vaporization of tissues [16–18]. In addition, thermal ablation technology is designed to destroy tumors without disrupting adjacent liver structures. These treatments have achieved acceptable outcomes in previous studies of liver tumors [12, 14, 19].

RFA

A large body of literature exists on the use of RFA for HCC and liver metastases. During the process of ablation, the needle is placed directly into the targeted tumor, and one or more electrodes are deployed from the tip of the needle to the tumor tissues. The heat and the friction generated by the radio energy through the ion produced by the needle generate heat and destroy the tumor tissues. A miniature thermometer coupled to the tip of the electrode allows continuous monitoring of tissue temperature. The power is automatically adjusted to keep the target temperature constant. As tissue temperature increases above 60 °C, cancer cell death occurs almost instantaneously [20].

Multiple ablations can overlap to reduce the chance of residual disease and/or local recurrence following ablation. The size of the ablated area depends mainly on the size of the electrode needle, the temperature generated in the tissues and the duration of the energy applied. A sharp boundary separates dead tissue and unaffected surrounding tissue [20–22].

MWA

MWA is an alternative method of inducing tissue thermal coagulation. Microwave magnetic fields make surrounding molecules rotate at high speed and frictional heating, resulting in tissue coagulation, dehydration, and necrosis. It involves placing needle electrodes directly into the targeted tumors. Each ablation produces a hyperechoic region surrounding the needle. Unlike RFA, MWA does not need to use a retractable tip that results in a tendency to be more elliptical and requires more courses of treatment for larger tumors. On the other hand, treatment sessions are usually shorter than that for RFA because an ablation is produced in 60 seconds with microwave therapy [23].

Currently, MWA is performed usually using a cooling shaft system that produces a maximum power of 100 W at 2450 MHz [24], while the conventional setting for ablation is 60–100 W output power, 120–300 seconds. If the hyperechoic microbubbles produced by heat do not completely cover the entire tumor, extended microwave emission is required until the desired ablative range is reached. After MWA treatment, needle burning is needed to prevent tracking of tumor cells [12, 15, 25].

Survival Outcomes after RFA for ICC

In previous studies, the technical success rate (i.e., complete ablation without local progression for at least 1 month) defined by the Interventional Radiology Reporting Standard [26] has been reported to be between 80% and 100% in ICC. However, local tumor progression rate after RFA was relatively high, which was reported to range from 8% to 50% [27–33], and the pooled rate in a meta-analysis was reported to be 21% (95% confidence interval [CI], 13–30%) [34]. The incidence of major complications observed after RFA was reported to be between 3.9% and 27% [14, 19, 29–32, 35].

In a meta-analysis on RFA for ICC, the pooled 1-, 3-, and 5-year survival rates were 82% (95% CI, 72–90%), 47% (28–65%) and 24% (11–40%), respectively. These results were comparable to the outcomes recently estimated using the SEER database [26, 34]. Amini et al. reported that in a review of 1232 patients who were selected from the SEER database, only 64 (5.2%) patients underwent ablative therapy alone. Interestingly, they noted that the median survival of patients who were treated with ablation therapy was 20 months, which was worse than the outcomes of patients who were treated with resection but better than the outcomes following radiation therapy alone [26]. A review from Shindoh et al. reported that although the outcomes mentioned above were likely to be influenced by the differences in the baseline characteristics of the patients in each group, RFA might confer a modest survival advantage compared with other nonsurgical treatment options [36].

More recently, an original article reported by Takahashi et al. demonstrated that the median overall survival after ICC ablation was 23.6 months (range: 7.4–122.5 months), and the estimated 1-, 3-, and 5-year survival rates were 95% (95% CI: 86–100%), 40% (21–76%) and 32% (15–70%), respectively. The median disease-free survival was 8.2 months (range: 1.1–70.4 months) [12]. Another study reported that an increased tumor stage was associated with worse outcomes following RFA. The use of RFA was associated with a significantly prolonged survival compared with no local therapy in patients with stage I disease (2.1 vs. 0.7 years, $P = 0.012$), whereas patients with stage IV disease demonstrated no survival benefit from RFA [11]. Of note, all patients who were diagnosed as having ICC from 2004 to 2015 in the National Cancer Database (NCDB) were analyzed in this article, and the tumor staging was according to the seventh edition of the American Joint Committee on Cancer (AJCC)/Union for International Cancer Control (UICC) staging system of ICC [37]. Figure 9.1 shows the features of an ICC tumor before and after ablation on contrast-enhanced magnetic resonance imaging (MRI).

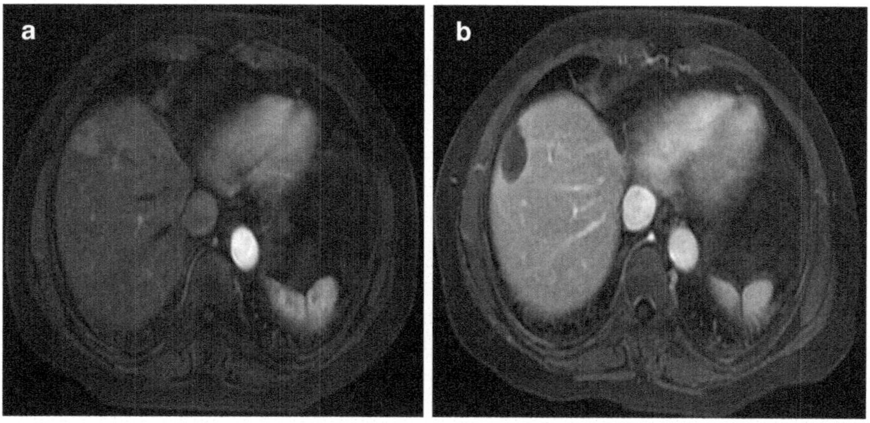

Fig. 9.1 A 59-year-old female patient who underwent left lateral lobectomy of the liver for a histopathologically proven ICC. Two years after the operation, a 1.6 cm recurrent lesion in the right lobe was identified by MRI (**a**). The nonenhancing area completely enveloped the ablated tumor at 2months after the ablation (**b**)

RFA Versus MWA in the Treatment of ICC

Compared with RFA, MWA may have several distinct advantages including less dependence on tissue conductivity, shorter ablation time, higher intratumoral temperature, and larger ablation area and homogeneity [35, 38, 39]. Up to now, only two original studies reported by Zhang et al. [15] and Yu et al. [25] have described the relatively detailed procedures and outcomes of MWA in ICC. There has been no report to compare the outcomes following RFA versus MWA within any independent study. The comparison of outcomes of these two procedures from 5 studies using either RFA or MWA for ICC is listed in Table 9.1.

Among these studies, a meta-analysis by Han et al. included 7 observational studies that comprised 84 ICC patients [27–33] through a comprehensive literature search on Ovid MEDLINE and EMBASE to identify the studies that reported data of overall survival, local tumor progression, and complications after RFA. The pooled 1-, 3-, and 5-year overall survival rates were 82% (95% CI: 72–90%), 47% (28–65%) and 24% (11–40%), respectively, as above-mentioned [34]. In an article by Zhang et al., a total of 107 patients with 171 ICC tumors (≤5 cm in size, tumor number≤3) underwent MWA. The median follow-up after MWA was 20.1 months (2.8–63.5 months). The median progression-free survival (PFS) after MWA was 8.9 months; and the PFS rates at 6, 12, 18, and 24 months after the treatment were 67.4%, 41.5%, 18.2%, and 8.7%, respectively. The median overall survival was

Table 9.1 Reported outcomes following RFA and MWA in ICC patients

Authors (country)	Treatment	Study design	*N*	Tumor size (cm)	Indication	OS (%)		
						1-year	3-year	5-year
Carrafiello, 2010 (Italy) [28]	RFA	Retrospective	6	1.0–5.8	Unresectable ICC	NA	–	–
Giorgio, 2011(Italy) [40]	RFA	Retrospective	10	2.4–5.5	Unresectable ICC	100	83	83
Han, 2015(South Korea) [34]	RFA	Meta-analysis	84	0.7–10	Unresectable/ recurrent ICC	82	47	24
Yu, 2011(China) [25]	MWA	Retrospective	15	1.3–9.9	Unresectable ICC	60	–	–
Zhang, 2018 (China) [15]	MWA	Retrospective	107	≤5	Unresectable/ recurrent ICC	93.5	39.6	7.9

RFA radiofrequency ablation, *MWA* microwave ablation; *N* number, *OS* overall survival, *NA* not available

28.0 months; and the overall survival rates at 1, 3, and 5 years after the treatment were 93.5%, 39.6%, and 7.9%, respectively [15]. In these two articles, the reported 1-year overall survival rate following RFA was lower than that after MWA, while RFA had a higher 3- and 5-year overall survival rates than MWA.

Complications Following Percutaneous Ablation

There are fewer reports on complications associated with percutaneous thermal ablation for ICC compared to HCC. In general, complications are classified as minor and major according to the clinical practice guidelines proposed by the Society of Interventional Radiology (SIR) [27]. Complications that require additional therapy, cause prolonged hospital stay, lead to permanent adverse sequelae, or result in death are evaluated as major complications. Others are considered as minor complications.

The following data are obtained by pooling 14 original studies about ICC [3, 12, 14, 15, 19, 27–33, 35, 40]. In 380 patients who were treated with percutaneous thermal ablation, major complications were registered in 5% (19/380) of patients. The mortality rate was 0.26% (1/380). Major complications included abdominal bleeding (1/380, 0.26%), needle-track cancer seeding (1/380, 0.26%), large biloma (2/380, 0.52%), biliary stricture (1/380, 0.26%), biliary fistula (1/380, 0.26%), pleural effusion with symptoms of dyspnea (3/380, 0.79%), hepatic failure (1/380, 0.26%), and liver abscess (9/380, 2.37%). One patient died of hepatic sepsis at 3.3 months after ablation despite percutaneous drainage and antibiotic therapy [29].

The minor complications included asymptomatic pleural effusion, mild bile duct dilation with or without jaundice, gallbladder wall thickening, a small amount of pleural effusion around the ablated area, small hematomas, minimal to moderate pain and fever, and increase in aminotransaminases. All minor complications resolved with conservative treatment. However, since the reported overall incidence of complications following ablation is low, percutaneous thermal ablation is generally considered safe for patients with ICC.

Ablation Versus Surgical Resection for ICC

Surgical resection is considered the first-line treatment for patients with localized ICC. The goals of surgery include achieving a margin-negative hepatic resection and performing a porta hepatis lymphadenectomy. However, the majority of patients present with advanced disease at diagnosis, and only about 30% of patients may be eligible for liver resection [41]. Surgical resection has been reported to provide a 5-year overall survival of 22–60% depending on specific clinicopathologic criteria [3, 4]. However, tumor recurrence rates after resection are high, ranging between 44% and 70% at 5 years after surgery [42, 43].

In most previous studies, the outcomes following ablative therapies were mainly investigated among patients who had unresectable ICC or recurrent ICC after initial surgery [3, 12, 14, 15, 19, 23, 27–35, 40, 44]. Prognostic factors associated with ablation treatment included tumor size, nodal invasion, and tumor differentiation. Given the different indications for treatment among patients receiving surgery or ablation, it is difficult to directly compare their long-term outcomes. There is only one original article, which has compared the outcomes of repeat hepatic resection versus thermal ablation for recurrent ICC [14]. Median survival time after repeated hepatic resection and thermal ablation therapy was 20.3 and 21.3 months, respectively. The 1-, 2-, and 3-year overall survival rates were 83.8%, 38.0% and 17.1% after repeated hepatic resection, and 69.8%, 37.3% and 20.5% after thermal ablation therapy (Table 9.2). Overall survival rates did not differ significantly between the two groups ($p = 0.996$), especially in patients with tumors less than 3 cm in size [14], suggesting that although

Table 9.2 Reported outcomes following RFA and surgical resection in ICC patients

Authors (country)	Treatment	*N*	Tumor size (cm)	3-year OS (%)	5-year OS (%)
Zhang, 2013(China) [14]	RFA + MWA	77	≤5	25	NA
	Repeated HR	32	≤5	17	NA
Wang, 2013 (China) [51]	HR	367	5.5	41	35
Saiura, 2011 (Japan) [52]	HR	44	5.7	56	43
Saxena, 2010 (Australia) [53]	HR	40	6.5	48	28
Zhang, 2018(China) [15]	MWA	107	≤5	39.6	7.9
Kim, 2011(South Korea) [29]	RFA	13	0.8–8.0	51	15
Xu, 2012(China) [19]	RFA + MWA	18	1.4–6.9	30	30

HR hepatic resection, *RFA* radiofrequency ablation, *MWA* microwave ablation, *N* number, *OS* overall survival *NA* not available ablation might be effective in selected patients with recurrent ICC, its indication should be limited according to tumor size [40].

Tumor size is an important factor associated with the therapeutic outcomes of ablation. The length of hospital stay, treatment cost, and risk of complications tend to be less with ablation than with hepatic resection. The incidence of major complications is also higher for hepatectomy compared to thermal ablation (46.9% vs. 3.9%) [14]. Post-ablation mortality is rare, whereas the perioperative mortality rates following resection of ICC range from 1.2% to over 7% [4, 45, 46]. Other studies have suggested that the overall survival rate after ablation for ICC is significantly higher compared to conservative treatments and comparable to that after radical resection in well-selected patients [47–50]. These results suggest that ablation may represent a less invasive alternative to surgical resection and is safe and effective for patients with recurrent ICC. While additional research is needed, ablation therapy may be considered a first-line treatment for selected patients with small recurrent ICC.

An important limitation of ablative techniques is the omission of regional, lymph node dissection. While not routinely performed for HCC, lymphadenectomy is an important component of accurate staging and locoregional control for patients with ICC. While less important for patients with recurrent ICC, the inability to perform lymph node evaluation limits the current application of percutaneous ablation to patients with otherwise resectable de novo ICC.

Combined Therapy

Because of the advanced stage at which most patients with ICC present, only a small proportion are suitable for radical surgical resection or complete therapeutic ablation. Combined multimodality therapy is an alternative approach to overcome some of these limitations. Unlike HCC, ICC has poor vascularity with a fibrotic characteristic, which leads to a limited survival benefit following transarterial chemoembolization (TACE) [54]. On the other hand, percutaneous thermal ablation in combination with TACE may provide improved outcomes. TACE can effectively decrease heat dispersion during thermal ablation by occluding bloodstream and consequently promote tumor ruin [55]. Meanwhile, thermal ablation may decrease the required chemotherapy dose of TACE and accordingly lessen side reaction and may also expand the ablation area and prolong progression-free survival. A study on microwave ablation combined with TACE for ICC demonstrated improved results compared to either TACE or ablation alone [56, 57].

Satellite lesions are often present in patients with ICC, which may preclude the ability to perform radical resection. Local thermal ablation combined with surgical resection is an option for patients with initially unresectable ICC. Although there is no sufficient data about ICC specifically, several studies in HCC have reported encouraging results. In a study by Choi et al., 53 patients with multifocal HCC received combined intraoperative RFA with hepatic resection. The cumulative survival rates at 1, 2,

3, 4, and 5 years were 87%, 83%, 80%, 68%, and 55%, respectively. Patients with smaller resected tumors (≤5 cm) demonstrated better survival results compared with those with larger tumor ($P = 0.004$). No procedure-related deaths occurred. They reported hepatectomy-related complications in 4 patients (4/53, 8%) and RFA-related complication only in 1 patient (1/53, 2%) [58]. However, current data on multimodality treatment in ICC, particularly percutaneous thermal ablation combined with surgical resection or other locoregional treatments are still lacking.

In clinical practice, patients with recurrent, metastatic, or unresectable ICC are often treated with systemic chemotherapy first. This approach prioritizes early systemic therapy for biologically aggressive cancer, ensures the absence of rapidly progressive disease, and potentially downsizes liver disease enabling the use of locoregional treatments. Percutaneous ablation, like other locoregional therapies, is most often considered in these patients who have demonstrated favorable tumor biology in order to optimize locoregional control and facilitate chemotherapy-free time.

Summary

Although percutaneous thermal ablation for ICC has been shown to have several distinct advantages, such as minimally invasiveness, easy to perform, repeatability, and cost-effectiveness [19], data for its efficacy remain limited [11]. Indeed, while the indications for ablation in HCC are well established (solitary lesion ≤5 cm, or no more than 3 lesions and each ≤3 cm), there remain no formal guidelines for the indications for percutaneous thermal ablation of ICC.

Based on the outcomes of retrospective data, percutaneous ablation appears safe and associated with acceptable locoregional control and survival outcomes for patients with recurrent or unresectable ICC. While ablation may be appropriate for some select patients with early stage disease, the inability to perform regional lymph node dissection prevents the wider adoption of ablation for patients with otherwise resectable disease. Although more high-quality data are needed, including prospective multicenter trials, percutaneous ablation is an important component of the multimodality treatment of patients with ICC, particularly at high-volume centers equipped with experienced multidisciplinary teams.

References

1. Lubezky N, Facciuto M, Harimoto N, Schwartz ME, Florman SS. Surgical treatment of intrahepatic cholangiocarcinoma in the USA. J Hepatobiliary Pancreat Sci. 2015;22(2):124–30.
2. Patel T. Increasing incidence and mortality of primary intrahepatic cholangiocarcinoma in the United States. Hepatology. 2001;33(6):1353–7.
3. Kamphues C, Seehofer D, Eisele RM, Denecke T, Pratschke J, Neumann UP, et al. Recurrent intrahepatic cholangiocarcinoma: single-center experience using repeated hepatectomy and radiofrequency ablation. J Hepatobiliary Pancreat Sci. 2010;17(4):509–15.

4. Endo I, Gonen M, Yopp AC, Dalal KM, Zhou Q, Klimstra D, et al. Intrahepatic cholangiocarcinoma: rising frequency, improved survival, and determinants of outcome after resection. Ann Surg. 2008;248(1):84–96.
5. Aljiffry M, Abdulelah A, Walsh M, Peltekian K, Alwayn I, Molinari M. Evidence-based approach to cholangiocarcinoma: a systematic review of the current literature. J Am Coll Surg. 2009;208(1):134–47.
6. Blechacz B, Gores GJ. Cholangiocarcinoma: advances in pathogenesis, diagnosis, and treatment. Hepatology. 2008;48(1):308–21.
7. McGahan JP, Browning PD, Brock JM, Tesluk H. Hepatic ablation using radiofrequency electrocautery. Investig Radiol. 1990;25(3):267–70.
8. Rossi S, Fornari F, Pathies C, Buscarini L. Thermal lesions induced by 480 KHz localized current field in Guinea pig and pig liver. Tumori. 1990;76(1):54–7.
9. Lau WY, Lai EC. The current role of radiofrequency ablation in the management of hepatocellular carcinoma: a systematic review. Ann Surg. 2009;249(1):20–5.
10. Widmann G, Schullian P, Haidu M, Bale R. Stereotactic radiofrequency ablation (SRFA) of liver lesions: technique effectiveness, safety, and interoperator performance. Cardiovasc Intervent Radiol. 2012;35(3):570–80.
11. Kolarich AR, Shah JL, George TJ Jr, Hughes SJ, Shaw CM, Geller BS, et al. Non-surgical management of patients with intrahepatic cholangiocarcinoma in the United States, 2004–2015: an NCDB analysis. J Gastrointest Oncol. 2018;9(3):536–45.
12. Takahashi EA, Kinsman KA, Schmit GD, Atwell TD, Schmitz JJ, Welch BT, et al. Thermal ablation of intrahepatic cholangiocarcinoma: safety, efficacy, and factors affecting local tumor progression. Abdom Radiol. 2018;43(12):3487–92.
13. Xu Y, Shen Q, Liu P, Xu Z, Wu P, Lu Z, et al. Microwave ablation for the treatment of hepatocellular carcinoma that met up-to-seven criteria: feasibility, local efficacy, and long-term outcomes. Abdom Radiol. 2017;27(9):3877–87.
14. Zhang SJ, Hu P, Wang N, Shen Q, Sun AX, Kuang M, et al. Thermal ablation versus repeated hepatic resection for recurrent intrahepatic cholangiocarcinoma. Ann Surg Oncol. 2013;20(11):3596–602.
15. Zhang K, Yu J, Yu X, Han Z, Cheng Z, Liu F, et al. Clinical and survival outcomes of percutaneous microwave ablation for intrahepatic cholangiocarcinoma. Int J Hyperth. 2018;34(3):292–7.
16. Dodd GD 3rd, Soulen MC, Kane RA, Livraghi T, Lees WR, Yamashita Y, et al. Minimally invasive treatment of malignant hepatic tumors: at the threshold of a major breakthrough. Radiographics. 2000;20(1):9–27.
17. Cline HE, Hynynen K, Watkins RD, Adams WJ, Schenck JF, Ettinger RH, et al. Focused US system for MR imaging-guided tumor ablation. Radiology. 1995;194(3):731–7.
18. Pennes HH. Analysis of tissue and arterial blood temperatures in the resting human forearm. J Appl Physiol. 1948;1(2):93–122.
19. Xu HX, Wang Y, Lu MD, Liu LN. Percutaneous ultrasound-guided thermal ablation for intrahepatic cholangiocarcinoma. Br J Radiol. 2012;85(1016):1078–84.
20. Lin SM. Recent advances in radiofrequency ablation in the treatment of hepatocellular carcinoma and metastatic liver cancers. Chang Gung Med J. 2009;32(1):22–32.
21. Hansler J, Frieser M, Tietz V, Uhlke D, Wissniowski TT, Bernatik T, et al. Percutaneous ultrasound-guided radiofrequency ablation (RFA) using saline-perfused (wet) needle electrodes for the treatment of hepatocellular carcinoma–long-term experience. Ultraschall Med. 2007;28(6):604–11.
22. Plasencia Martinez JM. Pulmonary radiofrequency ablation (Part 1): current state. Radiologia. 2015;57(4):275–86.
23. Liang P, Wang Y, Yu X, Dong B. Malignant liver tumors: treatment with percutaneous microwave ablation–complications among cohort of 1136 patients. Radiology. 2009;251(3):933–40.
24. Kuang M, Lu MD, Xie XY, Xu HX, Mo LQ, Liu GJ, et al. Liver cancer: increased microwave delivery to ablation zone with cooled-shaft antenna–experimental and clinical studies. Radiology. 2007;242(3):914–24.

25. Yu J, Liang P, Yu X, Liu F, Chen L, Wang Y. A comparison of microwave ablation and bipolar radiofrequency ablation both with an internally cooled probe: results in ex vivo and in vivo porcine livers. Eur J Radiol. 2011;79(1):124–30.
26. Goldberg SN, Grassi CJ, Cardella JF, Charboneau JW, Dodd GD 3rd, Dupuy DE, et al. Image-guided tumor ablation: standardization of terminology and reporting criteria. J Vasc Interv Radiol. 2009;20(7 Suppl):S377–90.
27. Chiou YY, Hwang JI, Chou YH, Wang HK, Chiang JH, Chang CY. Percutaneous ultrasound-guided radiofrequency ablation of intrahepatic cholangiocarcinoma. Kaohsiung J Med Sci. 2005;21(7):304–9.
28. Carrafiello G, Lagana D, Cotta E, Mangini M, Fontana F, Bandiera F, et al. Radiofrequency ablation of intrahepatic cholangiocarcinoma: preliminary experience. Cardiovasc Intervent Radiol. 2010;33(4):835–9.
29. Kim JH, Won HJ, Shin YM, Kim KA, Kim PN. Radiofrequency ablation for the treatment of primary intrahepatic cholangiocarcinoma. AJR Am J Roentgenol. 2011;196(2):W205–9.
30. Kim JH, Won HJ, Shin YM, Kim PN, Lee SG, Hwang S. Radiofrequency ablation for recurrent intrahepatic cholangiocarcinoma after curative resection. Eur J Radiol. 2011;80(3):e221–5.
31. Fu Y, Yang W, Wu W, Yan K, Xing BC, Chen MH. Radiofrequency ablation in the management of unresectable intrahepatic cholangiocarcinoma. AJR Am J Roentgenol. 2012;23(5):642–9.
32. Haidu M, Dobrozemsky G, Schullian P, Widmann G, Klaus A, Weiss H, et al. Stereotactic radiofrequency ablation of unresectable intrahepatic cholangiocarcinomas: a retrospective study. Cardiovasc Intervent Radiol. 2012;35(5):1074–82.
33. Butros SR, Shenoy-Bhangle A, Mueller PR, Arellano RS. Radiofrequency ablation of intrahepatic cholangiocarcinoma: feasability, local tumor control, and long-term outcome. Clin Imaging. 2014;38(4):490–4.
34. Han K, Ko HK, Kim KW, Won HJ, Shin YM, Kim PN. Radiofrequency ablation in the treatment of unresectable intrahepatic cholangiocarcinoma: systematic review and meta-analysis. J Vasc Interv Radiol. 2015;26(7):943–8.
35. Yu MA, Liang P, Yu XL, Cheng ZG, Han ZY, Liu FY, et al. Sonography-guided percutaneous microwave ablation of intrahepatic primary cholangiocarcinoma. Eur J Radiol. 2011;80(2):548–52.
36. Giorgio A, Gatti P, Matteucci P, Giorgio V. Ablative therapies for intrahepatic cholangiocarcinoma. Hepatobiliary Surg Nutr. 2018;7(3):192–4.. 37
37. Farges O, Fuks D, Le Treut YP, Azoulay D, Laurent A, Bachellier P, et al. AJCC 7th edition of TNM staging accurately discriminates outcomes of patients with resectable intrahepatic cholangiocarcinoma. Cancer. 2011;117(10):2170–7.
38. Wright AS, Sampson LA, Warner TF, Mahvi DM, Lee FT Jr. Radiofrequency versus microwave ablation in a hepatic porcine model. Radiology. 2005;236(1):132–9.
39. Vroomen L, Petre EN, Cornelis FH, Solomon SB, Srimathveeravalli G. Irreversible electroporation and thermal ablation of tumors in the liver, lung, kidney, and bone: what are the differences? Diagn Interv Imaging. 2017;98(9):609–17.
40. Giorgio A, Calisti G, DE Stefano G, Farella N, DI Sarno A, Amendola F, et al. Radiofrequency ablation for intrahepatic cholangiocarcinoma: retrospective analysis of a single-center experience. Anticancer Res. 2011;31(12):4575–80.
41. Park HM, Yun SP, Lee EC, Lee SD, Han SS, Kim SH, et al. Outcomes for patients with recurrent intrahepatic cholangiocarcinoma after surgery. Ann Surg Oncol. 2016;23(13):4392–400.
42. Ercolani G, Vetrone G, Grazi GL, Aramaki O, Cescon M, Ravaioli M, et al. Intrahepatic cholangiocarcinoma: primary liver resection and aggressive multimodal treatment of recurrence significantly prolong survival. Ann Surg. 2010;252(1):107–14.
43. Hyder O, Hatzaras I, Sotiropoulos GC, Paul A, Alexandrescu S, Marques H, et al. Recurrence after operative management of intrahepatic cholangiocarcinoma. Surgery. 2013;153(6):811–8.
44. Joo I, Lee JM, Yoon JH. Imaging diagnosis of intrahepatic and Perihilar cholangiocarcinoma: recent advances and challenges. Radiology. 2018;288(1):7–13.

45. Lang H, Sotiropoulos GC, Sgourakis G, Schmitz KJ, Paul A, Hilgard P, et al. Operations for intrahepatic cholangiocarcinoma: single-institution experience of 158 patients. J Am Coll Surg. 2009;208(2):218–28.
46. Jonas S, Thelen A, Benckert C, Biskup W, Neumann U, Rudolph B, et al. Extended liver resection for intrahepatic cholangiocarcinoma: a comparison of the prognostic accuracy of the fifth and sixth editions of the TNM classification. Ann Surg. 2009;249(2):303–9.
47. Wu ZF, Wu XY, Zhu N, Xu Z, Li WS, Zhang HB, et al. Prognosis after resection for hepatitis B virus-associated intrahepatic cholangiocarcinoma. World J Gastroenterol. 2015;21(3):935–43.
48. Jutric Z, Johnston WC, Hoen HM, Newell PH, Cassera MA, Hammill CW, et al. Impact of lymph node status in patients with intrahepatic cholangiocarcinoma treated by major hepatectomy: a review of the National Cancer Database. HPB. 2016;18(1):79–87.
49. Spolverato G, Yakoob MY, Kim Y, Alexandrescu S, Marques HP, Lamelas J, et al. The impact of surgical margin status on long-term outcome after resection for intrahepatic cholangiocarcinoma. Ann Surg Oncol. 2015;22(12):4020–8.
50. Park J, Kim MH, Kim KP, Park DH, Moon SH, Song TJ, et al. Natural history and prognostic factors of advanced cholangiocarcinoma without surgery, chemotherapy, or radiotherapy: a large-scale observational study. Gut Liver. 2009;3(4):298–305.
51. Wang Y, Li J, Xia Y, Gong R, Wang K, Yan Z, et al. Prognostic nomogram for intrahepatic cholangiocarcinoma after partial hepatectomy. J Clin Oncol. 2013;31(9):1188–95.
52. Saiura A, Yamamoto J, Kokudo N, Koga R, Seki M, Hiki N, et al. Intrahepatic cholangiocarcinoma: analysis of 44 consecutive resected cases including 5 cases with repeat resections. Am J Surg. 2011;201(2):203–8.
53. Saxena A, Chua TC, Sarkar A, Chu F, Morris DL. Clinicopathologic and treatment-related factors influencing recurrence and survival after hepatic resection of intrahepatic cholangiocarcinoma: a 19-year experience from an established Australian hepatobiliary unit. J Gastrointest Surg. 2010;14(7):1128–38.
54. Kim JH, Yoon HK, Sung KB, Ko GY, Gwon DI, Shin JH, et al. Transcatheter arterial chemoembolization or chemoinfusion for unresectable intrahepatic cholangiocarcinoma: clinical efficacy and factors influencing outcomes. Cancer. 2008;113(7):1614–22.
55. Seki T, Tamai T, Nakagawa T, Imamura M, Nishimura A, Yamashiki N, et al. Combination therapy with transcatheter arterial chemoembolization and percutaneous microwave coagulation therapy for hepatocellular carcinoma. Cancer. 2000;89(6):1245–51.
56. Yang GW, Zhao Q, Qian S, Zhu L, Qu XD, Zhang W, et al. Percutaneous microwave ablation combined with simultaneous transarterial chemoembolization for the treatment of advanced intrahepatic cholangiocarcinoma. Onco Targets Ther. 2015;8:1245–50.
57. Zhao Q, Qian S, Zhu L, Qu XD, Zhang W, Yan ZP, et al. Transcatheter arterial chemoembolization with gemcitabine and oxaliplatin for the treatment of advanced biliary tract cancer. Onco Targets Ther. 2015;8:595–600.
58. Choi D, Lim HK, Joh JW, Kim SJ, Kim MJ, Rhim H, et al. Combined hepatectomy and radiofrequency ablation for multifocal hepatocellular carcinomas: long-term follow-up results and prognostic factors. Ann Surg Oncol. 2007;14(12):3510–8.

Chapter 10
Transarterial Therapies

Susan Shamimi-Noori and Michael C. Soulen

Background

Intrahepatic cholangiocarcinoma (ICC) is the second most common primary hepatic malignancy. The incidence of ICC and associated mortality rates are rising [1, 2]. ICC is rapidly fatal with a median overall survival (OS) of <4 months without treatment [3]. The highest survival rates are observed among patients who undergo surgical resection, which increases the 5-year survival from approximately 10% to 20–40% [4]. However, only 20–40% of patients with ICC are surgical candidates [5].

Palliative systemic therapy with gemcitabine and cisplatin has become the standard of care first-line treatment based on two phase III trials of 493 patients with locally advanced (25%) or metastatic (75%) cholangiocarcinoma from intrahepatic (n = 108, 22%) extrahepatic (n = 149, 30%) gallbladder (n = 181, 37%) or ampullary (n = 24, 5%) primaries received either intravenous cisplatin followed by gemcitabine or gemcitabine alone. The median overall survival in the combination therapy group was 11.6 months compared to 8 months in the gemcitabine only group (HR 0.65, 95% CI0.54 to 0.78, $P < 0.001$). The median progression-free survival was also higher in the combination therapy group (8.8 months vs. 6.7 months, HR 0.64, 95% CI 0.54–0.78, $P < 0.001$) [6].

S. Shamimi-Noori (✉)
Division of Interventional Radiology, Department of Radiology, Hospital of the University of Pennsylvania, Philadelphia, PA, USA
e-mail: Susan.Shamimi-Noori@uphs.upenn.edu

M. C. Soulen
Division of Interventional Radiology, Department of Radiology, Hospital of the University of Pennsylvania, Philadelphia, PA, USA

Department of Radiology, Abramson Cancer Center, University of Pennsylvania, Philadelphia, PA, USA
e-mail: michael.soulen@uphs.upenn.edu

T. M. Pawlik et al. (eds.), *Intrahepatic Cholangiocarcinoma*,
https://doi.org/10.1007/978-3-030-22258-1_10

Locoregional therapy has shown promising results for the treatment of ICC in patients who are not surgical candidates. While percutaneous ablation may have a role in the treatment of patients with small tumors, its efficacy in larger tumors is less clear. Transarterial therapies have been shown to be safe and effective in the treatment of a variety of primary and secondary hepatic malignancies [7–14]. Due to the rarity of ICC, the available data on locoregional therapies is limited, based only on small retrospective studies [15, 16]. Therefore, the purpose of this chapter is to discuss the technical aspects of transarterial therapies, provide an overview of the available literature supporting their use, and discuss triaging patients among the available transarterial therapies.

Transarterial Therapy

While transarterial therapies can be used in a neoadjuvant approach to facilitate downstaging [17, 18], the more common goal of treatment is to provide locoregional control and potentially prolong overall survival (OS), especially when combined with effective systemic chemotherapy. Similar OS is observed among patients with and without the extrahepatic disease, and the major cause of mortality from ICC is liver failure or biliary compromise [19–21]. To that end, although high-quality evidence is lacking, effective locoregional treatments including transarterial therapies may improve both the quantity and quality of life through the prevention of local complications and reducing the burden of active disease.

The technical goal of transarterial therapy is to deliver concentrated antitumor therapy to hepatic tumors with sparing of surrounding liver parenchyma and with low systemic toxicity. Due to the dual blood supply of the liver, patients can undergo selective transarterial treatments with low complication rates. More recently, selective transarterial treatments have been shown to be safe even in select patients with portal vein thrombosis [21, 22]. Commonly used transarterial hepatic treatments for ICC include lipiodol-based chemoembolization, drug-eluting bead chemoembolization, and radioembolization.

Lipiodol-based chemoembolization, also known as conventional chemoembolization (cTACE), was described as early as 1980 for the treatment of hepatocellular carcinoma [23]. One or more chemotherapeutic agents are emulsified into an oil-based contrast and injected into the tumor arterial bed. While there is no standardized chemotherapeutic agent combination for chemoembolization of cholangiocarcinoma, a combination of doxorubicin, mitomycin-C, and cisplatin (if available) is commonly used. Gentamicin has also been used [24]. The oil-based emulsion penetrates the tumor capillary bed maintaining a high concentration of intratumoral chemotherapy [25]. Injection of the emulsion is followed by injection of a particulate agent such as gelatin sponge, polyvinyl alcohol, or trisacryl gelatin microspheres. These particles devascularize the tumor resulting in ischemia as well as preventing washout of the previously injected chemotherapeutic emulsion [26, 27].

The most common toxicity of lipiodol-based chemoembolization is post-embolization syndrome manifested by post-procedure pain, fevers, nausea, and vomiting. Symptoms are usually mild and patients are often discharged home within 24 hours of treatment. Post-embolization syndrome is manageable with oral anti-nausea and pain medications. The rate of post-embolization syndrome after chemoembolization has been reported between 30% and 65% [9, 20].

Emulsions can be unstable resulting in some systemic release of chemotherapy. Drug-eluting bead (DEB) chemoembolization (DEB-TACE) was developed with the aim of further limiting the systemic release of chemotherapy [28]. DEBs are microspheres loaded with chemotherapeutic agents. These beads are then injected into the hepatic tumor arterial supply. DEBs have treatment effect via two mechanisms: embolization and local controlled release of the chemotherapeutic agents. There are multiple DEBs in clinical use which can be loaded with a variety of chemotherapeutic agents, the most common of which are doxorubicin and irinotecan [26]. Lammer et al. have shown an improved systemic toxicity profile of DEB-TACE compared to cTACE. While DEB-TACE has been shown to be safe and effective for both primary and secondary liver cancers, a survival benefit over cTACE has not been demonstrated [29].

Transarterial radioembolization (TARE) of hepatic tumors was first described in the 1960s, however, its use has been further developed over the last two decades [30, 31]. This form of selective internal radiation therapy is delivered by intra-arterial injection of microspheres containing Yttrium-90, a radionuclide emitting beta radiation. While the radiosensitivity of hepatic tissue limits the ability to administer significant doses of external beam radiation, TARE allows tumoricidal radiation doses to be given with less radiation-induced injury to the surrounding liver [32]. There is also some embolic effect of the Yttrium-90 labeled microspheres; however, the main therapeutic mechanism is through radiation-induced cell death. Both resin and glass-based Yttrium-90 microspheres have been developed. Resin microspheres are granted full premarketing Food and Drug Administration approval for the treatment of colorectal metastases in conjunction with intrahepatic chemotherapy. Glass microspheres are approved by the Food and Drug Administration under a humanitarian device exemption for the treatment of unresectable hepatocellular carcinoma with and without portal vein occlusion in patients who can have appropriately positioned hepatic arterial catheters, and therefore, the use of glass microspheres currently requires institutional review board oversight in the United States [33]. Off-label use of both resin and glass microspheres has been studied in a variety of primary and secondary liver cancers. Fatigue is the most common adverse event of transarterial radioembolization and occurs in over half of patients [9].

Similar selection and exclusion criteria have been developed for all transarterial therapies. The purpose of stringent exclusion criteria is to reduce the risk of liver decompensation and other complications following treatment. Patient performance status (Eastern Cooperative Oncology Group (ECOG) score ≤ 2) and liver function reserve must be adequate. A serum total bilirubin level >3 is considered a contraindication to transarterial hepatic therapy. Patients with portal vein thrombosis and/or serum total bilirubin levels between 2 and 3 should be considered for selective sublobar or subsegmental arterial delivery of therapy. Caution is also advised in treatment of patients with a Child-Pugh B score greater than 8 or those with tumor occupying >50–70% of the total liver volume. Technical considerations such as the presence of large arterioportal or arteriovenous shunting, renal insufficiency and other confounding comorbidities should also be taken into account. With regards specifically toTARE, radiation exposure to adjacent organs (e.g., heart, lungs, etc.) and prior radiation therapies can limit the total dose administered. Planning hepatic arteriography, arterial infusion of technetium-99m micro-aggregated albumin, and subsequent lung and liver scintigraphy are performed as a separate procedure prior to radioembolization to evaluate for any dosimetric or anatomic contraindications and to calculate the appropriate treatment dose [34].

Evidence for Conventional Transarterial Chemoembolization (cTACE)

A large retrospective study of patients with unresectable ICC comparing cTACE using cisplatin (72 patients) to best supportive treatment (83 patients) showed a median overall survival of 12.2 months in the chemoembolization group compared to 3.3 months in the supportive care group. A statistically significant improvement in survival was observed both in patients with and without extrahepatic disease [35].

A retrospective multi-center series of 62 patients evaluated survival aftercTACE with triple chemotherapy (mitomycin-C, doxorubicin, cisplatin) in patients with either ICC or poorly differentiated adenocarcinoma. Median overall survival was 15 months from initial chemoembolization and 20 months from initial diagnosis. There was no statistically significant survival difference between patients with ICC and patients with poorly differentiated adenocarcinoma of unknown primary. Median OS was higher in patients who also received systemic chemotherapy compared to those who did not: 28 months vs. 16 months (HR 1.94, 95%CI 1.13–3.33, $p = 0.02$). Patients with extrahepatic disease had a lower median overall survival compared to those without extrahepatic disease; however, this was not statistically significant. Post-embolization syndrome occurred in 65% of patients and major complication rate was reported at 3% [20].

Promising results were seen in another retrospective case series of 17 patients with unresectable cholangiocarcinoma treated with cTACE using a triple chemotherapy regimen of mitomycin-C, doxorubicin, and cisplatin. Median OS from time of diagnosis was 23 months. Two out of 17 patients with previously unresectable disease underwent successful resection after chemoembolization. There was 1 major complication (6%) and 2 minor complications (12%) [36].

Vogl et al. sought to evaluate OS and local tumor control endpoints in patients with unresectable cholangiocarcinoma treated with cTACE using various chemotherapeutic agents. In this study of 115 patients, chemotherapeutic regimens used in a lipiodol-based emulsion included mitomycin-C alone (24 patients), gemcitabine alone (8 patients), mitomycin-C combined with gemcitabine (54 patients), and the combination of mitomycin-C, gemcitabine, and cisplatin (29 patients). No statistically significant difference was found among the different chemotherapy regimens and median OS for the entire group was 13 months. Using RECIST criteria, 8.7% of patients showed partial response, 57.4% showed stable disease, and 33.9% showed progressive disease at follow up. No major complications were reported and the rate of post-embolization syndrome was 13% [37].

Gemcitabine-based cTACE was retrospectively studied by Gusani et al. In this 42-patient study, median OS was 9.1 months from time of first treatment 45% of the patients had extrahepatic disease. Per RECIST criteria, stable disease was seen in 48% of patients and progressive disease in 15% of patients. Tumor response in 7 patients was not evaluable. Grade 3 or higher adverse events were reported in 7 patients (16.6%). It was also noted that the median OS was statistically higher in patients treated with gemcitabine-cisplatin and TACE compared to gemcitabine alone (13.8 months vs. 6.3 months, $p = 0.0005$) [38].

Herber et al. showed that cTACE can be effective in patients with large tumors. In a retrospective study of 15 patients with a mean tumor size of 10.8 ± 4.6 cm (range 2–18 cm), median OS was 16.3 months after cTACE using mitomycin-C as a single chemotherapeutic agent. According to RECIST criteria, 60% of patients showed stable disease, 6.7% of patients showed partial response, and 26.7% of patients showed progressive disease. There were two major complications. No deaths or acute liver failure was reported. Forty percent of patients experienced post-embolization syndrome [39].

Although the literature is limited to small prospective and retrospective case series, data shows that cTACE is safe and effective in the treatment of unresectable ICC. The most common adverse event is self-limited post-embolic syndrome. Median OS after conventional chemoembolization is promising with data suggesting improved outcomes compared to reported rates of systemic chemotherapy alone. Evidence for the use of cTACE in treatment of ICC is summarized in Table 10.1.

Evidence for Drug-Eluting Bead Transarterial Chemoembolization (DEB-TACE)

A prospective multi-institutional study of 24 patients with unresectable ICC showed a similar median OS among those treated with DEB-TACE versus cTACE. Median survival was reported at 17.5 months from date of diagnosis.41.7% of patients had extrahepatic disease. A total of 42 treatments were performed, the majority of which used irinotecan-loaded beads. Seven treatments used doxorubicin-loaded beads. Three patients (12.5%) underwent subsequent surgical resection. According to RECIST criteria, at 3 months, 20 patients (83%) showed stable disease and 2 patients (8%) showed either complete or partial response. The major complication

Table 10.1 Series reporting outcomes of cTACE for intrahepatic cholangiocarcinoma

Investigators (year)	Study design	Anticancer agents	# of patients in treatment group	Extrahepatic lesions	Previous systemic therapy	# of adverse events (grade ≥ 3)	Median OS	Reference #
Vogl et al. (2012)	Prospective	Mitomycin-based (± cisplatin, ± gemcitabine)	115	Excluded	–	0	13 months from initial cTACE	[37]
Park et al. (2011)	Retrospective	Cisplatin	72	$n = 39$ (54%)	Excluded	26	12.2 months from diagnosis	[35]
Kiefer et al. (2011)	Retrospective	Mitomycin-C, doxorubicin, cisplatin	62	$n = 19$ (31%)	$n = 18$ (29%)	5	15 months from initial cTACE, 20 months from diagnosis	[20]
Gusani et al. (2008)	Retrospective	Gemcitabine-based (± cisplatin, ± oxaliplatin)	42	$n = 19$(45%)	–	7	9.1 months from initial cTACE	[38]
Burger et al. (2005)	Retrospective	Mitomycin-C, doxorubicin, cisplatin	17	$n = 5$ (29%)	$n = 6$ (35%)	1	23 months from diagnosis	[36]
Herber et al. (2007)	Retrospective	Mitomycin-C	15	Excluded	$n = 4$ (27%)	2	16.3 months from initial cTACE	[39]

rate was reported at 9.5% and included hepatorenal syndrome resulting in death, sepsis attributed to a chest port infection, and liver failure which subsequently resolved [40].

Aliberti et al. prospectively evaluated 11 patients with unresectable ICC treated with DEB-TACE using doxorubicin-loaded beads. There was a 100% tumor response rate according to RECIST criteria and the median OS was reported as 13 months. All patients experienced symptoms of post embolic syndrome. One patient developed a hepatic abscess [41].

Another prospective study including 26 patients with unresectable ICC treated with DEB-TACE using irinotecan-eluting beads showed a similar median OS of 11.7 months. Forty-two percent of the patients had extrahepatic disease. Grade 3 or higher adverse events included post embolic syndrome, pleural empyema, liver abscess, and cholangitis, resulting in death. At 2 months, one patient had partial response according to RECIST criteria and was downstaged to surgery. Forty-two percent of patients had stable disease and 50% of patients had progressive disease [42].

The feasibility and safety of DEB-TACE using oxaliplatin-eluting beads in combination with systemic chemotherapy were retrospectively evaluated in 9 patients and compared to historical controls of patients treated with systemic chemotherapy alone. There was a significantly higher median OS in the DEB-TACE group (30 vs. 12.7 months; $p = 0.004$). At 3 months, 4 patients (44%) showed partial response and 5 patients (56%) showed stable disease according to RECIST criteria in the DEB-TACE group. All patients in the historical group showed progressive disease when reassessed between three and six cycles of treatment. Within the DEB-TACE group, no grade 4 adverse events were observed. Grade 3 adverse events included abdominal pain, cholangitis, and a hypertensive crisis [43]. Evidence for the use of DEB-TACE in treatment of ICC is summarized in Table 10.2.

Evidence for Transarterial Radioembolization (TARE)

Mouli et al. retrospectively reviewed 46 patients with ICC who received 92 radioembolization treatments at a single institution. Stratification occurred by performance status, solitary or multifocal tumors, tumor morphology (infiltrative or peripheral), and the presence/absence of portal vein thrombosis. Fatigue (54%), abdominal pain (28%), and nausea (13%) were the most common adverse events noted. Four patients developed grade 3 albumin toxicity, three patients developed grade 3 bilirubin toxicity, and one patient developed a gastroduodenal ulcer refractory to medical management. WHO imaging response was partial response in 11 patients (25%), stable disease in 33 patients (73%), and progressive disease in 1 patient (2%). EASL response was complete or partial response in 33 patients (73%) and stable disease in 12 patients (27%). Survival varied based on multiple patient and tumor characteristics. For example, the median OS was influenced by ECOG performance status (0, 1, and 2: 14.3 months, 7.2 months, and 9.9 months,

Table 10.2 Series reporting outcomes of DEB-TACE for intrahepatic cholangiocarcinoma

Investigators (year)	Study design	Anticancer agents	# of patients in treatment group	Extrahepatic lesions	Previous systemic therapy	# of adverse events (grade ≥ 3)	Median OS	Reference #
Kuhlmann et al. (2012)	Prospective	Irinotecan	26	$n = 11$ (42%)	$n = 5$ (19%)	11	11.7 months from initial DEB-TACE	[42]
Schiffman et al. (2011)	Prospective	Irinotecan (35 treatments); doxorubicin (7 treatments)	24	$n = 10$ (42%)	$n = 20$ (83%)	4	17.5 months from diagnosis	[40]
Aliberti et al. (2008)	Prospective	Doxorubicin	11	–	$n = 11$ (100%)	0	13 months unspecified time zero	[41]
Poggi et al. (2009)	Retrospective	Oxaliplatin DEB + systemic therapy	9	Excluded	$n = 9$ (100%)	11	30 months from initial DEB-TACE	[43]

respectively), tumor multifocality (solitary vs. multifocal: 14.6 months and 5.7 months, respectively), prior receipt of treatment (chemotherapy naïve vs. receipt of chemotherapy: 14.6 months and 5.7 months, respectively), absence of portal vein thrombosis (14.4 months and 5.3 months, respectively), tumor location (peripheral vs. infiltrative:15.6 months and 6.1 months, respectively), and disease burden (<25% vs. 25–50% liver involvement: 14.4 months vs. 5.3 months, respectively). Five patients were converted to resectable status [44].

In a prospective study of 25 patients with unresectable ICC treated with Y-90 resin microsphere TARE, the median OS was 9.3 months from first radioembolization procedure. Similar to Mouli et al., the authors found improved survival in patients with peripheral tumor type (rather than infiltrative) and in patients with better performance status. According to RECIST criteria, 24% of patients had partial response, 48% of patients had stable disease and 20% of patients had progressive disease. Fatigue and self-limited abdominal pain were again the most common clinical toxicities. Three patients developed grade 3 biochemical toxicities. One patient developed a self-limiting duodenal ulcer [45].

Another prospective study evaluated 24 patients with unresectable ICC treated with Y-90 glass microsphere TARE. The median OS was 14.9 months. Eight patients had limited extrahepatic disease and 9 patients had portal vein thrombosis. Per WHO criteria, there was a 27% partial response rate, 68% stable disease rate, and 5% progressive disease rate. Fatigue was reported in 75% of patients and abdominal pain reported in 42% of patients. Grade 3 or greater adverse events included bilirubin toxicity in 1 patient and a treatment-related gastroduodenal ulcer in 1 patient [46].

Rafi et al. prospectively evaluated 19 patients with unresectable chemorefractory ICC treated with Y-90 resin microsphere TARE. Eleven patients had extrahepatic disease. Median OS was 11.5 months after the first TARE. Survival was not statistically different between patients with and without extrahepatic disease. Toxicities of fatigue and abdominal pain were similar to that reported in other studies [47].

Another prospective study of 21 patients with unresectable chemorefractory ICC reported a median OS of 16.3 months from initial Y-90 resin microsphere TARE. Significantly improved OS was noted in patients found to have objective response based on modified mRECIST and EASL criteria [48].

A retrospective analysis was conducted to 33 patients treated with Y-90 resin microspheres and assessed at three-month intervals. Twelve patients had a partial response, 17 had stable disease, and 5 patients had disease progression after 3 months. The median time-to-progression was 9.8 months and the median OS was 22 months post-treatment. In addition, longer survival was observed in patients who were chemotherapy naïve (14.2 months vs. 11 months). Both survival and time-to-progression were prolonged in patients with a tumor burden ≤25% and in patients who had a response (partial response or stable disease) on imaging according to RECIST criteria [49].

A systematic review of 12 studies comprising 73 patients evaluated TARE in the treatment of unresectable ICC. The weighted median OS was 15.5 months. Tumor response was pooled and based on reported RECIST, modified RECIST, and

PERCIST criteria. At 3 months, weighted mean partial response was seen in 28% of patients and stable disease was seen in 54% of patients. Morbidity and mortality were reported in 8 of 12 studies. Overall, there was 1 mortality and 3 gastrointestinal ulcers reported. The most common morbidities were fatigue (33%), abdominal pain (28%), and nausea (25%). Seven patients were downstaged to surgery [50].

TARE has also shown potential in the treatment of recurrent postsurgical ICC. In a retrospective single-center study, Sulpice et al. reported on the treatment of recurrent mass-forming ICC following hepatectomy in 45 patients, 25 of whom recurred in the liver. Post recurrence, patients either had no therapy, systemic chemotherapy, repeat hepatectomy, TARE, or a combination of the three treatments. Repeat hepatectomy and TARE with Y-90 glass microspheres were associated with longer OS following recurrence. TARE was utilized in unresectable intrahepatic recurrences and could be used in combination with systemic chemotherapy. Median OS following recurrence was 13 months [51].

TARE in combination with chemotherapy has been shown to be effective for downstaging tumors to potential resection. In a retrospective study of 45 patients with unresectable ICC, 10 patients had single large ICCs that developed in noncirrhotic livers without the extrahepatic disease. After combination therapy with TARE and systemic chemotherapy, 8 of the 10 patients underwent surgical resection with curative intent. The 2 remaining patients had disease progression. Initial unresectability was due to hepatic vein tumor involvement within the functional liver remnant in 7 of the patients and portal vein tumor involvement within the functional liver remnant in 1 of the patients [17]. Evidence for the use of TARE in treatment of ICC is summarized in Table 10.3.

Triaging Patients Among Treatment Modalities

Little research is available to suggest the superiority of one transarterial therapy over the others. Indeed, multiple studies have shown no significant difference in long-term outcomes or radiographic tumor response, but similar toxicity rates, with different transarterial therapies. A multi-institutional retrospective study evaluated 198 patients treated with various transarterial therapies (cTACE, DEB-TACE, TARE, and bland arterial embolization). Median OS was 13.2 months and no significant difference based on the type of transarterial therapy administered. Overall, transarterial therapies were well tolerated. Complications occurred in 29.8% of patients with a major complication rate of 8.1% [52].

In a systematic review of 20 studies evaluating a total of 929 patients with unresectable cholangiocarcinoma treated with transarterial therapies, median OS was 12.4 months including was 12.5 months with TARE and 13 months with TACE [53].

Another meta-analysis of 20 studies including 657 patients treated with transarterial therapies for unresectable ICC also failed to show a difference in OS between therapeutic modalities. Median OS of the cohort was 14.5 months including 13.9 months, 12.4 months, and 12.3 months for TARE, cTACE, and DEB-TACE,

Table 10.3 Series reporting outcomes of TARE for intrahepatic cholangiocarcinoma

Investigators (year)	Study design	Type of Y90 microsphere	# of patients in treatment group	Extrahepatic lesions	Previous systemic therapy	# of adverse events (grade ¾)	Median OS	Reference #
Mouli et al. (2013)	Retrospective	Glass	46	*n* = 16 (35%)	*n* = 16 (35%)	8	Analysis performed based on various patient and tumor characteristics	[44]
Hoffman et al. (2012)	Retrospective	Resin	33	*n* = 8 (24%)	*n* = 27 (79%)	0	22 months from initial TARE	[49]
Saxena et al. (2010)	Prospective	Resin	25	*n* = 12 (48%)	*n* = 18 (72%)	3 biochemical events(clinical toxicity not graded)	9.3 months from initial TARE	[45]
Ibrahim et al. (2008)	Prospective	Glass	24	*n* = 8 (33%)	*n* = 7 (29%)	5 biochemical events(clinical toxicity not graded)	14.9 months from initial TARE	[46]
Camacho et al. (2014)	Prospective	Resin	21	–	*n* = 21 (100%)	–	16.3 months from initial TARE	[48]
Rafi et al. (2013)	Prospective	Resin	19	*n* = 11 (58%)	*n* = 19 (100%)	2	11.5 months from initial TARE	[47]

respectively. Response rates (complete or partial response) for TARE and cTACE were reported as 27.4% and 17.3%, respectively. Stable disease was reported as 54.8%, 46.9%, and 61.5% for TARE, cTACE, and DEB-TACE, respectively [54].

Until a large randomized controlled trial is completed, clinical decision making among transarterial techniques will depend on specific patient characteristics, provider experience, and patient goals of care. For example, radioembolization may have a lower immediate toxicity profile compared to chemoembolization [9]. Avoidance of severe post-embolization syndrome may be preferred in frail patients or patients who have other immediate post-procedure obligations such as the need to quickly return to employment or need to be a primary caregiver. The effect of post-embolization syndrome on short-term performance status may hinder a patient's ability to get concomitant systemic chemotherapy. On the other hand, the tumor response to radioembolization is usually not apparent until 3–4 months post-treatment, whereas the tumor response to chemoembolization is evaluated 1 month post-treatment. Some patients and referring oncologists prefer knowing treatment results earlier and may prefer increased short-term toxicity to a longer time to treatment evaluation [15].

Therefore, decision-making should be individualized and discussed in a multidisciplinary manner.

Chemoembolization should be used with caution in patients with prior biliary interventions such as bilioenteric anastomoses, biliary stents, or sphincterotomy. These patients are at high risk of liver abscess formation after chemoembolization, less so following radioembolization [55, 56]. Historically, portal vein thrombus has been a contraindication for chemoembolization; however, radioembolization has been shown to be safe and effective in select patients with portal vein thrombosis [57].

Due to the radiosensitivity of the liver, caution must be taken when radioembolization is used in patients who have received prior radiation therapy. If underlying liver function is within previously mentioned limits, chemoembolization is safe in previously radiated patients [15]. Radioembolization, however, may prove to be an efficacious treatment when used in combination with systemic chemotherapy. Certain chemotherapies, including gemcitabine and cisplatin, have been shown to be radiosensitizers [58]. Multiple prospective randomized controlled trials are currently underway which evaluate first-line therapy for unresectable cholangiocarcinoma.

Conclusion

In summary, available evidence shows that transarterial therapies are safe and effective in the palliative treatment of unresectable ICC. Specifically, evidence suggests a benefit of transarterial therapies for local tumor control and possibly survival with minimum impact on the quality of life. These therapies also have a role in downstaging tumors enabling surgical resection in a small proportion of patients. Other advantages of transarterial therapies include the high local hepatic concentration of the delivered therapeutic agent with low systemic toxicity as well as the minimally invasive nature of the treatments. Randomized controlled trials are needed to further elucidate how to triage patients among the different types of transarterial therapies as well as to elucidate the optimal treatment sequencing.

References

1. Khan SA, Toledano MB, Taylor-Robinson SD. Epidemiology, risk factors, and pathogenesis of cholangiocarcinoma. HPB. 2008;10(2):77–82.
2. Shaib YH, Davila JA, McGlynn K, El-Serag HB. Rising incidence of intrahepatic cholangiocarcinoma in the United States: a true increase? J Hepatol. 2004;40(3):472–7.
3. Park J, Kim M-H, Kim K, Park DH, Moon S-H, Song TJ, et al. Natural history and prognostic factors of advanced cholangiocarcinoma without surgery, chemotherapy, or radiotherapy: a large-scale observational study. Gut Liver. 2009;3(4):298–305.
4. Simo KA, Halpin LE, McBrier NM, Hessey JA, Baker E, Ross S, et al. Multimodality treatment of intrahepatic cholangiocarcinoma: a review: multimodality therapy of iCCA. J Surg Oncol. 2016;113(1):62–83.
5. Bridgewater J, Galle PR, Khan SA, Llovet JM, Park J-W, Patel T, et al. Guidelines for the diagnosis and management of intrahepatic cholangiocarcinoma. J Hepatol. 2014;60(6):1268–89.
6. Valle J, Furuse J, Jitlal M, Beare S, Mizuno N, Wasan H, et al. Cisplatin and gemcitabine for advanced biliary tract cancer: a meta-analysis of two randomized trials–PubMed –NCBI. Ann Oncol. 2014;25(2):391–8.
7. Lo C. Randomized controlled trial of transarterial lipiodol chemoembolization for unresectable hepatocellular carcinoma. Hepatology. 2002;35(5):1164–71.
8. Llovet JM, Real MI, Montaña X, Planas R, Coll S, Aponte J, et al. Arterial embolization or chemoembolization versus symptomatic treatment in patients with unresectable hepatocellular carcinoma: a randomized controlled trial. Lancet. 2002;359(9319):1734–9.
9. Salem R, Lewandowski RJ, Kulik L, Wang E, Riaz A, Ryu RK, et al. Radioembolization results in longer time-to-progression and reduced toxicity compared with chemoembolization in patients with hepatocellular carcinoma. Gastroenterology. 2011;140(2):497–507.e2.
10. Salem R, Lewandowski RJ, Mulcahy MF, Riaz A, Ryu RK, Ibrahim S, et al. Radioembolization for hepatocellular carcinoma using Yttrium-90 microspheres: a comprehensive report of long-term outcomes. Gastroenterology. 2010;138(1):52–64.
11. Kennedy A, Coldwell D, Sangro B, Wasan H, Salem R. Integrating radioembolization into the treatment paradigm for metastatic neuroendocrine tumors in the liver. Am J Clin Oncol. 2012;35(4):393–8.
12. Kennedy AS, Dezarn WA, McNeillie P, Coldwell D, Nutting C, Carter D, et al. Radioembolization for unresectable neuroendocrine hepatic metastases using resin 90Y-microspheres: early results in 148 patients. Am J Clin Oncol. 2008;31(3):271–9.
13. Ando E, Tanaka M, Yamashita F, Kuromatsu R, Yutani S, Fukumori K, et al. Hepatic arterial infusion chemotherapy for advanced hepatocellular carcinoma with portal vein tumor thrombosis: analysis of 48 cases. Cancer. 2002;95(3):588–95.
14. Vogl TJ, Zangos S, Eichler K, Yakoub D, Nabil M. Colorectal liver metastases: regional chemotherapy via transarterial chemoembolization (TACE) and hepatic chemoperfusion: an update. Eur Radiol. 2007;17(4):1025–34.
15. Currie B, Soulen M. Decision making: intra-arterial therapies for cholangiocarcinoma—TACE and TARE. Semin Interv Radiol. 2017;34(02):092–100.
16. National Comprehensive Cancer Network. Hepatobiliary Cancers (Version 1. 2018). Available at: https://www.nccn.org/professionals/physician_gls/PDF/hepatobiliary.pdf.Accessed September 8, 2018.

17. Rayar M, Sulpice L, Edeline J, Garin E, Levi Sandri GB, Meunier B, et al. Intra-arterial Yttrium-90 Radioembolization combined with systemic chemotherapy is a promising method for downstaging unresectable huge intrahepatic cholangiocarcinoma to surgical treatment. Ann Surg Oncol. 2015;22(9):3102–8.
18. Chua TC, Liauw W, Saxena A, Chu F, Glenn D, Chai A, et al. Systematic review of neoadjuvant transarterial chemoembolization for resectable hepatocellular carcinoma. Liver Int. 2010;30(2):166–74.
19. Seidensticker R, Seidensticker M, Doegen K, Mohnike K, Schütte K, Stübs P, et al. Extensive use of interventional therapies improves survival in Unresectable or recurrent intrahepatic cholangiocarcinoma. Gastroenterol Res Pract. 2016;2016:1–13.
20. Kiefer MV, Albert M, McNally M, Robertson M, Sun W, Fraker D, et al. Chemoembolization of intrahepatic cholangiocarcinoma with cisplatinum, doxorubicin, mitomycin C, ethiodol, and polyvinyl alcohol: a 2-center study. Cancer. 2011;117(7):1498–505.
21. Memon K, Kulik L, Lewandowski RJ, Mulcahy MF, Benson AB, Ganger D, et al. Radioembolization for hepatocellular carcinoma with portal vein thrombosis: impact of liver function on systemic treatment options at disease progression. J Hepatol. 2013;58(1):73–80.
22. Chern M-C, Chuang VP, Liang C-T, Lin ZH, Kuo T-M. Transcatheter arterial chemoembolization for advanced hepatocellular carcinoma with portal vein invasion: safety, efficacy, and prognostic factors. J Vasc Interv Radiol. 2014;25(1):32–40.
23. Yamada R, Nakatsuka H, Nakamura K, Sato M, Itami M, Kobayashi N, et al. Hepatic artery embolization in 32 patients with unresectable hepatoma. Osaka City Med J. 1980;26(2):81–96.
24. Ray CE, Edwards A, Smith MT, Leong S, Kondo K, Gipson M, et al. Meta-analysis of survival, complications, and imaging response following chemotherapy-based transarterial therapy in patients with unresectable intrahepatic cholangiocarcinoma. J Vasc Interv Radiol. 2013;24(8):1218–26.
25. Nakamura H, Hashimoto T, Oi H, Sawada S. Transcatheter oily chemoembolization of hepatocellular carcinoma. Radiology. 1989;170:783–6.
26. Savic LJ, Chapiro J, Geschwind J-FH. Intra-arterial embolotherapy for intrahepatic cholangiocarcinoma: update and future prospects. HepatoBiliary Surg Nutr. 2017;6(1):7–21.
27. Gaba RC, Lewandowski RJ, Hickey R, Baerlocher MO, Cohen EI, Dariushnia SR, et al. Transcatheter therapy for hepatic malignancy: standardization of terminology and reporting criteria. J Vasc Interv Radiol. 2016;27(4):457–73.
28. Hong K. New intra-arterial drug delivery system for the treatment of liver cancer: preclinical assessment in a rabbit model of liver cancer. Clin Cancer Res. 2006;12(8):2563–7.
29. Lammer J, Malagari K, Vogl T, Pilleul F, Denys A, et al. Prospective randomized study of doxorubicin-eluting bead embolization in the treatment of hepatocellular carcinoma: results of the PRECISION V study. Cardiovasc Intervent Radiol. 2010;33(1):41–52.
30. Ariel I. Treatment of inoperable primary pancreatic and liver cancer by the intra-arterial administration of radioactive isotopes (Y90 radiating microspheres). Ann Surg. 1965;162:267–78.
31. Salem R, Thurston KG. Radioembolization with Yttrium-90 microspheres: a state-of-the-art brachytherapy treatment for primary and secondary liver malignancies. J Vasc Interv Radiol. 2006;17(10):1571–93.
32. Lewandowski RJ, Geschwind J-F, Liapi E, Salem R. Transcatheter intraarterial therapies: rationale and overview. Radiology. 2011;259(3):641–57.
33. Salem R, Thurston KG. Radioembolization with 90Yttrium microspheres: a state-of-the-art brachytherapy treatment for primary and secondary liver malignancies. J Vasc Interv Radiol. 2006;17(8):1251–78.
34. Shamimi-Noori S, Gonsalves C, Shaw C. Metastatic liver disease: indications for Locoregional therapy and supporting data. Semin Interv Radiol. 2017;34(02):145–66.
35. Park S-Y, Kim JH, Yoon H-J, Lee I-S, Yoon H-K, Kim K-P. Transarterial chemoembolization versus supportive therapy in the palliative treatment of unresectable intrahepatic cholangiocarcinoma. Clin Radiol. 2011;66(4):322–8.

36. Burger I, Hong K, Schulick R, Georgiades C, Thuluvath P, Choti M, et al. Transcatheter arterial chemoembolization in unresectable cholangiocarcinoma: initial experience in a single institution. J Vasc Interv Radiol. 2005;16(3):353–61.
37. Vogl TJ, Naguib NNN, Nour-Eldin N-EA, Bechstein WO, Zeuzem S, Trojan J, et al. Transarterial chemoembolization in the treatment of patients with unresectable cholangiocarcinoma: results and prognostic factors governing treatment success. Int J Cancer. 2012;131(3):733–40.
38. Gusani NJ, Balaa FK, Steel JL, Geller DA, Marsh JW, Zajko AB, et al. Treatment of unresectable cholangiocarcinoma with gemcitabine-based Transcatheter Arterial Chemoembolization (TACE): a single-institution experience. J Gastrointest Surg. 2008;12(1):129–37.
39. Herber S, Otto G, Schneider J, Manzl N, Kummer I, Kanzler S, et al. Transarterial Chemoembolization (TACE) for inoperable intrahepatic cholangiocarcinoma. Cardiovasc Intervent Radiol. 2007;30(6):1156–65.
40. Schiffman SC, Metzger T, Dubel G, Andrasina T, Kralj I, Tatum C, et al. Precision hepatic arterial irinotecan therapy in the treatment of unresectable intrahepatic cholangiocellular carcinoma: optimal tolerance and prolonged overall survival. Ann Surg Oncol. 2011;18(2):431–8.
41. Aliberti C, Benea G, Tilli M, Fiorentini G. Chemoembolization (TACE) of unresectable intrahepatic cholangiocarcinoma with slow-release doxorubicin-eluting beads: preliminary results. Cardiovasc Intervent Radiol. 2008;31(5):883–8.
42. Kuhlmann JB, Euringer W, Spangenberg HC, Breidert M, Blum HE, Harder J, et al. Treatment of unresectable cholangiocarcinoma: conventional transarterial chemoembolization compared with drug-eluting bead transarterial chemoembolization and systemic chemotherapy. Eur J Gastroenterol Hepatol. 2012;24(4):437–43.
43. Poggi G, Amatu A, Montagna B, Quaretti P, Minoia C, Sottani C, et al. OEM-TACE: anew therapeutic approach in unresectable intrahepatic cholangiocarcinoma. Cardiovasc Intervent Radiol. 2009;32(6):1187–92.
44. Mouli S, Memon K, Baker T, Benson AB, Mulcahy MF, Gupta R, et al. Yttrium-90 radioembolization for intrahepatic cholangiocarcinoma: safety, response, and survival analysis. J Vasc Interv Radiol. 2013;24(8):1227–34.
45. Saxena A, Bester L, Chua TC, Chu FC, Morris DL. Yttrium-90 radiotherapy for unresectable intrahepatic cholangiocarcinoma: a preliminary assessment of this novel treatment option. Ann Surg Oncol. 2010;17(2):484–91.
46. Ibrahim SM, Mulcahy MF, Lewandowski RJ, Sato KT, Ryu RK, Masterson EJ, et al. Treatment of unresectable cholangiocarcinoma using yttrium-90 microspheres: results from a pilot study. Cancer. 2008;113(8):2119–28.
47. Rafi S, Piduru SM, El-Rayes B, Kauh JS, Kooby DA, Sarmiento JM, et al. Yttrium-90 radioembolization for unresectable standard-chemorefractory intrahepatic cholangiocarcinoma: survival, efficacy, and safety study. Cardiovasc Intervent Radiol. 2013;36(2):440–8.
48. Camacho JC, Kokabi N, Xing M, Prajapati HJ, El-Rayes B, Kim HS. Modified response evaluation criteria in solid tumors and European Association for the Study of the liver criteria using delayed-phase imaging at an early time point predict survival in patients with unresectable intrahepatic cholangiocarcinoma following Yttrium-90 radioembolization. J Vasc Interv Radiol. 2014;25(2):256–65.
49. Hoffmann R-T, Paprottka PM, Schön A, Bamberg F, Haug A, Dürr E-M, et al. Transarterial hepatic Yttrium-90 radioembolization in patients with unresectable intrahepatic cholangiocarcinoma: factors associated with prolonged survival. Cardiovasc Intervent Radiol. 2012;35(1):105–16.
50. Al-Adra DP, Gill RS, Axford SJ, Shi X, Kneteman N, Liau S-S. Treatment of unresectable intrahepatic cholangiocarcinoma with yttrium-90 radioembolization: a systematic review and pooled analysis. Eur J Surg Oncol EJSO. 2015;41(1):120–7.
51. Sulpice L, Rayar M, Boucher E, Pracht M, Meunier B, Boudjema K. Treatment of recurrent intrahepatic cholangiocarcinoma. Br J Surg. 2012;99(12):1711–7.

52. Hyder O, Marsh JW, Salem R, Petre EN, Kalva S, Liapi E, et al. Intra-arterial therapy for advanced intrahepatic cholangiocarcinoma: a multi-institutional analysis. Ann Surg Oncol. 2013;20(12):3779–86.
53. Yang L, Shan J, Shan L, Saxena A, Bester L, Morris DL. Trans-arterial embolization therapies for unresectable intrahepatic cholangiocarcinoma: a systematic review. 2015;6(5):19.
54. Boehm LM, Jayakrishnan TT, Miura JT, Zacharias AJ, Johnston FM, Turaga KK, et al. Comparative effectiveness of hepatic artery-based therapies for unresectable intrahepatic cholangiocarcinoma: hepatic artery therapy for unresectable ICC. J Surg Oncol. 2015;111(2):213–20.
55. Kim W, Clark TWI, Baum RA, Soulen MC. Risk factors for liver abscess formation after hepatic chemoembolization. J Vasc Interv Radiol. 2001;12(8):965–8.
56. Devulapalli KK, Fidelman N, Soulen MC, Miller M, Johnson MS, Addo E, et al. Y90 radioembolization for hepatic malignancy in patients with previous biliary intervention: multicenter analysis of hepatobiliary infections. Radiology. 2018;288(3):774–81.
57. Abouchaleh N, Gabr A, Ali R, Al Asadi A, Mora RA, Kallini JR, et al. Y90 radioembolization for locally advanced hepatocellular carcinoma with portal vein thrombosis: long-term outcomes in a 185-patient cohort. J Nucl Med. 2018;59(7):1042–8.
58. Boeckman HJ. Cisplatin sensitizes cancer cells to ionizing radiation via inhibition of nonhomologous end joining. Mol Cancer Res. 2005;3(5):277–85.

Chapter 11
Radiotherapy

Florence K. Keane and Theodore S. Hong

Introduction

Intrahepatic cholangiocarcinoma (ICC) is a rare and aggressive malignancy arising from intrahepatic biliary ducts. ICC accounted for approximately 15% of the 42,220 new diagnoses and 30,200 deaths from liver and intrahepatic bile duct cancer in the USA in 2018 [1]. The incidence of ICC has increased in the USA over the past 40 years [2, 3], in part due to improvements in diagnostic techniques distinguishing ICC from cancers of the unknown primary site, as well as other hepatic and bile duct malignancies [4]. In addition to advancements in diagnostic imaging, molecular profiling has also suggested that ICC is a distinct entity as compared with extrahepatic, perihilar, and gallbladder cancers [5, 6].

ICC is associated with a high risk of local tumor invasion, nodal and distant metastases, and the majority of patients present with disease too advanced for resection. Even for those patients who undergo resection, risk of recurrence remains high. Liver-directed radiotherapy, historically considered a palliative maneuver due to concerns over hepatic tolerance, has emerged as a valuable treatment modality in both the adjuvant and definitive setting. We will discuss the role of radiotherapy in the management of ICC, with a particular focus on advanced technologies of SBRT and charged particle therapy.

F. K. Keane · T. S. Hong (✉)
Department of Radiation Oncology, Massachusetts General Hospital, Boston, MA, USA
e-mail: fkeane@partners.org; tshong1@partners.org

T. M. Pawlik et al. (eds.), *Intrahepatic Cholangiocarcinoma*,
https://doi.org/10.1007/978-3-030-22258-1_11

Role of Adjuvant Radiotherapy

Resection remains the optimal definitive treatment for patients with ICC. However, outcomes after resection remain poor for the vast majority of patients. While a margin-negative (R0) resection is associated with 5-year overall survival as high as 63% [7], on average 5-year OS after resection ranges from 22% to 35% [8–10]. Factors associated with increased risk of recurrence after resection include tumor size, histologic grade, vascular invasion, biliary invasion, positive margins, and nodal metastasis [9, 11].

Randomized data on the role of adjuvant systemic therapy are complicated by the inclusion of patients with extrahepatic cholangiocarcinoma and gallbladder cancer in addition to those patients with the intrahepatic disease. Due to the relative rarity of these diagnoses, trials have also included patients with a variety of histologic features after resection, leading to the grouping of patients with R0 resections without nodal metastases in trials with patients with R1 resections and nodal involvement. Recently presented randomized trials of adjuvant chemotherapy have presented conflicting results. The BILCAP (adjuvant capecitabine for biliary tract cancer) trial [12], a randomized trial of adjuvant capecitabine after resection for completely resected cholangiocarcinoma or gallbladder cancer, was presented in abstract form in 2017 and showed an improvement in overall survival with the use of adjuvant capecitabine in the intent-to-treat analysis. Of note, only 18% of patients enrolled on this trial had intrahepatic cholangiocarcinoma, and the per-protocol analysis did not show a significant difference in survival. By contrast, the PRODIGE 12-ACCORD 18 Phase III trial [13] did not report an improvement in disease-free survival with adjuvant gemcitabine and oxaliplatin. The difference in outcomes may have been driven in part by the patient populations enrolled on each trial. The BILCAP trial included a less favorable patient population compared with the PRODIGE 12-ACCORD 18 trial, with lower rates of R0 resection (62% vs. 87%) and higher rates of nodal metastasis (54% vs. 37%). Randomized trials are ongoing, including the ACTICCA-1 trial, which will randomize patients with resected cholangiocarcinoma or gallbladder cancer to gemcitabine and cisplatin versus capecitabine alone.

There are no randomized data on adjuvant radiotherapy in biliary tract cancers, including ICC. A meta-analysis [14] of 20 studies including 6712 patients with intrahepatic cholangiocarcinoma, extrahepatic cholangiocarcinoma, and gallbladder cancer reported an improvement in overall survival with the use of adjuvant therapy after resection in patients with positive margins (OR 0.36, 95% CI 0.19–0.68) or nodal metastases (OR 0.49, 95% CI 0.30–0.80). Approximately, 27% of patients included in this meta-analysis received some form of adjuvant therapy, with options including chemotherapy alone, radiotherapy alone, or chemoradiotherapy. Patients with nodal metastases most often received chemotherapy or chemoradiotherapy, while those patients with involved margins were typically treated with radiotherapy alone. There was a larger benefit seen with the use of adjuvant chemotherapy or chemoradiotherapy as compared with radiotherapy alone, with the benefit of adjuvant radiotherapy alone seemingly limited to those patients with R1 resection. Of note, only one trial in this meta-analysis included patients with intrahepatic cholangiocarcinoma.

Retrospective single-institution series have reported a benefit with adjuvant radiotherapy in patients with ICC. For example, Jan et al. [15] reported a series of 373 patients with peripheral ICC treated between 1977 and 2001, of whom 63 received adjuvant radiotherapy. There was a significant improvement in median overall survival with the use of adjuvant radiotherapy (11.7 vs. 6.3 months, $p = 0.02$). A series of 90 patients with regional nodal metastases reported a median overall survival of 19.1 months with the use of adjuvant radiotherapy as compared to 9.5 months with observation alone [16].

Therefore, while there is not yet a consensus on the use of adjuvant therapy after resection in ICC, given the high risk of recurrence after resection, the NCCN guidelines currently recommend consideration of adjuvant therapy, specifically chemotherapy and/ or chemoradiotherapy, in patients with adverse risk factors including positive margins and nodal metastases. Although SWOG S0809 [17], a phase II trial of postoperative therapy in patients with high-risk resected extrahepatic cholangiocarcinoma and gallbladder cancer excluded patients with ICC, it does provide encouraging results and a potential framework for the incorporation of adjuvant therapy in the treatment of ICC. Eligible patients included those with high-risk features such as nodal metastases, pathologic T2–4 disease, or positive margins. Patients received four cycles of gemcitabine and cisplatin followed by radiotherapy with concurrent capecitabine. The at-risk nodal stations received a dose of 45 Gy, while the tumor bed receiving 54 to 59.4 Gy. Two-year OS was 65% with this regimen. Treatment was generally well tolerated, as 86% of patients were able to complete the full course of treatment. There was an increased risk of local failure (30%) in patients who did not receive radiotherapy or did not complete radiotherapy as per protocol, supporting the use of radiotherapy in these high-risk patients. At our institution, we favor clinical trial enrolment whenever feasible. For those patients with high-risk pathologic features after resection, we recommend multidisciplinary evaluation, with consideration of adjuvant chemotherapy followed by chemoradiotherapy as appropriate.

Definitive Radiotherapy

While a margin-negative resection is an optimal treatment for ICC, most patients are unresectable at the time of diagnosis due to tumor size, vascular/ biliary invasion or nodal metastasis [18]. Outcomes are often dismal for these patients, with median survival ranging from 3 to 9 months. Trials of both fluoropyrimidine-based and gemcitabine-based chemotherapy regimens showed an improvement in outcomes over best supportive care [19] and historical controls [20]. More recently, both the ABC (advanced biliary tract cancer)-02 trial [21] and the BT (biliary tract) 22 trial [22] demonstrated an improvement in survival with the use of gemcitabine and cisplatin over gemcitabine monotherapy in patients with locally advanced or metastatic disease. Nonetheless, despite advances in chemotherapy regimens, survival remains poor, with a median overall survival of approximately 11 months [23]. With the development of modern radiotherapy techniques, radiotherapy has emerged as a safe and effective option to improve outcomes in patients with locally advanced disease (Table 11.1).

Table 11.1 Outcomes after liver-directed radiotherapy for intrahepatic cholangiocarcinoma

Study	Design	Modality	Pts with IHCC	Prior liver-directed therapies	Tumor Size (range)	Multiple lesions	Dose (Gy)	Number of fractions (range)	1-year LC	1-year OS	Grade ≥ 3 toxicity
Hong et al., 2015 [29]	Phase II	Proton	39	45.8%	2.2–10.9 cm	12.8%	58 GyE (15.1–67.5 GyE)	15	94.1% at 2 years	46.5% at 2 years	7.7%
Tse et al., 2008 [34]	Phase I	Photon, SBRT	10	50%	172 (10–465) ml	**	36 (24–54)	6	65%	58%	2 transient biliary obstruction, 2 w/ decline to CP B
Goodman et al., 2010 [39]	Phase I	Photon, SBRT	5	NR	32.6 (0.8–146.4) ml	NR	18–30	1	77%***	71.4%***	None
Tao et al., 2016 [31]	Retrospective	Proton or IMRT	79	NR	2.2–17 cm	39%	58.05 (35–100)	3–30	81%	87%	15.2%*
Chen et al., 2010 [30]	Retrospective	Photon, 3D-CRT	35	42.9%	7.7 ± 3.2 cm	25.7%	50 (30–60)	25 (10–33)	32.2%	38.5%	8.6%
Mahadevan et al., 2015 [54]	Retrospective	Photon, SBRT	34^	73.4%	63.8 cm^3(5.9–500.1)	~23%	30 (10–45)	3 (1–5)	88%	58%	Four grade 3 toxicities
Ibarra et al., 2012 [36]	Retrospective	Photon, SBRT	11	50%	80.2 (31.6–818.5) ml	18.2%	36–60	1–10	50%	45%	7 patients
Barney et al., 2012 [55]	Retrospective	Photon, IMRT, or 3D-CRT	6	83.3%	16–412.4 ml	NR	55 (45–60)	3 or 5	100%	73%	1 grade 3, 1 grade 5 due to hepatic failure
Liu et al., 2013 [32]	Retrospective	Photon,3D-CRT	6	54***	8.8 (0.2–222.4) ml***	51%***	20–50	3–5	93%***	81.8%***	None
Dewas et al., 2012[37]	Retrospective	Photon, SBRT	6	50%	6.3 (3.6–11.2) cm	0%	45 (29–45)	3–4	100%	NR	NR

Sandler et al., 2016 [56]	Retrospective	Photon, SBRT	6	74%	2.7 cm (1–7.3)	NR	40 (25–50)	5	78***	59%***	16% long term
Lanciano et al., 2012 [57]	Retrospective	Photon, SBRT	4	36.7%***	25.3 (0.53–316) ml***	26.7%***	36–60	3	92%***	73%***	None
Goyal et al., 2010 [38]	Retrospective	Photon, SBRT	3	100%	384 (80–818)	0%	34 (24–45)	1–3	82% at 8 months	NR	None

Adapted from Keane et al. [58]. With permission from Elsevier

Abbreviations: *Pts* patients, *IHCC* intrahepatic cholangiocarcinoma, *LC* local control, *OS* overall survival, *NR* Not reported

*Toxicities may include some redundancies, may be due to progression in some instances

**All patients had tumor venous thrombosis or extrahepatic disease

***Results include patients with other primary liver cancers included in the publication

^Includes patients with both IHCC and hilar cholangiocarcinoma

Conformal Radiotherapy

Historically, limitations in imaging, tumor localization, radiotherapy planning, and delivery often required treatment of the entire liver, which was in turn associated with a significant risk of hepatotoxicity and radiation-induced liver disease (RILD). RILD, characterized by the development of anicteric hepatomegaly, ascites, and elevated LFTs (often with minimal increase in bilirubin), can occur as early as 2 weeks and as late as 4 months after hepatic radiotherapy. The risk of RILD directly correlates with the dose and volume of liver irradiated. For example, retrospective series reported a 10% rate of RILD in patients receiving 33 Gy in 1.5 Gy twice-daily fractions [24] and a 44% rate of RILD in patients receiving ≥35 Gy [25]. The risk of RILD also increases in patients with compromised hepatobiliary function [26, 27].

The development of conformal radiotherapy enabled assessment of the interaction between radiotherapy dose, target volume, hepatic volume, and toxicity. Multiple series have now demonstrated that partial hepatic tolerance to radiotherapy is quite high and delivery of tumoricidal doses of radiotherapy with minimal toxicity is feasible in carefully selected patients. Series of Phase I/II dose-escalation trials [26, 28] of hyperfractionated radiotherapy with concurrent chemotherapy conducted at the University of Michigan in patients with unresectable HCC or ICC established key metrics regarding hepatobiliary tolerance to radiotherapy. Patients were treated to a median dose of 58.5 Gy in twice-daily fractions (range 28.5–90 Gy). The maximum tolerated dose for each patient was based on a maximum of 10–15% risk of RILD as determined using a normal tissue complication probability (NTCP) model. The effective liver volume (Veff) parameter was used to facilitate comparison of dose between different radiotherapy plans. The Phase II trial enrolled 128 patients, 44 of whom had cholangiocarcinoma. Treatment was well tolerated, with a 4% rate of ≥3 RILD. Median overall survival was 13.3 months for patients with ICC, far superior to historical controls. There was a particular benefit to dose-escalation in the overall cohort, with median OS of 23.9 months in patients treated to ≥75 Gy versus 14.9 months in patients treated to <75 Gy ($p < 0.01$).

Retrospective and large-database series have also demonstrated an improvement in outcomes with the use of radiotherapy for unresectable ICC (Table 11.1) [29–32]. A retrospective series [30] of 84 patients with ICC treated with radiotherapy, arterially directed therapy (TACE), supportive care, or a combination thereof reported an improvement in outcomes with the use of radiotherapy as compared with TACE alone or supportive care alone. A total of 35 patients ($n = 41.7\%$) received radiotherapy, of whom 15 also received TACE. Radiotherapy was associated with a significant improvement in OS in the overall cohort (9.5 vs. 5.1 months, $p = 0.003$), as well as in the subgroup of patients with central tumors (13.3 vs. 3.5 months). A SEER analysis [33] of 3839 patients with IHCC treated between 1988 and 2003 with resection (25%), resection and adjuvant radiotherapy (7%), radiotherapy alone (10%) or no treatment (58%) reported a 4 month improvement in median survival with the use of radiotherapy as compared with no treatment (7 vs. 3 months, $p < 0.01$). The usual limitations of large-database series, including the lack of data on systemic therapies and comorbidities, must be considered when assessing this study, but in the context of other series and Phase II trials, it does provide additional support for consideration of radiotherapy for unresectable ICC.

Stereotactic Body Radiotherapy and Hypofractionated Radiotherapy

Stereotactic body radiotherapy (SBRT) or stereotactic ablative radiotherapy (SABR) delivers high doses of radiotherapy with rapid fall-off through the use of rigid immobilization, precise tumor localization, and multiple conformal beams. While there are no randomized trials of SBRT in unresectable ICC, multiple Phase II single-arm trials and retrospective series have demonstrated its safety and efficacy for the treatment of primary hepatic tumors [34–39]. Of note, hypofractionated radiotherapy employs similar rigid immobilization, localization and highly conformal beam arrangements as SBRT, but fractionates treatment over a longer course, typically 15 fractions. Given the large size of many primary hepatic tumors, hypofractionated radiotherapy is often employed instead of SBRT and will also be discussed herein. As in systemic therapy, the available data often include a variety of intrahepatic tumors, including hepatocellular carcinoma and ICC.

A Phase I dose-escalation trial of six-fraction SBRT conducted at Princess Margaret Cancer Center [34] enrolled 41 patients with primary hepatic tumors, of whom 10 had IHCC. Fifty percent of patients with ICC had received prior therapy, including chemotherapy, resection, and ablative therapy. Radiotherapy dose was selected based on the risk of toxicity as determined by the effective liver dose parameter (Veff) and NTCP model, with a median dose of 36 Gy (range 24–54 Gy). Treatment was well tolerated, and two patients with ICC and eight patients with HCC developed grade 3 elevation in liver enzymes, but there were no grade 4 or 5 events. Survival was also encouraging, with a median OS of 15 months.

Retrospective series have also provided support for the role of ablative doses of radiotherapy in the treatment of ICC, with improvements in local control and overall survival without significant toxicity. Tao et al. [31] published a series of 79 patients with unresectable IHCC treated with dose-escalated definitive radiotherapy to a median dose of 58.05 Gy (range 35–100 Gy), corresponding to a median biologic equivalent dose of 80.5 Gy (range 43.75–180 Gy). Nearly 90% of patients received chemotherapy prior to radiotherapy, 63% received concurrent chemotherapy, and 47% received adjuvant chemotherapy. There was not a significant difference in the use of chemotherapy by radiotherapy dose. Patients were treated with both photon ($n = 54$, 68%) and proton beam therapy ($n = 25$, 32%). To facilitate dose-escalation while still meeting standard constraints for organs at risk, the authors incorporated a simultaneous integrated boost to the gross tumor volume of 75 Gy in 15 fractions or 100 Gy in 25 fractions. There was a significant improvement in 3-year overall survival with BED >80.5 Gy (73% vs. 38%, $p = 0.017$) and

3-year local control (78% vs. 45%, $p = 0.04$). Three patients were hospitalized within 90 days of completion of treatment, but there were no cases of radiation-induced liver disease. There were seven instances of biliary stenosis (9%) but these were thought to be due to disease progression.

Charged Particle Therapy

Charged particle therapy, including proton beam therapy and carbon ion therapy, is characterized by rapid energy absorption and steep dose fall-off. The minimal exit dose of proton beam therapy is particularly appealing when considering the need to deliver a tumoricidal dose of radiotherapy while maximizing sparing of uninvolved hepatic parenchyma. Similar to SBRT, while there are no randomized data for charged particle therapy in primary hepatic tumors, a Phase II trial and retrospective data have provided encouraging results regarding its efficacy and safety.

The University of Tsukuba [40] reported the largest series to date of proton therapy in primary liver tumors, including 318 patients with HCC who were treated between 2001 and 2007. There were only five grade ≥3 toxicities. While this trial did not include patients with ICC, the safety data regarding the role of proton therapy in the treatment of hepatic tumors are encouraging, particularly given the inclusion of patients with Child-Pugh B cirrhosis. Overall survival was 44.6% for the overall cohort. A retrospective series [41] of proton therapy for the treatment 28 patients with cholangiocarcinoma included six patients with ICC. Patients were treated to a median dose of 69.2 GyE, with significant improvement in local control with doses >70 Gy (1-year local control 82.1% vs. 22.2%).

While these retrospective data were encouraging, there were limited prospective data regarding both photon radiotherapy and charged particle therapy in ICC. A Phase II multi-institutional trial [29] of hypofractionated, dose-escalated proton beam therapy conducted at Massachusetts General Hospital and M.D. Anderson Cancer Center enrolled 83 patients with localized, unresectable HCC ($n = 44$), ICC ($n = 37$), and mixed HCC/ICC ($n = 2$). The majority of patients with ICC received systemic therapy prior to trial enrollment ($n = 24$, 61.5%). For patients with ICC, median tumor dimension was 6.0 cm (range 2.2–10.9 cm), 12.8% had multiple tumors, and 28.2% had tumor vascular thrombosis. The dose was 58.05 GyE in 15 fractions for tumors within 2 cm of the porta hepatis and 67.5 GyE in 15fractions for tumors more than 2 cm from the porta hepatis. Doses were de-escalated as needed to ensure mean liver dose ≤24 GyE. For patients with IHCC, median radiotherapy dose was 58.05 GyE, and the mean dose to the uninvolved liver was 21.4 GyE (range 3.2–29.5 GyE). Local control at 2-years was 94.1% for ICC, with only two local failures. Four additional local failures occurred after 2 years. Of note, all patients with local failures received less than 60 GyE. Median OS for ICC was 22.5 months, with 2-year OS of 46.5%. The rate of grade 3 treatment-related toxicities was 3.6% in the overall cohort and 7.7% in patients with IHCC. There were no grade 4 or 5 toxicities.

These impressive outcomes, particularly given the advanced disease of the patients enrolled, demonstrate the value of radiotherapy for the treatment of unresectable ICC.

Optimal timing of radiotherapy with systemic therapy for ICC remains an open question. With the publication of ABC-02 and BT-22 trials, cisplatin and gemcitabine were established as the standard of care for metastatic and locally advanced cholangiocarcinoma. Of note, the median overall survival in the gemcitabine and cisplatin arm on ABC-02 was 11.2 months, as compared to 22.5 months in the Phase II trial [29] discussed above. While this difference is likely driven in part by the significant proportion of metastatic patients included on ABC-02 (~75%), given the excellent outcomes seen with radiotherapy in this population further study is needed. NRG GI-001, a currently enrolling Phase III trial, will randomize patients with unresectable ICC to systemic therapy with gemcitabine and cisplatin followed by radiotherapy to systemic therapy alone.

Radiotherapy Treatment Planning and Delivery

Treatment of intrahepatic cholangiocarcinoma with radiotherapy is complex and requires careful patient selection, rigid immobilization, careful delineation of targets and organs at risk, and rigorous quality assurance.

Prior to radiotherapy planning, three fiducial markers are placed in the liver around the target lesion. These markers are critical for treatment planning and delivery and facilitate motion assessment as well as patient set-up and treatment delivery. Biopsy can also be obtained if needed at the time of fiducial placement.

Patients are then simulated in the supine position with arms up and immobilized with custom immobilization, which may include vacuum bags or thermoplastic devices, with or without a body frame. The variable contrast enhancement patterns of intrahepatic cholangiocarcinoma on CT and MRI can complicate target identification (Figs. 11.1 and 11.2). Incorporation of multiphasic imaging with arterial, portal venous and delayed phases is critical to ensure complete identification of the tumor [42–45]. For example, while some tumors are characterized by arterial enhancement and rapid venous washout, similar to HCC, other lesions have delayed enhancement on CT [46], or are better identified with MRI. Consensus guidelines for contouring of HCC recommend contouring the gross tumor volume (GTV) across all phases of imaging [47]. While there are not yet consensus guidelines for contouring of ICC, we recommend the same principle as HCC be applied here. Technically, arterial phase images are obtained immediately after peak aortic enhancement as determined by bolus tracking, typically 30–35 seconds after the infusion begins. Portal venous images are obtained 70–75 seconds after the infusion begins, and delayed phase images are obtained 3 minutes after portal venous phase images. Of note, for those patients who are treated with proton therapy, we obtain the 4DCT prior to the multiphasic contrast scan to avoid any impact of the increased density of intravenous contrast on treatment planning.

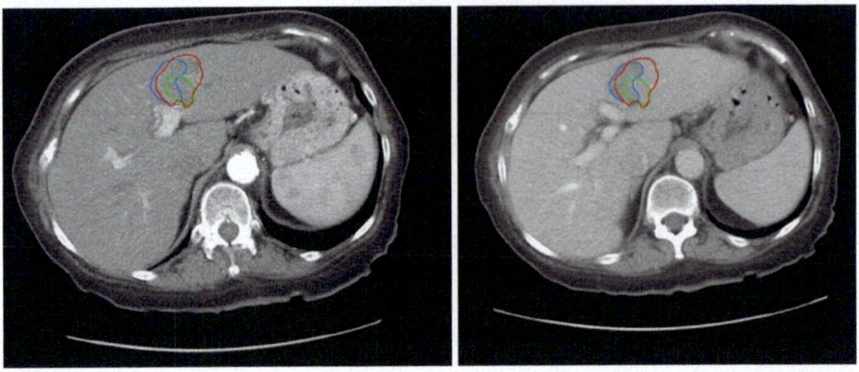

Fig. 11.1 Intrahepatic cholangiocarcinoma with variable enhancement patterns in the arterial phase (left) and portal venous phase (right). There is a lack of overlap with between gross tumor volumes on arterial (red), portal venous (blue), and delayed (green phases)

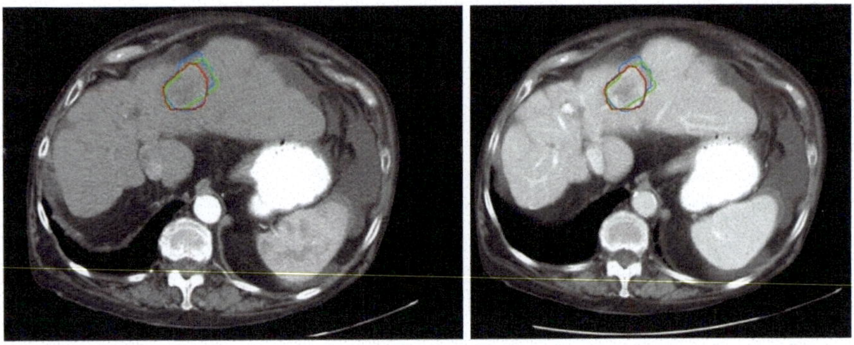

Fig. 11.2 Intrahepatic cholangiocarcinoma with variable enhancement patterns in the arterial phase (left) and portal venous phase (right). There is a lack of overlap with between gross tumor volumes on arterial (red), portal venous (blue), and delayed (green phases)

While the use of MR-based simulation is increasing, many centers continue to rely on CT simulation with a fusion of relevant MR sequences. Accurate fusions of MR sequences with the planning CT is critical, as suboptimal fusions can result in target misidentification [47]. For those centers without MR-based simulation, alignment of MR-compatible fiducial markers or performing MRI in the treatment position are two possible techniques for improving the accuracy and ease of fusions.

A 4-dimensional (4D) CT is also performed during the simulation for assessment of both target and hepatic motion [48, 49]. For those patients who do not require respiratory gating, the average phase CT is used as the baseline CT for planning. For those patients with significant tumor motion, respiratory gating is employed, with treatment delivered during expiratory phases. Active breathing control and abdominal compression have also been explored to reduce motion and may be used based on the policy of individual treatment centers [34, 48, 50–53].

While consensus guidelines are not yet available for ICC, the ongoing protocol NRG GI001, a randomized Phase III trial of cisplatin and gemcitabine with or without hypofractionated radiotherapy, provides information on treatment planning. In addition to the gross tumor volume (GTV), which is defined as the parenchymal and nodal disease as seen on multiphasic CT imaging and /or MRI, an internal target volume (ITV) must also be delineated based on the 4DCT. A clinical target volume (CTV) may be delineated at physician preference based on clinical concerns. The planning target volume (PTV) varies based on patient immobilization, treatment modality (photons vs. protons), and onboard imaging. The minimum PTV, as defined on NRG GI001, is 4 mm. When selecting the prescription dose, assessment of the organs at risk, specifically the dose to the porta hepatis and the average dose to the liver, is critical. Peripheral tumors, defined as >2 cm from the porta hepatis may be treated to a maximum dose of 67.5 Gy (or GyE) in 15 fractions, assuming that the mean liver dose is ≤22 Gy. Central tumors, within 2 cm of the porta hepatis, may be treated to a maximum dose of 58.05 Gy (or GyE) in 15 fractions. The volume of liver receiving 10 Gy should be less than 80%, and at least 700 cc of the uninvolved liver should be spared. Constraints are also specified for the spinal cord, stomach, small bowel, esophagus, and kidneys.

Treatment delivery requires onboard imaging prior to and during treatment. Onboard cone beam CT as available on linear accelerators can be used to assess fiducial and soft tissue position prior to treatment, in-between treatment fields, and after completion of each fraction. Fiducials may also be tracked during treatment with onboard kV imaging, which is particularly helpful in the treatment of patients with respiratory gating.

Future Directions

While single-arm Phase II trial and retrospective series have provided encouraging data on the use of radiotherapy in ICC, prospective randomized trials are critical. As discussed above, NRG GI001 is currently randomizing patients with unresectable ICC to systemic therapy alone versus systemic therapy followed by hypofractionated radiotherapy. Patients will receive their cycles of cisplatin plus gemcitabine followed by restaging and stratification based on tumor size and number of lesions, then randomized to an additional five cycles of chemotherapy versus one cycle of chemotherapy, radiotherapy, then four cycles of chemotherapy. Maintenance gemcitabine is permitted. The ABC-07 trial, a Phase II trial, will randomize patients with advanced biliary tract cancer to cisplatin plus gemcitabine with or without SBRT. Successful completion of these trials is critical to definitively establish the role of liver-directed radiotherapy for biliary tract cancers.

Summary

The role of liver-directed radiotherapy in intrahepatic cholangiocarcinoma has evolved from a strictly palliative treatment to a valuable component in the management of both the adjuvant and definitive IHCC. Data on modern liver-directed radiotherapy have demonstrated its safety and efficacy. Careful assessment of patient comorbidities and disease extent is required to determine the optimal combination of therapies for patients with ICC. Prospective randomized trials are needed to determine the optimal timing of radiotherapy and integration with systemic therapy.

References

1. Siegel RL, Miller KD, Jemal A. Cancer statistics, 2018. CA Cancer J Clin. 2018;68(1):7–30.
2. Shaib YH, Davila JA, McGlynn K, El-Serag HB. Rising incidence of intrahepatic cholangiocarcinoma in the United States: a true increase? J Hepatol. 2004;40(3):472–7.
3. Patel T. Increasing incidence and mortality of primary intrahepatic cholangiocarcinoma in the United States. Hepatology. 2001;33(6):1353–7.
4. Saha SK, Zhu AX, Fuchs CS, Brooks GA. Forty-year trends in cholangiocarcinoma incidence in the U.S.: intrahepatic disease on the rise. Oncologist. 2016;21(5):594–9.
5. Borger DR, Tanabe KK, Fan KC, Lopez HU, Fantin VR, Straley KS, et al. Frequent mutation of isocitrate dehydrogenase (IDH)1 and IDH2 in cholangiocarcinoma identified through broad-based tumor genotyping. Oncologist. 2012;17(1):72–9.
6. Zhu AX, Borger DR, Kim Y, Cosgrove D, Ejaz A, Alexandrescu S, et al. Genomic profiling of intrahepatic cholangiocarcinoma: refining prognosis and identifying therapeutic targets. Ann Surg Oncol. 2014;21(12):3827–34.
7. DeOliveira ML, Cunningham SC, Cameron JL, Kamangar F, Winter JM, Lillemoe KD, et al. Cholangiocarcinoma: thirty-one-year experience with 564 patients at a single institution. Ann Surg. 2007;245(5):755–62.
8. Maithel SK, Gamblin TC, Kamel I, Corona-Villalobos CP, Thomas M, Pawlik TM. Multidisciplinary approaches to intrahepatic cholangiocarcinoma. Cancer. 2013;119(22):3929–42.
9. Spolverato G, Vitale A, Cucchetti A, Popescu I, Marques HP, Aldrighetti L, et al. Can hepatic resection provide a long-term cure for patients with intrahepatic cholangiocarcinoma? Cancer. 2015;121(22):3998–4006.
10. Mavros MN, Economopoulos KP, Alexiou VG, Pawlik TM. Treatment and prognosis for patients with intrahepatic cholangiocarcinoma: systematic review and meta-analysis. JAMA Surg. 2014;149(6):565–74.
11. Wang Y, Li J, Xia Y, Gong R, Wang K, Yan Z, et al. Prognostic nomogram for intrahepatic cholangiocarcinoma after partial hepatectomy. J Clin Oncol. 2013;31(9):1188–95.
12. Primrose JN, Fox R, Palmer DH, Prasad R, Mirza D, Anthoney DA, et al. Adjuvant capecitabine for biliary tract cancer: the BILCAP randomized study. J Clin Oncol. 2017;35(15_suppl):4006.
13. Edeline J, Bonnetain F, Phelip JM, Watelet J, Hammel P, Joly J-P, et al. Gemox versus surveillance following surgery of localized biliary tract cancer: results of the PRODIGE 12-ACCORD 18 (UNICANCER GI) phase III trial. J Clin Oncol. 2017;35(4_suppl):225.
14. Horgan AM, Amir E, Walter T, Knox JJ. Adjuvant therapy in the treatment of biliary tract cancer: a systematic review and meta-analysis. J Clin Oncol. 2012;30(16):1934–40.

15. Jan YY, Yeh CN, Yeh TS, Chen TC. Prognostic analysis of surgical treatment of peripheral cholangiocarcinoma: two decades of experience at Chang Gung Memorial Hospital. World J Gastroenterol (WJG). 2005;11(12):1779–84.
16. Jiang W, Zeng ZC, Tang ZY, Fan J, Zhou J, Zeng MS, et al. Benefit of radiotherapy for 90 patients with resected intrahepatic cholangiocarcinoma and concurrent lymph node metastases. J Cancer Res Clin Oncol. 2010;136(9):1323–31.
17. Ben-Josef E, Guthrie KA, El-Khoueiry AB, Corless CL, Zalupski MM, Lowy AM, et al. SWOG S0809: a phase II intergroup trial of adjuvant Capecitabine and gemcitabine followed by radiotherapy and concurrent Capecitabine in extrahepatic cholangiocarcinoma and gallbladder carcinoma. J Clin Oncol. 2015;33(24):2617–22.
18. Endo I, Gonen M, Yopp AC, Dalal KM, Zhou Q, Klimstra D, et al. Intrahepatic cholangiocarcinoma: rising frequency, improved survival, and determinants of outcome after resection. Ann Surg. 2008;248(1):84–96.
19. Glimelius B, Hoffman K, Sjoden PO, Jacobsson G, Sellstrom H, Enander LK, et al. Chemotherapy improves survival and quality of life in advanced pancreatic and biliary cancer. AnnOncol. 1996;7(6):593–600.
20. Dingle BH, Rumble RB, Brouwers MC, Cancer Care Ontario's Program in Evidence-Based Care's Gastrointestinal Cancer Disease Site G. The role of gemcitabine in the treatment of cholangiocarcinoma and gallbladder cancer: a systematic review. Can J Gastroenterol. 2005;19(12):711–6.
21. Valle J, Wasan H, Palmer DH, Cunningham D, Anthoney A, Maraveyas A, et al. Cisplatin plus gemcitabine versus gemcitabine for biliary tract cancer. N Engl J Med. 2010;362(14):1273–81.
22. Okusaka T, Nakachi K, Fukutomi A, Mizuno N, Ohkawa S, Funakoshi A, et al. Gemcitabine alone or in combination with cisplatin in patients with biliary tract cancer: a comparative multicentre study in Japan. Br J Cancer. 2010;103(4):469–74.
23. Valle JW, Furuse J, Jitlal M, Beare S, Mizuno N, Wasan H, et al. Cisplatin and gemcitabine for advanced biliary tract cancer: a meta-analysis of two randomized trials. AnnOncol. 2014;25(2):391–8.
24. Russell AH, Clyde C, Wasserman TH, Turner SS, Rotman M. Accelerated hyperfractionated hepatic irradiation in the management of patients with liver metastases: results of the RTOG dose escalating protocol. Int J Radiat Oncol Biol Phys. 1993;27(1):117–23.
25. Ingold JA, Reed GB, Kaplan HS, Bagshaw MA. Radiation hepatitis. Am J Roentgenol Radium Therapy, Nucl Med. 1965;93:200–8.
26. Ben-Josef E, Normolle D, Ensminger WD, Walker S, Tatro D, Ten Haken RK, et al. Phase II trial of high-dose conformal radiation therapy with concurrent hepatic artery floxuridine for unresectable intrahepatic malignancies. J Clin Oncol. 2005;23(34):8739–47.
27. Jung J, Yoon SM, Kim SY, Cho B, Park JH, Kim SS, et al. Radiation-induced liver disease after stereotactic body radiotherapy for small hepatocellular carcinoma: clinical and dose-volumetric parameters. Radiat Oncol. 2013;8:249.
28. Dawson LA, McGinn CJ, Normolle D, Haken RKT, Walker S, Ensminger W, et al. Escalated focal liver radiation and concurrent hepatic artery fluorodeoxyuridine for unresectable intrahepatic malignancies. J Clin Oncol. 2000;18(11):2210–8.
29. Hong TS, Wo JY, Beow YY, Ben-Josef E, McDonnell E, Blaskowsky LS, et al. A multi-institutional phase II study of high dose hypofractionated proton beam therapy in patients with localized, unresectable hepatocellular carcinoma and intrahepatic cholangiocarcinoma. J Clin Oncol. 2015;34(5):460–8.
30. Chen YX, Zeng ZC, Tang ZY, Fan J, Zhou J, Jiang W, et al. Determining the role of external beam radiotherapy in unresectable intrahepatic cholangiocarcinoma: a retrospective analysis of 84 patients. BMC Cancer. 2010;10:492.
31. Tao R, Krishnan S, Bhosale PR, Javle MM, Aloia TA, Shroff RT, et al. Ablative radiotherapy doses lead to a substantial prolongation of survival in patients with inoperable intrahepatic cholangiocarcinoma: a retrospective dose-response analysis. J Clin Oncol. 2016;34(3):219–26.

32. Liu E, Stenmark MH, Schipper MJ, Balter JM, Kessler ML, Caoili EM, et al. Stereotactic body radiation therapy for primary and metastatic liver tumors. Transl Oncol. 2013;6(4):442–6.
33. Shinohara ET, Mitra N, Guo M, Metz JM. Radiotherapy is associated with improved survival in adjuvant and palliative treatment of extrahepatic cholangiocarcinomas. Int J Radiat Oncol Biol Phys. 2009;74(4):1191–8.
34. Tse RV, Hawkins M, Lockwood G, Kim JJ, Cummings B, Knox J, et al. Phase I study of individualized stereotactic body radiotherapy for hepatocellular carcinoma and intrahepatic cholangiocarcinoma. J Clin Oncol. 2008;26(4):657–64.
35. Bujold A, Massey CA, Kim JJ, Brierley J, Cho C, Wong RK, et al. Sequential phase I and II trials of stereotactic body radiotherapy for locally advanced hepatocellular carcinoma. J Clin Oncol. 2013;31(13):1631–9.
36. Ibarra RA, Rojas D, Snyder L, Yao M, Fabien J, Milano M, et al. Multicenter results of stereotactic body radiotherapy (SBRT) for non-resectable primary liver tumors. Acta Oncol. 2012;51(5):575–83.
37. Dewas S, Bibault JE, Mirabel X, Fumagalli I, Kramar A, Jarraya H, et al. Prognostic factors affecting local control of hepatic tumors treated by stereotactic body radiation therapy. Radiat Oncol. 2012;7:166.
38. Goyal K, Einstein D, Yao M, Kunos C, Barton F, Singh D, et al. Cyberknife stereotactic body radiation therapy for nonresectable tumors of the liver: preliminary results. HPB Surg. 2010;2010
39. Goodman KA, Wiegner EA, Maturen KE, Zhang Z, Mo Q, Yang G, et al. Dose-escalation study of single-fraction stereotactic body radiotherapy for liver malignancies. Int J Radiat Oncol Biol Phys. 2010;78(2):486–93.
40. Nakayama H, Sugahara S, Tokita M, Fukuda K, Mizumoto M, Abei M, et al. Proton beam therapy for hepatocellular carcinoma: the University of Tsukuba experience. Cancer. 2009;115(23):5499–506.
41. Makita C, Nakamura T, Takada A, Takayama K, Suzuki M, Ishikawa Y, et al. Clinical outcomes and toxicity of proton beam therapy for advanced cholangiocarcinoma. Radiat Oncol. 2014;9:26.
42. Kim TK, Choi BI, Han JK, Jang HJ, Cho SG, Han MC. Peripheral cholangiocarcinoma of the liver: two-phase spiral CT findings. Radiology. 1997;204(2):539–43.
43. Niska J, Keane FK, Wolfgang J, Hahn PF, Wo JY, Zhu AX, et al. Impact of IV contrast enhancement phase on target definition for hepatocellular carcinoma(HCC) and intrahepatic cholangiocarcinoma(IHC): observations from patients enrolled on a prospective phase II trial. PractRadiatOncol. 2015;6(1):e9–16.
44. Valls C, Guma A, Puig I, Sanchez A, Andia E, Serrano T, et al. Intrahepatic peripheral cholangiocarcinoma: CT evaluation. Abdom Imaging. 2000;25(5):490–6.
45. Miura F, Okazumi S, Takayama W, Asano T, Makino H, Shuto K, et al. Hemodynamics of intrahepatic cholangiocarcinoma: evaluation with single-level dynamic CT during hepatic arteriography. Abdom Imaging. 2004;29(4):467–71.
46. Kim SA, Lee JM, Lee KB, Kim SH, Yoon SH, Han JK, et al. Intrahepatic mass-forming cholangiocarcinomas: enhancement patterns at multiphasic CT, with special emphasis on arterial enhancement pattern–correlation with clinicopathologic findings. Radiology. 2011;260(1):148–57.
47. Hong TS, Bosch WR, Krishnan S, Kim TK, Mamon HJ, Shyn P, et al. Interobserver variability in target definition for hepatocellular carcinoma with and without portal vein thrombus: radiation therapy oncology group consensus guidelines. Int J Radiat Oncol Biol Phys. 2014;89(4):804–13.
48. Heinzerling JH, Anderson JF, Papiez L, Boike T, Chien S, Zhang G, et al. Four-dimensional computed tomography scan analysis of tumor and organ motion at varying levels of abdominal compression during stereotactic treatment of lung and liver. Int J Radiat Oncol Biol Phys. 2008;70(5):1571–8.

49. Langen KM, Jones DT. Organ motion and its management. Int J Radiat Oncol Biol Phys. 2001;50(1):265–78.
50. Blomgren H, Lax I, Naslund I, Svanstrom R. Stereotactic high dose fraction radiation therapy of extracranial tumors using an accelerator. Clinical experience of the first thirty-one patients. Acta Oncol. 1995;34(6):861–70.
51. Wong JW, Sharpe MB, Jaffray DA, Kini VR, Robertson JM, Stromberg JS, et al. The use of active breathing control (ABC) to reduce margin for breathing motion. Int J Radiat Oncol Biol Phys. 1999;44(4):911–9.
52. Case RB, Sonke JJ, Moseley DJ, Kim J, Brock KK, Dawson LA. Inter- and intrafraction variability in liver position in non-breath-hold stereotactic body radiotherapy. Int J Radiat Oncol Biol Phys. 2009;75(1):302–8.
53. Eccles CL, Dawson LA, Moseley JL, Brock KK. Interfraction liver shape variability and impact on GTV position during liver stereotactic radiotherapy using abdominal compression. Int J Radiat Oncol Biol Phys. 2011;80(3):938–46.
54. Mahadevan A, Dagoglu N, Mancias J, Raven K, Khwaja K, Tseng JF, et al. Stereotactic body radiotherapy (SBRT) for intrahepatic and hilar cholangiocarcinoma. J Cancer. 2015;6(11):1099–104.
55. Barney BM, Olivier KR, Miller RC, Haddock MG. Clinical outcomes and toxicity using stereotactic body radiotherapy (SBRT) for advanced cholangiocarcinoma. Radiat Oncol. 2012;7:67.
56. Sandler KA, Veruttipong D, Agopian VG, Finn RS, Hong JC, Kaldas FM, et al. Stereotactic body radiotherapy (SBRT) for locally advanced extrahepatic and intrahepatic cholangiocarcinoma. Adv Radiat Oncol. 2016;1(4):237–43.
57. Lanciano R, Lamond J, Yang J, Feng J, Arrigo S, Good M, et al. Stereotactic body radiation therapy for patients with heavily pretreated liver metastases and liver tumors. Front Oncol. 2012;2:23.
58. Keane F, Zhu A, ong T H. Radiotherapy for biliary tract cancers. Semin Radiat Oncol. 2018;28(4):342–50.

Chapter 12
Molecular Pathogenesis: From Inflammation and Cholestasis to a Microenvironment-Driven Tumor

Eleonora Milani, Mario Strazzabosco, Luca Fabris, and Massimiliano Cadamuro

Introduction

Intrahepatic cholangiocarcinoma (iCCA) is a primary hepatobiliary malignancy resulting from the neoplastic transformation of different epithelial cell types, such as the cholangiocyte, the progenitor stem cell abutting the canals of Hering, and even the hepatocyte. Regardless of the cell origin, a distinctive feature of this epithelial cancer is the accumulation of a dense fibro-inflammatory stroma (the so-called tumor reactive stroma, TRS) closely surrounding the tumor duct cells, encompassing

E. Milani
Department of Molecular Medicine, University of Padua, Padua, Italy
e-mail: eleonora.milani.1@studenti.unipd.it

M. Strazzabosco
International Center for Digestive Health (ICDH), University of Milano-Bicocca, Milano, Italy

Section of Digestive Diseases, Department of Internal Medicine, Yale University, New Haven, CT, USA
e-mail: mario.strazzabosco@yale.edu

L. Fabris (✉)
Department of Molecular Medicine, University of Padua, Padua, Italy

International Center for Digestive Health (ICDH), University of Milano-Bicocca, Milano, Italy

Section of Digestive Diseases, Department of Internal Medicine, Yale University, New Haven, CT, USA
e-mail: luca.fabris@unipd.it

M. Cadamuro
Department of Molecular Medicine, University of Padua, Padua, Italy

International Center for Digestive Health (ICDH), University of Milano-Bicocca, Milano, Italy
e-mail: massimiliano.cadamuro@unipd.it

T. M. Pawlik et al. (eds.), *Intrahepatic Cholangiocarcinoma*,
https://doi.org/10.1007/978-3-030-22258-1_12

different cell populations, among which are activated fibroblasts, inflammatory cells, immune cells, and endothelial cells [1]. Evidence is mounting that a mutual exchange of multiple paracrine signals between the stromal and cancer cells boosts tumor development, overgrowth, and invasion [2, 3]. Based on these findings, iCCA has become paradigmatic of the Paget's theory, which in the nineteenth century, first addressed the importance of the tissue background (formerly recognized as "the soil") to induce and foster neoplastic transformation (behaving as "the seed"). From this viewpoint, two fundamental pathomechanisms have been pinpointed as pivotal triggers of the events culminating with the malignant transformation of the biliary epithelium, including biliary/liver inflammation – often in conjunction with periductal fibrosis and cholestasis. Both chronic inflammation and cholestasis variably occur in a number of disease conditions, not necessarily evolving to liver cirrhosis, which include primary cholangiopathies, parasitic infestations, and metabolic disorders, all known to bear an increased risk to develop iCCA. Among chronic cholangiopathies, primary sclerosing cholangitis (PSC) and the fibropolycystic liver diseases are well-characterized pre-malignant conditions of iCCA associated with a prominent peribiliary fibrotic reaction [1]. In PSC, biliary fibrosis is accompanied by a progressive bile duct loss, while in fibropolycystic liver diseases, such as Caroli's disease (CD) and congenital hepatic fibrosis (CHF), progressive fibrous stroma accumulation develops in conjunction with a dysgenetic overgrowth of the bile ducts. Chronic infestation with liver flukes (*Opisthorchis viverrini* and *Clonorchis sinensis*), which are endemic in Eastern Asia, correlates with cholangiocarcinogenesis through mechanical irritation and excretion of toxic metabolites for the biliary epithelium, leading to inflammation, periductal fibrosis and proliferative response [4]. Recent studies have also highlighted the strong association of iCCA with metabolic conditions. Obesity, diabetes and non-alcoholic fatty liver disease (NAFLD), are all conditions characterized by a chronic, low-grade inflammatory response caused by insulin resistance, which is emerging as a risk factor for different epithelial malignancies [5].

In this chapter, we will first highlight the molecular underpinnings of the oncogenic effects related to inflammation and cholestasis. We review the different pathways and genetic anomalies related to these pathogenetic mechanisms, which are mostly relevant for iCCA pathogenesis. Then, we discuss the complex role of the tumor microenvironment in sustaining iCCA invasiveness, along with a systematic overview of the main cell types by which it is populated and the paracrine factors mediating their deleterious interplay.

Inflammation

Malignant transformation of biliary epithelial cells generally occurs in the setting of chronic inflammation, where high levels of a plethora of cytokines, chemokines, growth factors, and reactive oxygen species (ROS) induce molecular changes and dysregulation in proliferation, apoptosis, survival, and senescence signaling [1] (Fig. 12.1). iCCA frequently develops in liver disease conditions characterized by

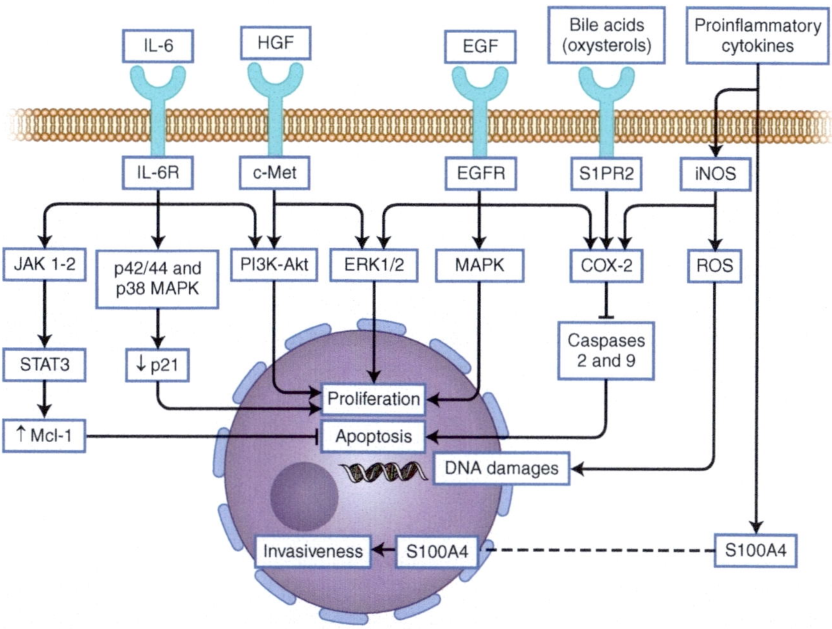

Fig. 12.1 Main intracellular pathways involved in iCCA carcinogenesis. Proliferation, apoptosis, malignant transformation, and cancer invasiveness are driven by numerous signal pathways typically activated in chronic inflammation and cholestasis, involving pro-inflammatory cytokines (i.e., IL-6), growth factors (i.e., EGF, and HGF), DAMP (S100A4), and bile acids. IL-6 interleukin-6, HGF hepatocyte growth factor, EGF epidermal growth factor, DAMP damage-associated molecular patterns, S1PR2 sphingosine-1-phosphate receptor 2, iNOS inducible nitric oxide synthases, IL-6R interleukin-6 receptor, MAPK mitogen-activated protein kinase, PI3K phosphatidylinositol-3-Kinase, ERK extracellular receptor kinase, COX cyclooxygenase, ROS reactive oxygen species, STAT signal transducer and activator of transcription, Mcl-1 Myeloid cell leukemia 1

different degrees of inflammation, such as intrahepatic lithiasis, intraductal parasitic infection, PSC, and CHF/CD. As such, several inflammatory mediators play a key role in bile ducts carcinogenesis.

Interleukin (IL)-6 is the principal cytokine of the IL-6 family and is a key mediator involved in the pathogenesis of CCA. IL-6 controls several pathways involved in cell proliferation and survival acting both in an autocrine and paracrine manner [6]. This cytokine is secreted at high levels by CCA cells and its signal is transduced through the binding to a heterodimer composed by the specific receptor IL-6R and by a low-affinity co-receptor gp80/130. IL-6 stimulates cancer cell proliferation through the stimulation of the mitogen-activated protein kinases (MAPK) pathway, ERK1/2 (also known as p42/44), and p38, which in turn promotes the downregulation of cyclin-dependent kinase inhibitor p21$^{WAF1/CIP1}$, a major cell cycle regulator and a typical marker of senescence [7]. IL-6 can also influence resistance to apoptosis in malignant cholangiocytes through the phosphorylation of the Janus kinases

(JAK)-1 and -2, leading to the phosphorylation of signal transducer and activator of transcription (STAT) proteins, in particular, of STAT3. Thus, phosphorylated STAT3 undergoes translocation into the nucleus, where it acts as a transcriptional factor upregulating the expression of several genes, including Myeloid Cell Leukemia-1 (Mcl-1), an anti-apoptotic protein belonging to the Bcl2 family, responsible for the resistance to tumor-necrosis-factor-related apoptosis-inducing ligand (TRAIL) [8]. Notably, this mechanism could be further sustained by another member of the IL-6 family, the leukemia inhibitory factor (LIF), expressed by both tumor cholangiocytes and inflammatory cells, that can be involved in inducing the strong chemoresistance typically affecting iCCA [9]. Under normal conditions, the IL-6-STAT3 signaling pathway is inhibited by suppressors of cytokine signaling 3 (SOCS-3), whereas this negative feedback is epigenetically silenced in CCA [10].

Hepatocyte growth factor (HGF) is a multifunctional growth factor secreted by several cell types, that could also stimulate malignant cell proliferation via its receptor c-MET; c-MET is overexpressed in tumor tissues and leads to the upregulation of a variety of signaling pathways, including phosphatidylinositol-4,5-bisphosphate 3-kinase (PI3K), STAT3, and Ras-MAPK. MET activation unfolds a broad invasive-growth program, that involves cell proliferation and survival, cell motility and scattering, branching morphogenesis, and angiogenesis [11]. MET amplification has been detected in 7% of iCCA and appears to be associated with poor clinical outcome, as well as increased resistance to MET inhibitors and acquired resistance to epidermal growth factor receptor (EGFR) and c-erb-B2/HER2 (ERBB2) inhibitors [12]. EGFR is overexpressed in 16% of CCA, with a marked prevalence in iCCA (around 30%), and is another factor relevant to cholangiocarcinogenesis. EGFR phosphorylation facilitates the downstream activation of the p38 MAPK, and of ERK1/2, responsible for the dysregulation of cell proliferation and cell-cell interactions. Another member of EGFR family, ERBB2, is overexpressed by malignant cholangiocytes (particularly ERBB2 amplifications are found to enrich in fluke-related CCAs) and contributes to CCA development by stimulating cancer cell proliferation. Interestingly, ERBB2, together with a wide range of cytokines and mitogens, including IL-6, HGF, EGF, and also bile acids, sustains cyclooxygenase (COX)-2 production, which in turn is involved in the activation of IL-6 receptor favoring a self-sustaining autocrine loop [13].

Whereas COX-1 is constitutively expressed by many cell types and regulates several physiological responses, COX-2 and its product, prostaglandin E_2(PGE_2), are increased in CCA, where these factors play a major role in shaping several malignant features. The COX2/PGE_2 axis interferes with apoptosis, either by upregulating Mcl-1 or by inhibiting caspase-2 and -9, two effectors of the pro-apoptotic cascade. Furthermore, the role of COX2 in cholangiocarcinogenesis is further confirmed by studying the effects on CCA growth of celecoxib, a selective COX2 inhibitor. Upon celecoxib treatment, CCA cells show an arrest at the G_1-S checkpoint in the cell cycle progression, while increasing the expression levels of the cdk inhibitors p21 and p27 [14]. In chronic cholangiopathies, COX2 activation is also stimulated by the *ex-novo* expression of inducible nitric oxide synthase (iNOS). This results in the accumulation of high local concentrations of nitric oxide (NO) and of reactive nitrogen oxide species (RNOS), responsible for the accumulation of DNA damages due to the generation of mutagenic compounds such as 8-oxo-7,8-dihydro-2′-deoxyguanosine (8-oxo-dG) and 8-nitro guanine. Moreover, mutagenic effects caused by RNOS accumulation depend on the inactivation DNA repair enzyme, such as 8-oxo-deoxyguanine DNA glycosylase 1 (hOGG1), through the nitrosylation of tyrosine and cysteine residues [15]. Several genetic mutations involving driver oncogenes (i.e., KRAS), tumor suppressor (i.e., p53, p16^{INK4a}, SMAD4, and APC) and chromatin-remodeling genes (i.e., ARID1A, PBRM1, and BAP1) have been reported in iCCA by next generation sequencing. Of note, inactivation of p53, a tumor suppressor gene regulating the balance between cell proliferation and apoptosis, is the most frequent genetic abnormality detected in iCCA (21.7–76%), while KRAS mutations are less common (9–17% of iCCA) [16]. Furthermore, a variety of fibroblast growth factor receptor 2 (FGFR2) gene fusion products have been noted in 10–16% of iCCA, highlighting the paramount importance of FGFR pathways in cholangiocarcinogenesis. Epigenetic modifications are inflammatory-related conditions of growing interest in the development of CCA; in particular, somatic mutations in isocitrate dehydrogenases (IDH)-1 and -2 have been detected in up to 25% of iCCA and their pro-oncogenic effects depend on the production of the oncometabolite 2-hydroxyglutarate (2-HG) which increases DNA methylation, thereby perturbing gene expression[17]. About 7% of iCCA are characterized by genetic inactivation of ARID1A that interacts with the switching defective/sucrose non-fermenting (SWI/SNF) chromatin-remodeling complex to inhibit the nuclear activity of the highly related transcriptional regulators yes-associated protein (YAP) and its transcriptional coactivator with PDZ-binding motif (TAZ). This inhibitory interaction is an alternative to YAP/TAZ association with TEAD leading to transcription of genes controlling cell fate plasticity, gain of stemness properties, and tumorigenesis [18]. Interestingly, the association between ARID1A–SWI/SNF and YAP/TAZ is influenced by mechanical stress derived from the cell microenvironment and may represent the molecular link by which an abnormally remodeled extracellular matrix (ECM) may exert pro-tumorigenic effects (see below) (Table 12.1).

Another protein recently found to be critically involved in CCA progression is S100A4 (also known as fibroblast-specific protein-1), a cytoskeletal calcium-binding protein, whose nuclear expression in malignant cholangiocytes has been shown to enhance tumor invasiveness and metastasis [19]. Usually localized in the cytoplasm of mesenchymal cells, following stimulation with IL1β, S100A4 may enter into the nucleus by undergoing SUMOylation, a post-translational mechanism similar to ubiquitination involved in multiple processes, among which gene transcription regulation, as demonstrated in human chondrocytes, or nuclear translocation. S100A4 nuclearization leads to the activation of the small GTPase Cdc-42 and Rho-A, the secretion of active matrix metalloproteinase (MMP)-9, and the expression of transmembrane metalloproteases MT-1-MMP, responsible for the formation of *invadopodia* (dynamic actin-based protrusions that degrade extracellular matrix) and thus enabling tumor cell invasion into the stromal microenvironment [20].

Table 12.1 List of gene mutations and signaling perturbations featuring iCCA

Gene/pathway alteration	Functional role
IL-6/IL-6R (gp130) overexpression	Cell proliferation, apoptosis resistance
HGF/c-MET amplification	Cell proliferation, survival, motility
EGFR overexpression	Cell proliferation, cell adhesion
HER2 amplification	Cell morphogenesis, development, and proliferation
KRAS mutations	Cell proliferation
BRAF mutations	Cell proliferation, secretion and differentiation
COX-2 overexpression	Cell proliferation, survival
Mcl-1 downregulation	Apoptosis
SWI-SNF complex inactivation	Cell differentiation
YAP/TAZ overexpression	Cell proliferation, survival, adhesion, migration
Hedgehog (Hh) overexpression	Development, cell migration
Notch overexpression	Cell proliferation, survival, migration, angiogenesis
p53 mutations	Cell cycle arrest, apoptosis, senescence, DNA repair
p21 $^{WAF1/CIP1}$and p27^{KIP1}downregulation	Negative cell cycle regulation
p16^{INK4a}, DPC4/Smad4 and APC inactivation	Cell cycle deceleration, cell attachment
FGFR2 rearrangements	Cell proliferation, differentiation and angiogenesis
IDH1–2 mutations	Altered methylation status and survival
MMP overexpression	ECM remodeling, cell migration
VEGF overexpression	Angiogenesis and lymphangiogenesis
PDGF-D overexpression	Lymphangiogenesis

IL interleukin, *HGF* hepatocyte growth factor, *EGF* epidermal growth factor, *HER* human epidermal growth factor receptor 2, *COX* cyclooxygenase, *YAP* yes-associated protein, *TAZ* transcriptional coactivator with PDZ-binding motif, *FGFR* fibroblast growth factor receptor, *IDH* Isocitrate dehydrogenase, *MMP* metalloproteinase, *VEGF* vascular endothelial growth factor, *PDGF* platelet-derived growth factor

Cholestasis

Cholestasis is another well-established risk factor for iCCA development along with chronic inflammation. The conjugated bile acids (CBA) and oxysterols, contained in the bile in high concentrations, stimulate production and secretion of several growth factors. CBAs promote tumorigenesis by acting as pro-proliferative agents, as well as by interfering with apoptosis. CBAs interact with sphingosine 1-phosphate receptor 2 (S1PR2) to activate ERK1/2 and Akt signaling; this modulatory axis activates the transcription factor nuclear factor kappa B (NF-kB) that unleashes IL-6 and COX-2 production. Moreover, CBAs may activate EGFR via a TNFα-dependent mechanism resulting in a mitogenic effect of cholangiocytes. CCA overgrowth is also promoted by the CBA-induced downregulation of the bile acid receptor farnesoid X-activated receptor (FXR), which instead, is upregulated by free bile acids [21]. Increased intracellular concentrations of CBAs contribute to resistance to apoptosis by inducing the overexpression of Mcl-1, which blocks the activation of the pro-apoptotic caspase cascade [22]. In contrast, increased levels of oxysterols, a product of cholesterol oxidation, promote carcinogenesis, and recently, oxysterols activate the developmental pathway of Hedgehog (Hh) by binding the extracellular domain of Smoothened, a G protein-coupled receptor transducing Hh signals [23]. The Sonic Hh variant is overexpressed by human CCA cells, whereby it modulates the cell cycle checkpoints and the migratory capabilities of malignant cells [24]. This interesting observation links cholestasis with a corruption of morphogenetic signaling ultimately leading to cancer as a perturbed developmental process.

Besides Hh, other morphogenetic pathways critically involved in liver embryogenesis and liver repair are often dysregulated in malignant cholangiocytes and have been implicated as fundamental players for cholangiocarcinogenesis. Recent studies have demonstrated that Notch1 orchestrates a pathologic transdifferentiation of hepatocytes into neoplastic cholangiocyte-like cells precursors of iCCA. Notch1 is overexpressed in iCCA tissue, and it is activated by its interaction with Jagged1 and Jagged2 ligands through a cell-cell contact. Upon ligand binding, Notch receptor undergoes two proteolytic cleavages operated by the metallo-endopeptidase containing a disintegrin and metalloprotease (ADAM) and γ-secretase leading to release of the Notch intracellular domain (NICD). NICD enters the nucleus and acts as transcriptional factor for many developmental genes, among which hairy and enhancer of split (Hes)-1, Hes-5, and Hairy/enhancer of split related with YRPW motif (Hey)-1, involved in cell fate determination, proliferation, migration, apoptosis, and angiogenesis [25]. In experimental cholestasis (3,5-diethoxycarbonyl-1,4-dihydrocollidine, DDC treatment), Notch activation is instrumental for biliary repair [26]. Moreover, using a mouse model of iCCA generated by the hydrodynamic transfection of the active form of Notch1 (NICD) and of the oncogene K-Ras^{V12D}, combined with cell-fate tracing techniques, iCCA originates from transdifferentiating hepatocytes. Treatment with different MEK inhibitors (U0126, PD901, and Selumetinib) induces iCCA regression by reducing proliferation and stimulating apoptosis [27]. Taking a similar approach, in which Notch2$^{flox/flox}$ mice were transfected with active forms of AKT and YAP, the absence of Notch2 prevents the neoplastic transformation of hepatocytes to iCCA generating in turn, hepatocellular adenoma-like lesions [28]. Overall, these findings suggest that persistent activation of both Hh and Notch signaling occurring in chronic cholestasis can exert potent oncogenic effects on the biliary epithelium.

Role of the Tumor Microenvironment in Inducing iCCA Invasiveness

The exuberant generation of a desmoplastic stroma, the TRS, is a characteristic trait of iCCA. TRS is composed of several cell elements lying in strict contact with each other, encompassing cancer-associated fibroblasts (CAF), tumor-associated macrophages (TAM), immune cells, lymphatic endothelial cells (LEC), assembled within an abnormal remodeled ECM consisting of collagen, glycoproteins, and

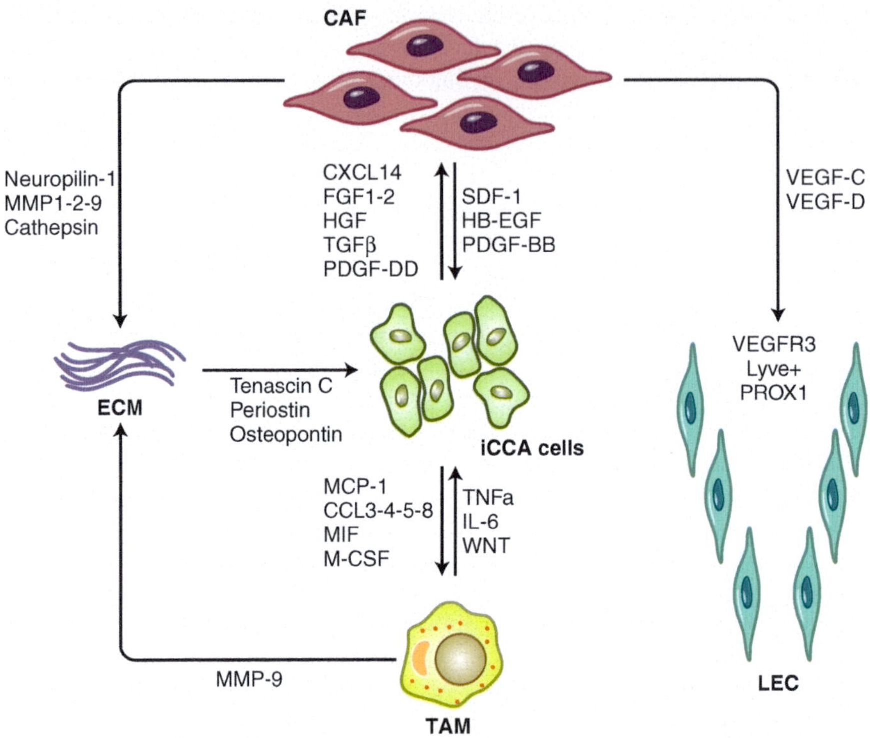

Fig. 12.2 Paracrine and autocrine factors mediating the complex interplay between neoplastic and stromal compartment in iCCA. Within the tumor microenvironment, multiple cell types densely surround the neoplastic bile ducts and provide them with several peptides stimulating the main malignant properties of CCA. On the other hand, malignant cholangiocytes are main drivers involved in the recruitment and activation of cells populating the TRS (CAF, TAM, and LEC, among others). iCCA intrahepatic cholangiocarcinoma, CAF cancer-associated fibroblast, TAM tumor-associated macrophage, LEC lymphatic endothelial cell, ECM extracellular matrix, FGF fibroblast growth factor, TGF transforming growth factor, HGF hepatocyte growth factor, MCP1 monocyte chemoattractant protein 1, MIF macrophage migration inhibitory factor, M-CSF monocyte colony stimulating factor, TNF tumor necrosis factor, IL interleukin, SDF stromal cell-derived factor, MMP metalloproteinase, VEGF vascular endothelial growth factor, PDGF platelet-derived growth factor

proteoglycans [29]. An intense cross talk mediated by a multitude of autocrine and paracrine cues occurs between the malignant and the stromal component and contribute to the acquisition of the hallmarks of cancer (Fig. 12.2).

CAFs

CAFs are the most represented cell population within the TRS. CAFs are a type of perpetually activated myofibroblasts, characterized by the expression of α-smooth muscle actin (SMA), vimentin, S1000A4, and fibroblasts activation protein (FAP) and are supposed to originate from different cell sources, including hepatic stellate cells (HSC), portal fibroblasts (PF), or bone marrow-derived mesenchymal cells. Once attracted nearby the malignant ducts, CAFs are activated by a broad range of cytokines, chemokines and growth factors largely produced from both CCA and inflammatory cells [30–32]. The most prominent are C-C motif chemokine ligand 2 (CCL2), C-X-C motif chemokine 14 (CXCL14), stromal cell-derived factor (SDF-1) fibroblast growth factor (FGF) 1-2, transforming growth factor (TGF)-β, insulin-like growth factor (IGF)-1, HGF, granulocyte-macrophage colony stimulating factor (GM-CSF)-1, and platelet-derived growth factors (PDGF). A stand-alone role is played by PDGF-DD. PDGF-DD is, in fact, overexpressed by neoplastic cholangiocytes under hypoxic conditions and binds to its cognate receptor, PDGFRβ, expressed by CAF, to activate both a proliferative ERK1/2-dependent pathway and a pro-migratory cascade, mediated by the activation of Rho-GTPases (in particular, Rac-1 and Cdc42) and by the phosphorylation of JNK [33]. Once within the tumor microenvironment, CAFs sustain cancer progression by releasing a plethora of cues, in particular, SDF-1, PDGF-BB, heparin-binding (HB)-EGF, and TGFβ, which molds the malignant behavior of tumor cholangiocytes by affecting their proliferation, survival, migration, and invasiveness.

SDF-1, also known as CXCL12, is a chemokine that, working in concert with the HGF/c-MET axis, binds to its specific receptor CXCR4 expressed by malignant cholangiocytes to activate ERK1/2 and PI3K/Akt pathways, providing them with a proliferative advantage. Notably, tumor cholangiocytes are hyper-responsive to SDF-1, as they overexpress CXCR4 upon the joint effect of TNFα secreted by TAM and HGF derived from the CAF themselves [30]. SDF-1 confers also a survival advantage to CCA cells by upregulating the expression of the anti-apoptotic protein Bcl-2 [34]. PDGF-BB is another member of the PDGF family suffice to stimulate pro-migratory and proliferative functions in CCA cells, together with an enhanced resistance to apoptosis. PDGF-BB is also able to inhibit the release of TRAIL, a regulator of apoptotic cellular responses, by activating the Hh signaling. Specifically, the interaction between PDGF-BB and its receptor PDGFRβ (also expressed by CCA cells) results in increased intracellular levels of cyclic adenosine monophosphate (cAMP), which stimulate the PKA-dependent translocation of Smoothened to the plasma membrane, followed by glioma-associated oncogene (GLI) activation, ultimately responsible for Hh stimulation [35].

HB-EGF is a growth factor copiously produced by CAF that supports tumor growth and metastasization through a paracrine loop. HB-EGF is a ligand for EGFR, whose activation is one of the most frequent phenotypic changes underlying CCA development. Activation of the HB-EGF/EGFR axis on one side stimulates the ERK1/2 and STAT3 pathways, while on the other, unfolds a β-catenin-mediated transcriptional program, proficient in cell migration and invasion. Of note, EGFR expression promotes TGFβ production by CCA cells, which further stimulates HB-EGF synthesis, in a self-perpetuating autocrine loop [36].

Moreover, CAFs act on the tumor microenvironment by displaying strong ECM modifying capabilities mediated by the production of multiple proteins, encompassing neuropilin-1, several MMPs (MMP-1, MMP-2, and MMP-9), cathepsins, and plasminogen activators, which remodel qualitatively and quantitatively the ECM scaffold through the modulation of integrin expression and changes in the collagen composition. This pathological remodeling results in an increased ECM stiffness that is essential for the activation of intracellular mechanosensors by which cells decipher structural changes of their microenvironment to assume a more aggressive malignant phenotype. In fact, a stiffer ECM activates YAP/TAZ [37] to induce a range of pro-oncogenic effects, such as cell proliferation, gain of stem cell-like properties, and invasive functions [29].

ECM ability to support cancer aggressiveness is also sustained by the aberrant deposition by CAFs and by other inflammatory cells of tenascin-C and periostin, two structural proteins acting as modulators of integrin-mediated pathways, which impinge upon CCA cell proliferation and invasion [30]. Besides effects on tumor cells and ECM, CAF favor TRS crowding by recruiting other stromal cell elements, in particular, inflammatory cells and endothelial cells, ultimately aiding the tumor spread.

TAMs

TAMs are the most represented immune cell population within the CCA microenvironment. TAMs mainly originate from circulating monocytes and are engaged nearby the tumor area by a variety of soluble factors secreted by either neoplastic or stromal cells, such as monocyte chemoattractant protein (MCP)-1, CCL3, CCL4, CCL5, CCL8, macrophage migration inhibitory protein-1α, vascular endothelial growth factor (VEGF), and M-CSF [31]. Once recruited into the TRS, monocytes can trans-differentiate prevalently into M2 macrophages, characterized by the constitutive expression of CCL17, CCL18, IL1α, IL6, IL10, and Arginase-1 under the control of PGE_2, IL-2, IL-10, and TGFβ [29]. In CCA, TAMs closely cooperate with CAF to generate a milieu tolerant to tumor growth and invasion, both by suppressing anti-tumor functions exerted by T cells and M1 macrophages, and by promoting tumor cell proliferation, migration, and apoptosis resistance, ECM remodeling, and angiogenesis. Several soluble factors underpin pro-tumorigenic effects of TAMs, including TNFα, IL6, and MMP-9. TNFα is in fact abundantly produced by lipopolysaccharide (LPS)-activated macrophages located at the tumor edge, and foster epithelial-to-mesenchymal-transition (EMT)-like phenotypic changes in CCA cells, resulting in the downregulation of epithelial markers, such as cytokeratin (K) 7 and 19, E-cadherin, and EpCAM, and upregulation of mesenchymal markers, such as N-cadherin, and vimentin, via a Snail and ZEB2-mediated processes [38]. Moreover, the activation of the TNFα-specific receptor TNFR2 stimulates the production by macrophages of MMPs, in particular, of MMP-9. MMP-9 secretion is stimulated by the activation of NF-kB, Akt, and MAPK signaling responsible for the activation of COX2 that, through PGE_2, acts as a trigger for MMP-9 secretion and activation [39]. MMPs secreted by TAMs are fundamental for the breakdown of the basement membrane, mainly composed by laminin, and of the surrounding matrix favoring intravasation of neoplastic cells and their metastatization. In addition, TAMs are a source of IL-6 and may activate morphogenetic pathways, such as the WNT/β--catenin signaling. In particular, Wnt3 produced by LPS-activated macrophages binds to its receptor Frizzle, whose stimulation leads to nuclear translocation of β-catenin, where it can regulate expression of oncogenes, such as c-Myc and cyclin D1 [40].

Immune Cells

During cancer growth, tumor cells progressively develop skills to avoid immune surveillance by activating a range of stratagems, including the expression of tumor-specific antigens, upregulation of immune checkpoint molecules, or secretory abilities to suppress proliferation of $CD4^+$ and $CD8^+$ lymphocyte proliferation [41]. Antagonizing mechanisms regulating escape from tumor immune response has become one of the most promising approaches for the treatment of malignancies with strong resistance to conventional chemotherapeutic agents or without alternative treatments, as the case of CCA. The blockade of the programmed-death cell protein (PD) receptor and ligand (PD-1/PD-L1) axis is one of the most valuable strategies in this context, as shown in both hematologic and solid neoplasms, including Hodgkin's lymphoma, non-small-cell lung cancer (NSCLC), renal cell carcinoma (RCC), and bladder cancer. Under physiological conditions, the interaction between PD-1, expressed on activated T and B cells, and PD-L1, expressed by macrophages and lymphocytes, induces $CD8^+$ cell exhaustion, controls tolerance, and attenuates immune response, reducing T cell activation and empowering the immunosuppressive functions of regulatory T cells (Tregs). In the tumor microenvironment, persistent overexpression of PD-1/PD-L1 correlates with poor disease outcome [42]. Cytokines, such as IFNγ and TNFα, abundantly released in the tumor microenvironment, upregulate PD-L1 expression not only on T, B, and endothelial cells but also on tumor cells, leading to PD-1 activation. PD-1 is usually expressed by tumor-infiltrating lymphocytes (TIL) to induce T cell exhaustion, and consequently loss of their ability to produce pro-inflammatory cytokines and cytolitic molecules [43]. Noteworthy, effectiveness of PD-L1 antibodies, such as pembrolizumab, has been tested in several clinical trials for patients with advanced iCCA and histological evidence of a dense TIL accumulation, with encouraging results [44].

LECs

Another structural component that is crucial for the TRS functions is the lymphatic network that develops in and around the neoplastic scar, and importantly, its extent correlates with a worse outcome and a shorter disease-free and overall survival in iCCA [45]. On a physiological ground, the function of the lymphatic system is to regulate fluid homeostasis, facilitate interstitial protein transport, and sustain immunological functions. Lymphatic vessels are composed by a thin layer of LEC, surrounded by a discontinuous wall of αSMA$^+$ mural cells, equipped with fenestrations, enabling immune cell migration, and with valves, to direct progression of the lymphatic fluid flux. LECs are characterized by the expression of several specific proteins, among which lymphatic vessel endothelial hyaluronan receptor-1 (Lyve-1), the sialoprotein podoplanin (PDPN), and the transcription factor prospero homeobox 1 (PROX1), together with VEGFR3, the cognate receptor for the main pro-lymphangiogenic growth factors, VEGF-C and VEGF-D, and by the co-receptor neuropilin-1. Besides, LECs express major histocompatibility complex class (MCH) I and II, sharing with professional antigen-presenting cells (APC) the ability to dictate self-tolerance [46]. In addition, LECs are a source of chemokines (i.e., CCL-19 and CCL-21) and express adhesion molecules, i.e. macrophage mannose receptor (MR), and common lymphatic endothelial and vascular endothelial receptor-1 (CLEVER-1), which facilitate leukocyte trafficking and transmigration [47]. Unfortunately, the flipside of this vast expression of adhesion molecules enabling cell trafficking is that they may favor tumor cell intravasation and thus, lymphatic metastasis. Similar to what happens with other solid cancer types, including melanoma, lung, colon, and breast cancer, lymphatic dissemination is the major route for tumor spread in iCCA, and the assessment of lymph node involvement is a critical step towards tumor staging and therapeutic patient stratification. In contrast with hepatocellular carcinoma (HCC) associated with a rich, newly formed blood vessel bed, which is a diagnostic hallmark, iCCA is characterized by a prominent tumor-associated lymphangiogenesis, which correlates with tumor progression (45). Among the main lymphangiogenic growth factors, VEGF-C is the most extensively studied. Upon VEGF-C stimulation, VEGFR-3 leads to the activation of PI3K/Akt and ERK pathways, which promote LEC proliferation, survival, and vascular assembly and sprouting. Of note, PI3K, the upstream activator of Akt, has been shown to interact directly with VEGFR-3 and to elicit LEC tube formation and migration, via a Rho GTPase Rac1-mediated pathway [48]. Angiopoietins (Ang-1 and Ang-2), and their cognate receptor Tie-2, are a further lymphangiogenic system regulating the endothelial layer stability, but with opposite roles. Whereas Ang-1 stimulates vascular stabilization and maturation in a paracrine manner, Ang-2 acts through an autocrine loop to induce vessel destabilization and disruption as prerequisite for vascular sprouting [49]. Different PDGF family members, as shown in CCA for PDGF-D, strongly cooperate to tumor-associated lymphangiogenesis. Besides promoting CAF migration and activation [33], tumor cell-derived PDGF-D enables CAF to produce VEGF-A and VEGF-C. In turn, VEGF-A and VEGF-C, by interacting with their receptors VEGFR-2 and VEGFR-3 expressed by LECs, kindle LEC migration and gathering into highly branched vascular structures, where they also enhance the endothelial permeability to make lymphatic vessels proficient to cancer cell invasion [50]. Tumor-associated lymphangiogenesis is a research area worth being further explored in order to identify new therapeutic avenues aimed at preventing iCCA spread.

Conclusion

In the last few years, increasing efforts have been made to unravel the complex landscape of molecular mechanisms promoting iCCA development, growth, and dissemination. Based on these findings, it is becoming clear that chronic inflammation and cholestasis occurring in several pre-malignant liver disease conditions are often associated with a perturbation of intracellular pathways controlled by driver oncogenes found to be strongly associated with iCCA. Beyond tumorigenesis, a critical component driving tumor progression is then the development of a highly dynamic TRS, acting as an engine that oversees and enhances numerous pro-invasive features of malignant cholangiocytes. Inside this multicellular compartment, where cell interactions are supported by an abnormally remodeled ECM, CAF work in concert with innate and adaptive immune cells, including TAM and TIL, to shape a microenvironment with a proclivity to cancer spread. In this setting, lymphatic vessels behave as a preferential route of dissemination. Given the wide heterogeneity of the tumor microenvironment in iCCA, it represents a challenge to derive relevant populations for basic research and drug discovery and may serve as a model that can be translated also to other epithelial tumors characterized by abundant desmoplasia, such as pancreatic or breast carcinomas.

Acknowledgments M.C. was supported by Fondazione Cariplo, Grant No. 2014-1099; L.F. was supported by the University of Padua, Progetti di Ricerca di Dipartimento (PRID) 2017.

Conflict of Interest Statement Authors have nothing to disclose.

References

1. Banales JM, Cardinale V, Carpino G, Marzioni M, Andersen JB, Invernizzi P, et al. Expert consensus document: cholangiocarcinoma: current knowledge and future perspectives consensus statement from the European Network for the Study of Cholangiocarcinoma (ENS-CCA). Nat Rev Gastroenterol Hepatol. 2016;13:261–80.
2. Cadamuro M, Stecca T, Brivio S, Mariotti V, Fiorotto R, Spirli C, et al. The deleterious interplay between tumor epithelia and stroma in cholangiocarcinoma. Biochim Biophys Acta Mol basis Dis. 2018;1864:1435–43.
3. Brivio S, Cadamuro M, Fabris L, Strazzabosco M. Molecular mechanisms driving cholangiocarcinoma invasiveness: an overview. Gene Expr. 2018;18:31–50.
4. Gupta A, Dixon E. Epidemiology and risk factors: intrahepatic cholangiocarcinoma. Hepatobiliary Surg Nutr. 2017;6(2):101–4.
5. Weroha SJ, Haluska P. The insulin-like growth factor system in cancer. Endocrinol Metab Clin N Am. 2012;41:335–50.
6. Berthiaume EP, Wands J. The molecular pathogenesis of cholangiocarcinoma. Semin Liver Dis. 2004;24:127–37.
7. Tadlock L, Patel T. Involvement of p38 mitogen-activated protein kinase signaling in transformed growth of a cholangiocarcinoma cell line. Hepatology. 2001;33(1):43–51.

8. Isomoto H, Kobayashi S, Werneburg NW, Bronk SF, Guicciardi ME, Frank DA, et al. Interleukin 6 upregulates myeloid cell leukemia-1 expression through a STAT3 pathway in cholangiocarcinoma cells. Hepatology. 2005;42(6):1329–38.
9. Morton SD, Cadamuro M, Brivio S, Vismara M, Stecca T, Massani M, et al. Leukemia inhibitory factor protects cholangiocarcinoma cells from drug-induced apoptosis via a PI3K/AKT-dependent Mcl-1 activation. Oncotarget. 2015;6(28):26052–64.
10. Isomoto H, Mott JL, Kobayashi S, Werneburg NW, Bronk SF, Haan S, et al. Sustained IL-6/STAT-3 signaling in cholangiocarcinoma cells due to SOCS-3 epigenetic silencing. Gastroenterology. 2007;132(1):384–96.
11. Comoglio PM, Giordano S, Trusolino L. Drug development of MET inhibitors: targeting oncogene addiction and expedience. Nat Rev Drug Discov. 2008;7:504–16.
12. Appleman LJ. MET signaling pathway: a rational target for cancer therapy. J Clin Oncol. 2011;29(36):4837–8.
13. Fava G, Lorenzini I. Molecular pathogenesis of cholangiocarcinoma. Dig Dis. 2014;32(5): 564–9.
14. Wu T. Cyclooxygenase-2 and prostaglandin signaling in cholangiocarcinoma. Biochim Biophys Acta (Rev Cancer). 2005;1755(2):135–50.
15. Jaiswal M, LaRusso NF, Burgart LJ, Gores GJ. Inflammatory cytokines induce DNA damage and inhibit DNA repair in cholangiocarcinoma cells by a nitric oxide-dependent mechanism. Cancer Res. 2000;60(1):184–90.
16. Blechacz B, Gores GJ. Cholangiocarcinoma: advances in pathogenesis, diagnosis, and treatment. Hepatology. 2008;48:308–21.
17. Wang P, Dong Q, Zhang C, Kuan PF, Liu Y, Jeck WR, et al. Mutations in isocitrate dehydrogenase 1 and 2 occur frequently in intrahepatic cholangiocarcinomas and share hypermethylation targets with glioblastomas. Oncogene. 2013;32(25):3091–100.
18. Chang L, Azzolin L, Di Biagio D, Zanconato F, Battilana G, Lucon Xiccato R, et al. The SWI/SNF complex is a mechanoregulated inhibitor of YAP and TAZ. Nature. 2018;563(7730):265–9.
19. Fabris L, Cadamuro M, Moserle L, Dziura J, Cong X, Sambado L, et al. Nuclear expression of S100A4 calcium-binding protein increases cholangiocarcinoma invasiveness and metastasization. Hepatology. 2011;54(3):890–9.
20. Cadamuro M, Spagnuolo G, Sambado L, Indraccolo S, Nardo G, Rosato A, et al. Low-dose paclitaxel reduces S100A4 nuclear import to inhibit invasion and hematogenous metastasis of cholangiocarcinoma. Cancer Res. 2016;76(16):4775–84.
21. Liu R, Zhao R, Zhou X, Liang X, Campbell DJW, Zhang X, et al. Conjugated bile acids promote cholangiocarcinoma cell invasive growth through activation of sphingosine 1-phosphate receptor 2. Hepatology. 2014;60(3):908–18.
22. Yoon J, Werneburg NW, Higuchi H, Canbay AE, Kaufmann SH, Akgul C, et al. Bile acids inhibit Mcl-1 protein turnover via anEpidermal Growth Factor Receptor/Raf-1-dependent Mechanism. Cancer Res. 2002;62(22):6500–5.
23. Nedelcu D, Liu J, Xu Y, Jao C, Salic A. Oxysterol binding to the extracellular domain of smoothened in hedgehog signaling. Nat Chem Biol. 2013;9(9):557–64.
24. El Khatib M, Kalnytska A, Palagani V, Kossatz U, Manns MP, Malek NP, et al. Inhibition of hedgehog signaling attenuates carcinogenesis in vitro and increases necrosis of cholangiocellular carcinoma. Hepatology. 2013;57(3):1035–45.
25. Zhou Q, Wang Y, Peng B, Liang L, Li J. The roles of Notch1 expression in the migration of intrahepatic cholangiocarcinoma. BMC Cancer. 2013;13(1):1.
26. Morell CM, Fiorotto R, Fabris L, Strazzabosco M. Notch signaling beyond liver development: emerging concepts in liver repair and oncogenesis. Clin Res Hepatol Gastroenterol. 2013;37:447–54.
27. Dong M, Liu X, Evert K, Utpatel K, Peters M, Zhang S, et al. Efficacy of MEK inhibition in a K-Ras-driven cholangiocarcinoma preclinical model. Cell Death Dis. 2018;9(2)
28. Wang J, Dong M, Xu Z, Song X, Zhang S, Qiao Y, et al. Notch2 controls hepatocyte-derived cholangiocarcinoma formation in mice. Oncogene. 2018;37(24):3229–42.

29. Brivio S, Cadamuro M, Strazzabosco M, Fabris L. Tumor reactive stroma in cholangiocarcinoma: The fuel behind cancer aggressiveness. World J Hepatol. 2017;9(9):455–68.
30. Sirica AE. The role of cancer-associated myofibroblasts in intrahepatic cholangiocarcinoma. Nat Rev Gastroenterol Hepatol. 2012;9:44–54.
31. Gentilini A, Pastore M, Marra F, Raggi C. The role of stroma in cholangiocarcinoma: the intriguing interplay between fibroblastic component, immune cell subsets, and tumor epithelium. Int J Mol Sci. 2018;19
32. Pinto C, Giordano DM, Maroni L, Marzioni M. Role of inflammation and proinflammatory cytokines in cholangiocyte pathophysiology. Biochim Biophys Acta Mol basis Dis. 2018;1864:1270–8.
33. Cadamuro M, Nardo G, Indraccolo S, Dall'Olmo L, Sambado L, Moserle L, et al. Platelet-derived growth factor-D and Rho GTPases regulate recruitment of cancer-associated fibroblasts in cholangiocarcinoma. Hepatology. 2013;58(3):1042–53.
34. Gentilini A, Rombouts K, Galastri S, Caligiuri A, Mingarelli E, Mello T, et al. Role of the stromal-derived factor-1 (SDF-1)-CXCR4 axis in the interaction between hepatic stellate cells and cholangiocarcinoma. J Hepatol. 2012;57(4):813–20.
35. Fingas CD, Bronk SF, Werneburg NW, Mott JL, Guicciardi ME, Cazanave SC, et al. Myofibroblast-derived PDGF-BB promotes hedgehog survival signaling in cholangiocarcinoma cells. Hepatology. 2011;54(6):2076–88.
36. Clapéron A, Mergey M, Aoudjehane L, Ho-Bouldoires THN, Wendum D, Prignon A, et al. Hepatic myofibroblasts promote the progression of human cholangiocarcinoma through activation of epidermal growth factor receptor. Hepatology. 2013;58(6):2001–11.
37. Zanconato F, Cordenonsi M, Piccolo S. YAP/TAZ at the roots of cancer. Cancer Cell. 2016;29(6):783–803.
38. Techasen A, Namwat N, Loilome W, Duangkumpha K, Puapairoj A, Saya H, et al. Tumor necrosis factor-α modulates epithelial mesenchymal transition mediators ZEB2 and S100A4 to promote cholangiocarcinoma progression. J Hepatobiliary Pancreat Sci. 2014;21(9):703–11.
39. Tanimura Y, Kokuryo T, Tsunoda N, Yamazaki Y, Oda K, Nimura Y, et al. Tumor necrosis factor α promotes invasiveness of cholangiocarcinoma cells via its receptor, TNFR2. Cancer Lett. 2005;219(2):205–13.
40. Loilome W, Bungkanjana P, Techasen A, Namwat N, Yongvanit P, Puapairoj A, et al. Activated macrophages promote Wnt/β-catenin signaling in cholangiocarcinoma cells. Tumor Biol. 2014;35(6):5357–67.
41. Hanahan D, Weinberg RA. Hallmarks of cancer: the next generation. Cell. 2011;144:646–74.
42. Gao Q, Wang XY, Qiu SJ, Yamato I, Sho M, Nakajima Y, et al. Overexpression of PD-L1 significantly associates with tumor aggressiveness and postoperative recurrence in human hepatocellular carcinoma. Clin Cancer Res. 2009;15(3):971–9.
43. Ohaegbulam KC, Assal A, Lazar-Molnar E, Yao Y, Zang X. Human cancer immunotherapy with antibodies to the PD-1 and PD-L1 pathway. Trends Mol Med. 2015;21:24–33.
44. Fontugne J, Augustin J, Pujals A, Compagnon P, Rousseau B, Luciani A, et al. PD-L1 expression in perihilar and intrahepatic cholangiocarcinoma. Oncotarget [Internet]. 2017;8(15). Available from: http://www.oncotarget.com/fulltext/15602.
45. Thelen A, Scholz A, Weichert W, Wiedenmann B, Neuhaus P, Gener R, et al. Tumor-associated angiogenesis and lymphangiogenesis correlate with progression of intrahepatic cholangiocarcinoma. Am J Gastroenterol. 2010;105(5):1123–32.
46. Tewalt EF, Cohen JN, Rouhani SJ, Engelhard VH. Lymphatic endothelial cells – key players in regulation of tolerance and immunity. Front Immunol. 2012;3(SEP):1–6.
47. Irjala H, Alanen K, Grénman R, Heikkilä P, Joensuu H, Jalkanen S. Mannose receptor (MR) and common lymphatic endothelial and vascular endothelial receptor (CLEVER)-1 direct the binding of cancer cells to the lymph vessel endothelium. Cancer Res. 2003;63(15):4671–6.
48. Zheng W, Aspelund A, Alitalo K. Lymphangiogenic factors, mechanisms, and applications. J Clin Investig. 2014;124:878–87.

49. Augustin HG, Young Koh G, Thurston G, Alitalo K. Control of vascular morphogenesis and homeostasis through the angiopoietin – Tie system. Nat Rev Mol Cell Biol. 2009;10(3):165–77.
50. Cadamuro M, Brivio S, Mertens J, et al. Platelet-derived growth factor-D enables liver Myofibroblasts to promote tumor Lymphangiogenesis in cholangiocarcinoma. J Hepatol. 2018;70(4):700–9.

Chapter 13
Clinical Trials and Novel/Emerging Treatment

Jonathan D. Mizrahi, Reham Abdel-Wahab, and Milind Javle

Introduction

Intrahepatic cholangiocarcinoma (ICC) is increasing in incidence and presents a therapeutic challenge, as most patients present at an advanced unresectable stage and face an adverse prognosis. Recent next-generation sequencing studies indicate that these tumors are enriched with several actionable mutations, perhaps more than other gastrointestinal cancers. Morphologically, these tumors are diverse and may be mass-forming, intraductal or periductal [1]. Therefore, the traditional, "one-size-fits-all" approach is not ideal for this cancer. Historically, liver-directed approaches have been more commonly used in hepatocellular cancer, while systemic chemotherapy remains the primary approach for the advanced stage of ICC. This paradigm has fortunately begun to change, and patients with ICC now have multiple treatment options including liver-directed and targeted therapies based on underlying mutational profile.

J. D. Mizrahi
Division of Cancer Medicine, The University of Texas MD Anderson Cancer Center, Houston, TX, USA
e-mail: JDMizrahi@mdanderson.org

R. Abdel-Wahab
Department of Gastrointestinal Medical Oncology, The University of Texas MD Anderson Cancer Center, Houston, TX, USA

Clinical Oncology Department, Faculty of Medicine, Assiut University, Asyut, Egypt
e-mail: RAAli@mdanderson.org

M. Javle (✉)
Department of Gastrointestinal Medical Oncology, The University of Texas MD Anderson Cancer Center, Houston, TX, USA
e-mail: mjavle@mdanderson.org

T. M. Pawlik et al. (eds.), *Intrahepatic Cholangiocarcinoma*,
https://doi.org/10.1007/978-3-030-22258-1_13

Liver-Directed Locoregional Therapies

Over two-thirds of ICC patients have unresectable disease at diagnosis and 71% of patients who undergo curative-intent resection develop postoperative disease recurrence. Local or regional recurrence after surgery occurs in 85% of the patients [2]. The role of locoregional therapies in ICC, including transarterial chemoembolization (TACE), transarterial radioembolization, hepatic artery infusion (HAI), radiation therapy, and radiofrequency (RFA), is still controversial and have not been evaluated in prospective randomized control trials. These therapies are reviewed below.

Radiation Therapy

With the remarkable advances in the radiotherapy technology, radiation therapy is now safe and effective for patients with ICC, particularly for those with an adequate liver reserve and without advanced primary sclerosing cholangitis (PSC). The use of radiotherapy for ICC can be in the adjuvant or advanced disease setting. Given the positive results of the adjuvant therapy for biliary cancer (BILCAP) trial, which showed improved overall survival with capecitabine as compared with placebo, chemotherapy after surgical resection of ICC is preferred [3]. A large retrospective review of 3839 ICC patients from the Surveillance, Epidemiology, and End Results (SEER) indicated however that surgery followed by adjuvant radiotherapy results in a significantly higher overall survival (OS) compared with surgery alone ($P = 0.01$). Similarly, patients treated with definitive radiotherapy (without resection) had a higher OS than patients who did not receive any radiation in this study [4]. Zheng et al. compared the treatment outcome of ICC treated with hepatectomy with postoperative radiotherapy for close margin (group A), hepatectomy without adjuvant radiotherapy for close margin (group B), and hepatectomy with a wide margin. This study showed that adjuvant radiotherapy for close surgical margin improved the 3-year OS, progression-free survival (PFS) and extrahepatic recurrence (55%, 44%, and 43%, respectively) as compared with 20%, 10%, and 65% in group B ($P = 0.01$, 0.03, and 0.007, respectively) [5]. Additionally, a meta-analysis of 11 studies with 226 unresectable or recurrent CCA patients was performed to evaluate the role of stereotactic body radiation therapy (SBRT). The median OS was 13.6 months with 53.8% pooled 1-year OS, 81.8% 1-year local recurrence rate, <10% grade 3 acute toxicity, and 10–20% late toxicity [6]. Studies investigating the role of radiation in ICC are summarized in Table 13.1 [7–12]. High doses of radiation can be safely delivered safely for ICC and in a study conducted at MD Anderson Cancer Center, dose correlated with longer OS and higher local control rate. Doses more than 80.5 Gy result in the median OS of 30 months and a 3-year OS with local control rate of 73% and 78%, respectively [13]. Novel approaches including high-dose hypofractionated proton therapy may be another promising modality for ICC. In a

Table 13.1 Clinical studies of locoregional therapy of unresectable ICC

Authors	Year	Country	Patients $N = ()$	Treatment sessions median (range)	Therapeutic agents	Median OS (months)	1-year OS rate (%)	DCR $N = (\%)$
cTACE								
Burger et al. [31]	2005	USA	17	2 (1–4)	Cisplatin	23	NA	NA
Herber et al. [29]	2007	Germany	15	3.9 (1–15)	Mitomycin-C	21.1	51.3%	10 (66.7%)
Gusani et al. [30]	2008	USA	42	3.5 (1–16)	Gemcitabine ($n = 18$) Gemcitabine/cisplatin ($n = 14$) Gemciatbine/cisplatin followed by oxaliplatin ($n = 4$) Gemcitabine followed by oxaliplatin ($n = 4$) Gemcitabine followed by cisplatin ($n = 2$)	Overall (9.1) Gemcitabine (6.3) Gemcitabine/cisplatin (13.8)	NA	20 (571%)[a]
Kim et al. [27]	2008	Republic of Korea	49	3 (1–17)	Cisplatin	10	46%	42 (55%)
Park et al. [26]	2011	Republic of Korea	72	2.5 (1–17)	Cisplatin	12.2	51%	59 (89.4%)[b]
Kiefer et al. [28]	2011	USA	62	2 (1–4)	Cisplatin/doxorubicin/mitomycin-C	15	61%	34 (75.6%)[c]
Vogl et al. [25]	2012	Germany	115	7.1 (3–30)	Gemcitabine ($n = 8$) Mitomycin-C ($n = 24$) Gemcitabine/mitomycin-C ($n = 54$) Gemcitabine/mitomycin-C/cisplatin ($n = 29$)	13	52%	76 (66.1%)

(continued)

Table 13.1 (continued)

Authors	Year	Country	Patients $N = ()$	Treatment sessions median (range)	Therapeutic agents	Median OS (months)	1-year OS rate (%)	DCR $N = (\%)$
DEB-TACE								
Poggi et al. [33]	2009	Italy	9	NA	Oxaliplatin eluting microspheres	30	NA	9 (100%)
Schiffman et al. [32]	2011	USA	24	NA	Doxorubicin ($n = 7$ sessions) Irinotecan ($n = 35$ sessions)	17.5	NA	22 (92%)
Aliberti et al. [34]	2017	Italy	127	NA	DEB doxorubicin ($n = 109$) LIF doxorubicin ($n = 18$)	DEBDOX: 14.3 LIFDOX: 13	NA	All: 120 (95%) DEBDOX: 103 (95%) LIFDOX: 15 (85%)
Y-90 radioembolization								
Ibrahim et al. [42]	2008	USA	24	1–2	–	14.9	NA	21 (95.5%)[d]
Saxena et al. [40]	2010	Australia	25	1–2	–	9.3	40%	17 (72%)[e]
Hoffmann et al. [43]	2012	Germany	33	1–2	–	22	NA	29 (87.9%)
Soydal et al. [38]	2016	Turkey	16	1–2	–	9.6	NA	NA
Shaker et al. [39]	2018	USA	17	1–2	–	33.6	NA	NA
Reimer et al. [41]	2018	Germany	21	1–2	–	15	NA	10 (47.6%)
Hepatic artery infusion								
Tanaka et al. [48]	2002	Japan	11	51 (12–84)	Fluorouracil	26	91%	9 (82%)
Shitara et al. [45]	2008	Japan	20	8 (2–46)	Mitomycin-C/degradable starch microspheres	14.1	NA	18 (90%)
Jarnagin et al. [46]	2009	USA	26	7 (2–25)	Floxuridine	NA	NA	25 (96.1%)
Inaba et al. [47]	2011	Japan	13	NA	Gemcitabine	12.8	NA	1 (7.7%)
Ghiringhelli et al. [50]	2013	France	12	7 (2–15)	Gemcitabine/oxaliplatin	20.3	NA	11 (91.7%)
Massani et al. [49]	2015	Italy	11	6	Fluorouracil/oxaliplatin	17.6	NA	7 (63.6%)

Radiation therapy (Rth)								
Jiang et al. [8]	2010	China	90	50 Gy (34–60)	Surgery + adjuvant Rth (n = 24) Surgery alone (n = 66)	Rth: 19.1 Surgery alone: 9.5	Rth: 68.8% Surgery alone: 43.2%	Rth: 18 (65%)
Barney et al. [11]	2012	USA	10	45-60Gy	SBRT	NA	73%	10 (100%)
Jia et al. [7]	2015	China	38	56.8 Gy (50–60)	Surgery + adjuvant IMRT (*n* = 14) Surgery alone (*n* = 24)	IMRT group: 21.8 Surgery alone group: 15	NA	NA
Mahadevan et al. [10]	2015	USA	34	30 Gy (10–45)	SBRT	17	58%	NA
Liu et al. [9]	2017	Taiwan	15	45 Gy (25–60)	SBRT	12.6	50.3%	12 (80%)
Shen et al. [12]	2017	China	28	45 Gy (36–54)	SBRT	15	57.1%	25 (89.3%)
Radiofrequency								
Kim et al.	2011	Republic of Korea	20 recurrent	1–2	RFA	27.4	70%	–
Kim et al.	2011	Republic of Korea	13 1ry lesions	1–2	RFA	38.5	85%	–
Haidu et al.	2011	Austria	11	1–2	Stereotactic RFA	60	91%	–
Giorgio et al. [63]	2011	Italy	10	NA	RFA	NA	100%	–
Xu et al.	2012	Shanghai	18	NA	RFA	8.8	36.3%	–
Fu et al.	2012	China	17	1–2	RFA	33	84.6%	–
Butros et al.	2014	USA	7	1–2	RFA	38.5	100%	–

[a]Response was not evaluated in 7 patients
[b]Response was not evaluated in 6 patients
[c]Response was not evaluated in 17 patients
[d]Response was not evaluated in 1 patient
[e]Response was not evaluated in 3 patients

single-arm, phase II, multi-institutional study, 92 patients with hepatocellular cancer or ICC received 15 fractions of proton therapy to a maximum total dose of 67.5 Gy equivalent [14]. With a median follow-up among survivors of 20 months, the local control rate at 2 years was 94.1% for ICC with an OS rate at 2 years of 46.5%. These studies indicate that radiation therapy is an attractive option for patients with ICC, both as adjuvant therapy for margin-positive and for locally advanced unresectable cases.

Liver Transplantation

While surgical resection of early-stage ICC remains the consensus treatment of choice, the role of liver transplantation in the management of this malignancy remains controversial. The potential benefits of transplant include replacement of underlying hepatobiliary pathology such as primary sclerosing cholangitis and cirrhosis with a healthy liver. The Mayo Clinic developed a protocol for the treatment of small extrahepatic and hilar cholangiocarcinoma involving neoadjuvant chemoradiation followed by liver transplantation, which is now the standard of care for a subset of extrahepatic CCA [15]. Five-year survival rates among these highly selected patients who treated per protocol were reported to be as high as 65–70% [16]. Unfortunately, most of the reported outcomes of patients with ICC undergoing liver transplant have been less encouraging with high recurrence rates and low OS.

Goldstein et al. reported a single institution study of liver transplantation with adjuvant radiation therapy and chemotherapy [17]. Fourteen patients were confirmed to have cholangiocarcinoma on post-transplant pathology, 8 of whom had ICC. The 1-year survival rate was reported to be 53% with a disease-free survival of 40% and 33% at 1 year and 2 years, respectively. In a larger retrospective analysis, the 1-year and 5-year survival rates of European patients who underwent liver transplantation between 1968 and 2000 for ICC were reported as 58% and 29%, respectively [18]. More recently, Becker et al. analyzed 280 patients in the United Network for Organ Sharing/Organ Procurement and Transplantation Network patient database who underwent liver transplantation for a diagnosis of cholangiocarcinoma [19]. They found a 5-year survival rate of 38% in patients who were transplanted after the year 2000. In the subgroup of patients who were known to have cholangiocarcinoma prior to liver transplantation, the authors reported a 5-year survival rate of 68%. This analysis did not assess outcomes by tumor location (i.e., intrahepatic vs. extrahepatic). In 2016, a retrospective international multicenter study evaluated patients with cirrhosis who received a liver transplant and were incidentally noted on explant to have ICC [20]. Of the patients who were considered to have "very early" ICC (single lesion ≤2 cm in size), 5-year cumulative recurrence risk was 18%, compared to 61% of patients with more advanced ICC. Notably, almost half of patients found to have ICC on explant did not have any suspicious hepatic lesions prior to surgery.

Whether these outcomes can be improved with better patient selection is an essential question regarding the future role of liver transplantation in the treatment of ICC. Hong et al. described the experience at the University of California Los Angeles with transplant in patients with cholangiocarcinoma who would otherwise not be eligible by the standards set by the Mayo Clinic [21]. Twenty-five patients underwent liver transplantation for ICC compared with 12 patients who underwent partial hepatectomy. On multivariate analysis, risk factors for reduced overall survival included partial hepatectomy rather than transplant, perineural invasion, hilar rather than intrahepatic tumor and multifocal tumors. Interestingly, tumor size, defined as ≥5 cm for ICC, was not found to be associated with worsened survival. The same authors used their experience with liver transplantation in cholangiocarcinoma to create a predictive scoring model of recurrence risk [22]. The 5-year recurrence-free survival was 78%, 19%, and 0% for patients in the low-risk, intermediate-risk, and high-risk groups, respectively.

Recently, our group investigated the role of a liver transplant for ICC in patients who had experienced disease response or stability for 6 months or more with systemic chemotherapy. Twenty-one patients were referred for evaluation and 12 patients were accepted, of whom six patients have undergone liver transplantation for ICC. Three patients received livers from extended criteria deceased donors that would otherwise have been discarded, two from domino living donors and one from a standard criteria liver donor. The median duration from diagnosis to transplantation was 26 months and median follow-up from transplantation was 36 months. All patients received neoadjuvant chemotherapy while awaiting liver transplantation. Overall survival was 100% at 1 year, 83% at 3 and 5 years. Three patients developed the recurrent disease at a median of 7·6 months after transplantation, with 50% recurrence-free survival at 5 years [23, 24].

In summary, the role of liver transplantation in the treatment of patients with unresectable ICC remains unclear. However, the above data suggest there may be a role for neoadjuvant therapy in improving outcomes of patients receiving liver transplantation.

Transarterial Chemoembolization (TACE)

Although TACE is ideally used for hypervascular tumors like hepatocellular carcinoma (HCC), hepatobiliary angiography identified that ICCs are relatively hypervascular tumors as compared to the normal liver parenchyma. The concept of conventional TACE (cTACE) is to deliver chemotherapeutic agents directly into the tumor feeding artery. Several studies have evaluated the efficacy and safety of cTACE in the treatment of CCA [25–31]. All trials included locally advanced unresectable CCA patients with ECOG PS ≤ 1. The range of median overall survival was 9–23 months and the procedure was tolerable. Although the results were promising, these studies included both ICC and extrahepatic CCA, making the evaluation of cTACE efficacy in ICC challenging. (Table 13.1) Moreover, drug-eluting bead TACE (DEB-TACE) is similar to cTACE but allows delivery of a higher dose of chemotherapeutic agents directly inside the tumor with less systemic toxicity and more tumor necrosis. Experience with DEB-TACE in ICC is limited but supports its efficacy and safety [32–34]. (Table 13.1) A retrospective review of three independent prospective studies compared the efficacy and safety of cTACE with mitomycin-C ($n = 10$), DEB-TACE with irinotecan ($n = 26$), and systemic therapy with gemcitabine and oxaliplatin ($n = 31$) for ICC. This study showed that the PFS and OS with DEB-TACE (3.9 and 11.7 months, respectively) were higher when compared with cTACE (1.8 and 5.7 months, respectively). Furthermore, this survival outcome was similar to that with systemic chemotherapy (6.2 and 11 months, respectively) [35].

Furthermore, due to a high rate of postoperative recurrence, the role of adjuvant TACE has been evaluated. Wu et al. retrospectively reviewed 114 ICC surgically resected patients of whom 75 were treated with adjuvant TACE. The study results showed that adjuvant TACE significantly improved the OS rate in patients who had poor prognostic factors including tumor size ≥5 cm and advanced stage [36].

Radioembolization

Radioembolization represents internal radiation therapy using Yttrium-90 (Y-90) microspheres, which emits a high dose of lethal beta radiations up to 120 Gy. While, both TACE and Y-90 delivered through the hepatic artery, Y-90, unlike TACE, is a non-occlusive procedure and its effect depends upon free radical release that can lead to apoptosis. While TACE is contraindicated in the presence of portal vein thrombosis, radioembolization can be safely performed in this setting. Moreover, radioembolization can be used for bilobar disease but each lobe is treated separately with at least 4 weeks gap between sessions [37]. Recent studies regarding the role of Y-90 in ICC are summarized in Table 13.1 [38–43]. A systematic review of 7 prospective case series and 5 retrospective cohort studies, which included 298 unresectable ICC patients concluded that the median OS in patients treated with Y-90 is 15.5 months with 82% overall response rate (ORR) [44]. This survival rate is similar to the reported survival rate of systemic chemotherapy and TACE. Thus, radioembolization should be considered one of the treatment approaches for ICC.

Hepatic Artery Infusion

Hepatic arterial infusion (HAI) chemotherapy is feasible in ICC and has followed the experience of treating colorectal cancer liver metastases. Although several chemotherapeutic agents can be infused through the hepatic artery, floxuridine is the most commonly used drug due to its short half-life, 95% extraction rate during the "first-pass" through the liver, low toxicity when combined with dexamethasone and extensive multicenter experience [45–50]. (Table 13.1) A meta-analysis of 20 studies included 657 unresectable ICC patients and compared the treatment outcome of HAI ($n = 62$), TACE ($n = 431$), DEB-TACE ($n = 37$), and yttrium-90 radioembolization ($n = 127$). The OS among HAI treated group was 22.8 months as compared with 13.9 months with Y-90, 12.4 months with cTACE and 12.3 months with DEB-TACE. The ORR was 56.9%, 27.4%, and 17.3% with HAI, Y-90, and TACE, respectively. While 61.5% of DEB-TACE treated patients had SD, none experienced CR or PR [51].

A retrospective analysis of 525 ICC patients revealed that HAI combined with systemic chemotherapy led to a higher OS benefit over chemotherapy alone (30.8 vs. 18.4 months, respectively) ($P < 0.001$) and the difference was maintained in patients with lymph node involvement [52]. Prospective trials of HAI are limited but suggest the feasibility of this approach along with systemic therapies [53].

Radiofrequency Ablation

Radiofrequency ablation is an effective locoregional treatment approach that can be used for the treatment of small ICC with 80–100% reported success rates [54]. A systematic review and a meta-analysis of 7 observational studies included 84 ICC patients showed that RFA associated with 1-, 3-, and 5-year OS rates of 82%, 47%, and 24%, respectively [55]. A previous study showed that complete ablation could be achieved with RFA session in lesions ≤3.4 cm in size. However, modern stereotactic RFA allows complete ablation of larger tumors with one session. Recently, stereotactic RFA used for treating 52 unresectable ICC lesions in 17 patients. Lesions up to 10 cm were completely ablated within one session with a median OS of 60 months [56]. A summary of the previously published studies of RFA in ICC has been summarized in Table 13.1 [57–63]. However, the majority of these studies included both primary and recurrent ICC lesions.

In summary, the concept of using liver-directed therapies for ICC is attractive as can provide effective locoregional control without systemic toxicities. However, majority of the evidence in this regard is retrospective and future multicenter randomized clinical trials are warranted to examine the efficacy of different modalities. Institutional expertise, tumor location, vascularity, and underlying liver function play a key role in the selection of the optimal approach.

Systemic and Targeted Therapy

Systemic Chemotherapy

Patients with advanced cholangiocarcinoma (CCA) have limited chemotherapeutic options. Gemcitabine and cisplatin is currently the worldwide standard first-line therapy for advanced CCA based on the randomized, controlled, phase III ABC-02 study, which enrolled 410 patients with locally advanced or metastatic biliary tract cancer, of those 241 patients (58.8%) were cholangiocarcinoma. In this trial, the median OS with the combination therapy was 11.7 months as compared with 8.1 months with gemcitabine alone Hazard ratio (HR) = 0.64, $P < 0.001$. Also, the PFS was 8 and 5 months, respectively (HR = 0.63, $P < 0.001$) [64]. A meta-analysis of 104 trials comprising 2810 biliary tract cancer (BTC) patients confirms the superiority of gemcitabine and platinum-based chemotherapy over other chemotherapeutic agents [65]. Recently, Shroff et al. reported the phase II study results of gemcitabine, cisplatin, and nab-paclitaxel for advanced BTC. Among the 60 treated patients, 38 had advanced unresectable ICC. Median follow-up was 12.2 months and median PFS 11.8 months. Partial response and disease control rates were 43% and 84%, respectively. Median OS was 19.2 months (95% CI, 13.2 to not estimable). Grade ≥ 3 toxicities occurred in 57% of patients, and 18% withdrew owing to toxicities. Neutropenia was the most common toxicity (32%).

Second-line systemic approaches for this disease with gemcitabine or fluoropyrimidine-based regimens including gemcitabine plus capecitabine, gemcitabine plus oxaliplatin, gemcitabine plus fluoropyrimidine, fluoropyrimidine with cisplatin, or oxaliplatin (FOLFOX) or irinotecan (FOLFIRI), or single-agent gemcitabine, fluorouracil, or capecitabine have limited efficacy with an average PFS of 3 months [66]. A systematic review of 14 phase II clinical trials, 9 retrospective cohort studies, and two case reports has been pooled and analyzed to identify the best second-line therapy for BTC and they concluded that there is no strong evidence to support one regimen over others [67]. This raises the great unmet need for prospective randomized controlled trials to explore a better combination treatment approaches for this cancer.

Targeted Therapy

Recently, next-generation sequencing (NGS) has indicated that ICC is enriched with a relatively high number of actionable mutations and has been a focus of intensive drug development. Promising anti-tumor activity has been noted with novel targeted therapies directed against fibroblast growth factor receptor 2 fusion (*FGFR*), isocitrate dehydrogenase-1 (*IDH1*) and *IDH2*, *BAP1*, *BRAF V600E* mutations, and *Her2/neu* amplification. A summary of the targeted therapy clinical trials is depicted in Table 13.2 [68–107].

IDH-1 and IDH-2 Pathway

Mutations in *IDH*1 and 2 have been identified in approximately 10–40% of ICC patients as compared with 3–4% of extrahepatic CCA [108, 109]. The prognostic significance of *IDH* mutations remains controversial. Majority of the retrospective data do not show any significant correlation between *IDH* mutations and patient

Table 13.2 Clinical studies of novel targeted therapies for advanced and metastatic Cholangiocarcinoma

Author	Year	Patients (*N*)	Agents	Trial phase	Line of therapy	Study arms	OS (months)	PFS (months)	RR (%)
FGFR									
BGJ398									
Javle et al. [74]	2018	61	Alone	II	Second	Single	NA	5.8	14.8
IDH									
AG-120									
Burris et al. [69]	2015	20	Alone	I	NA	Single	5	NA	5
EGFR									
Cetuximab									
Borbath et al. [68]	2013	44	With GEM	II	First	Single	13.5	NA	20.4
Gruenberger et al. [72]	2010	30	With GEMOX			Single	15.2	88	63
Malka et al. [78]	2014	150				I: GEMOX II: GEMOX + cetuximab	I: 12.4 II: 11	I: 5.3 II: 6	I: 29 II: 23
Chen et al. [70]	2015	122				I: GEMOX II: GEMOX + cetuximab	I: 9.8 II: 10.6	I:4.1 II:6.7	I:15 II:27
Paule et al. [79]	2007	9			Second	Single	7	4	22
Rubovszky et al. [81]	2013	34	With GEMCAP		Any line	Single	15.7	8.6	17.6

(continued)

Table 13.2 (continued)

Author	Year	Patients (*N*)	Agents	Trial phase	Line of therapy	Study arms	OS (months)	PFS (months)	RR (%)
Panitumumab									
Hezel et al. [73]	2014	31	With GEMOX	II	First	Single in KRAS wild type	20.3	10.6	45
Leone et al. [77]	2016	89				I: GEMOX II: GEMCOX + panitumumab In KRAS wild type	I: 10.2 II: 9.9	I: 4.4 II: 5.3	I:18.2 II: 26.7
Sohal et al. [82]	2013	35	With GEM-IRINO			Single in KRAS wild type	12.9	9.7	31.4
Vogel et al. [83]	2015	93	With GEMCIS			I: GEMCIS II: GEMCIS + panitumumab In KRAS wild type	I: 21.4 II: 12.8	I: 8.2 II: 6.7	I: 39 II: 45
Jensen et al. [75]	2012	46	With GEMOX-CAP		Any line	Single	10	8.3	33
Erlotinib									
Lee et al. [76]	2012	268	With GEMOX	III	First	I: GEMOX II: GEMOX + erlotinib	I: 9.5 II: 9.5	I: 4.2 II: 5.8	I: 16 II: 30
Chiorean et al. [71]	2012	11	With docetaxel	II		Single	5.7	NA	NA
Philip et al. [80]	2006	42	Alone		Any line	Single	7.5	2.6	8
HER2									
Lapatinib									
Ramanathan et al. [90]	2009	17	Alone	II	Any line	Single	5.2	1.8	0

Afatinib									
Moehler et al. [87]	2015	9	With GEMCIS	I	First	Single	7.7	5.2	NA
VGFR									
Bevacizumab									
Lyer et al. [99]	2018	50	With GEMCAP	II	First	Single	10.2	8.1	72
Zhu et al. [93]	2010	35	With GEMOX		Any line	Single	12.7	7	40
Sorafenib									
Luo et al. [106]	2017	44	Alone	Prospective		Single	5.7	3.2	53.9
El-Khoureiry et al. [85]	2012	31	Alone	II	First	Single	9	3	0
Moehler et al. [88]	2014	102	With GEM			I: GEM + sorafenib II: GEM	I: 8.4 II: 11.2	I: 3 II: 4.9	I: 8 II: 6
Lee et al. [86]	2013	39	With GEMCIS			Single	14.4	6.5	12[a]
Bengala et al. [84]	2010	46	Alone		Second	Single	4.4	2.3	32.6
Sunitinib									
Yi et al. [92]	2012	56	Alone	I	Second	Single	4.8	1.7	9
Neuzillet et al. [89]	2017	53	Alone	II		Single	9.6	5.2	15
Vanderanib									
Santoro et al. [91]	2015	173	Alone	II	First	Single	7.5	3.4	4
Cediranib									
Valle et al. [100]	2015	124	With GEMCIS	II/III	First	I: GEMCIS + cediranib II: GEMCIS	I: 14.1 II: 11.9	I: 8 II: 7.4	I: 44 II: 19
Regorafenib									
Sun et al. [105]	2017	37	Alone	II	Second	Single	5.6	3.6	10.7
Other less recognized pathways									
MAPK									

(continued)

Table 13.2 (continued)

Author	Year	Patients (*N*)	Agents	Trial phase	Line of therapy	Study arms	OS (months)	PFS (months)	RR (%)
Selumetinib									
Bridgewater et al. [96]	2016	12	With GEMCIS	I	First	Single	NA	6.4	37.5[b]
Bekaii-Saab et al. [95]	2011	28	Alone	II	Any line	Single	9.8	3.7	12
Trametinib									
Loka et al. [98].	2015	20	Alone	II	Second	Single	NA	2.4	5
Binimetinib									
Lowery et al. [107]	2015	12	With GEMCIS	I	First	Single	9.1	6.4	50
MK-2206									
Ahn et al. [94]	2015	8	Alone	II	Second	Single	3.5	1.7	0
c-MET									
Cabozanitib									
Goyal et al. [97]	2017	19	Alone	II	Second	Single	5.2	1.8	0
Combined targeted therapy									
Lubner et al. [103]	2010	49	Bevacizumab + erlotinib	II	First	Single	9.9	4.4	12[c]
El-Khoueiry et al. [101]	2014	34	Sorafenib + erlotinib			Single	6	2	6
Jensen et al. [102]	2015	88	Gemox-CAP + panitumumab versus bevacizumab			I: Gemox-CAP + panitumumab II: Gemox-CAP + bevacizumab	I: 9.5 II: 12.3	I: 6.1 II: 8.2	I: 46 II: 18
Shroff et al. [104]	2017	25	Pazopanib + trametinib	Ib	Second	Single	6.4	3.6	5[d]

[a]Response was not evaluated in 6 patients
[b]Response was not evaluated in 4 patients
[c]Response was not evaluated in 4 patients
[d]Response was not evaluated in 5 patients

survival [110–112]. Burris et al. [69] conducted a phase I dose escalation and expansion clinical trial to assess safety and tolerability to AG-120 in *IDH1* mutant ICC. Among 73 enrolled patients, 6% had partial response, 56% had stable disease, with 40% 6-months PFS [113]. This agent is now being investigated in a placebo-controlled phase III trial.

DNA Repair Gene Pathway

DNA repair mechanisms are essential for maintaining genomic stability. Dysregulation of DNA repair pathway is often associated with the accumulation of several GAs and higher tumor mutational burden (TMB). In a recent report on 422 BTCs who underwent mutational profiling, DNA repair genes mutations occurred in 45.2% ICC. In this trial, DNA repair genes were defined as 'direct' DNA repair genes (*ATM, ATR, BRCA1, BRCA2, FANCA, FANCD2, MLH1, MSH2, MSH6, PALB2, POLD1, POLE, PRKDC, RAD50*, and *SLX4*) and "caretaker" genes (*BAP1, CDK12, KMT2C/MLL3, TP53,* and *BLM*). Direct DNA repair gene alterations were associated with a high tumor mutation burden (TMB) [114].

Poly (ADP-ribose) polymerases (PARPs), a family of proteins including PARP1 and PARP2, are activated by DNA damage and facilitate DNA repair [115]. PARP inhibition (PARPi) has been an effective therapeutic strategy against tumors associated with DNA repair genes mutations. The preliminary results of a phase I study of PARPi (veliparib) in combination with capecitabine and oxaliplatin for 17 solid tumor patients included 6 cholangiocarcinoma patients of whom 3 (50%) experienced stable disease [116].

Preclinical and clinical studies noted that highly mutated tumors harbor neoantigens, which make them more responsive to immune checkpoint inhibitors [117–119]. PARP inhibitors alone or with checkpoint inhibitors are being investigated in ICC.

Fibroblast Growth Factor Receptor Pathway

FGFR is a complex pathway that consists of 4 FGFR transmembrane receptors (*FGFR1*, *FGFR2*, *FGFR3*, and *FGFR4*) and 18 *FGF* ligands. Dysregulation of the FGFR pathway including fusion, amplification, and mutation has been reported in ICC, with a relatively high incidence of *FGFR2* fusions in ICC (10–16%). FGFR mutated ICC may represent a specific disease phenotype, with a younger patient population and having a relatively indolent disease course [110]. Currently, several *FGFR*-specific targeted agents are being investigated in ICC including infigratinib (BGJ398), TAS-120, ARQ087, pemigatinib (INCB54828), JNJ425756493, and PRN1371. Sixty-one patients with FGFR2 fusion (n = 48), mutation (n = 8), or amplification (n = 3) were treated with infigratinib [74]. The overall response rate was 14.8% (18.8% FGFR2 fusions only), disease control rate was 75.4% (83.3% FGFR2 fusions only), and the estimated median progression-free survival was

5.8 months. Grade 3 or 4 treatment-related adverse events occurred in 25 patients (41%) and included hyperphosphatemia (16.4%), stomatitis (6.6%), and palmar-plantar erythrodysesthesia (4.9%).

EGFR and BRAF Mutations

Genetic aberrations in Epidermal Growth Factor Receptor (*EGFR*), *BRAF*, and *Her2/neu* have been identified in BTC and are relatively uncommon in ICC (0–2%). EGFR overexpression, on the other hand, has been reported in 11–27% of ICC [120]. EGFR inhibitors including erlotinib, cetuximab, and panitumumab alone or in combination with systemic chemotherapy have been investigated in several phase II trials [68–83]. One phase III trial that investigated the addition of erlotinib to gemcitabine and oxaliplatin showed an improved response rate without a survival benefit. However, subgroup analysis showed that the improvement in response correlated with tumor *KRAS* status, only *KRAS* wt benefited from erlotinib [121]. Dabrafenib, a *BRAF V600E* mutation blockade, has been administrated in combination with trametinib, MEK inhibitor, for *BRAF V600E* mutated patients with a promising response [122, 123]. Currently, there is an ongoing trial to study the efficacy of this combination on rare tumors including BTC (NCT02034110) [124].

Vascular Endothelial Growth Factor Pathway

Prior studies showed that 54% of ICC patients have *VEGF* overexpression and this may be an important target in this cancer. However, single-agent VGFR inhibitors including sorafenib, sunitinib, and vandetanib failed to show any encouraging survival benefit in BTC patients. Recently, ABC-03 trial compared the efficacy of gemcitabine and cisplatin with and without cediranib, a VGFR 1–3 inhibitor. The addition of cediranib improved the overall response rate (44% vs. 19%, $P = 0.004$) without any survival benefit. Further studies are required to identify predictive biomarkers for VEGF inhibitors for better patient allocation in clinical trials [120]. Lubner et al. treated 53 eligible patients with BTC in a multicenter trial of bevacizumab with erlotinib [103]. Of 49 evaluable patients, six (12%) had a confirmed partial response. Stable disease was documented in another 25 patients (51%). Rash was the most common grade 3 toxicity. Four patients had grade 4 toxicities. Median OS was 9.9 months, and time to treatment progression was 4.4 months indicating that VEGFR-directed therapies have potential benefit in this cancer.

Chromatin Remolding Pathway

Genetic aberrations in chromatin remolding genes comprising *BAP1*, *ARID1A*, *PBRM,* and *MLL* have been noted in ICC [110]. *BAP1* mutation in cholangiocarcinoma associated with aggressive disease and poor response to standard systemic therapy and exploring BAP-1 targeted agents such as EZH2 inhibitors may have therapeutic value [125]. Preclinical studies have indicated the efficacy of histone deacetylase inhibitors such as vorinostat in CCA models although clinical efficacy has yet to be demonstrated [126].

Immunotherapy

The role of immunotherapy in cancer treatment continues to progress and enormous strides have been made in melanoma, renal cell carcinoma, urothelial cancer and non-small cell lung cancer [127, 128]. Therapeutic strategies across various tumor types that harness patient innate and acquired immune systems have included immune checkpoint inhibitors, vaccines, and cytotoxic T lymphocyte therapy. Immune checkpoint inhibitors, including anti-PD-(L)1 and anti-CTLA-4 antibodies, have been particularly exciting in their propensities to lead to prolonged, durable responses in a subset of patients [129]. Predictive factors include TMB, PDL-1 expression and tumor immune infiltration [130].

Among BTCs, ICCs have fewer CD8+ T lymphocytes than extrahepatic CCAs and gallbladder cancers [131]. Higher levels of infiltrating CD8+ T lymphocytes have been shown to portend a more favorable prognosis in patients with colorectal cancer and pancreatic cancer [132, 133]. A meta-analysis of 12 studies with over 2300 patients by Wang et al. did note a positive association between intraepithelial CD8+, CD4+, and Foxp3+ T lymphocytes and OS in BTC patients, though this data was not broken down by disease subtype [134].

In addition to the prognostic value of the immune infiltrate of malignancy, there is also a predictive value in regards to response to checkpoint inhibition. In particular, tumors that possess what has been termed an "immune-inflamed phenotype" are characterized by numerous infiltrating immune cells and a higher likelihood of response to checkpoint inhibition [135]. Conversely, there is evidence that patients whose tumors have fewer infiltrating CD8+ T lymphocytes do not respond as well to checkpoint inhibition [136].

In May 2017, the FDA granted accelerated approval to pembrolizumab for the treatment of patients with cancers who harbor high microsatellite instability (MSI-H) or mismatch repair deficiency (dMMR) in the metastatic, pre-treated setting. While this approval indeed applies to patients with cholangiocarcinoma, the incidence of MSI-H or dMMR in this population is very low, having been reported as low as 1% and as high as 10% [137, 138]. The KEYNOTE-158 trial assessed response to pembrolizumab among 21 patients with non-colorectal MSI-H tumors, of whom 3 had cholangiocarcinomas. The overall response rate among the non-colorectal tumor patients was 42.9% with a disease control rate of 66.7% [139].

Recently, at the European Society of Medical Oncology (ESMO) annual meeting, KEYNOTE-158 was presented. A total of 104 patients with BTC were treated with single-agent pembrolizumab. The overall response rate was 5.8%: 17 pts. (16%) had stable disease and the median PFS was 2.0 months while the median OS was 9.1 months. The available data suggest that treatment with single-agent checkpoint inhibitors in patients with advanced cholangiocarcinoma have very modest clinical efficacy in an unselected population and should not be considered in the absence of MSI-H or outside a clinical trial setting.

The role of vaccine therapy and adoptive immunotherapy with cytotoxic T lymphocytes (CTLs) for cholangiocarcinoma constitute alternative avenues of immunotherapy with heavy research interest. Peptide and dendritic cell vaccines rely on the patient's intrinsic immune system to activate an anti-tumor response, while adoptive immunotherapy strategies, including CTLs, aim to expand reactive T-cells in the laboratory prior to re-infusion into the patient.

A number of peptide and dendritic cell vaccines targeting antigens such as WT1 and MUC1 among others have been developed and studied in phase I and II trials. Aruga et al. performed a phase I trial utilizing a four-peptide vaccine developed from cancer-testis antigens that are commonly expressed in cholangiocarcinoma [140]. The vaccine was administered weekly until disease progression in nine patients with advanced, pre-treated BTC. It was well tolerated with median PFS and OS similar to what is seen with cytotoxic chemotherapy. Notably, seven of the nine patients were found to have peptide-specific T-cell responses as assessed by analysis of peripheral T-cells. Early phase trials combining vaccines with chemotherapy in either the metastatic or adjuvant setting have yielded mixed results [141, 142]. Kida et al. analyzed tumor and peripheral blood samples from patients with BTCs, nine of whom had ICCs, in order to assess the best candidates for tumor-associated antigens as targets for immunotherapy [143]. By studying the tumor-infiltrating lymphocytes and peripheral lymphocytes from the patient samples and comparing these to controls without BTCs, the authors found a number of potential epitopes that may be suitable for vaccine therapy. Furthermore, they concluded that patients with high peripheral blood lymphocyte counts, indicating a robust baseline immune system, were the ones who benefited most from immunotherapy.

The efficacy of adoptive immunotherapy in ICC with ex-vivo expansion of cytotoxic T lymphocytes and subsequent re-introduction to the patient has been studied in the setting of adjuvant therapy after surgical resection [142]. Shimizu et al. found that combination of this adoptive immunotherapy approach combined with postoperative dendritic cell vaccine yielded a median PFS increase from 7.7 months to 18.3 months and a median OS increase from 17.4 months to 31.9 months when compared to surgery alone. An ongoing clinical trial at the National Cancer Institute is assessing the efficacy of infusing tumor-infiltrating cytotoxic T lymphocytes expanded ex vivo with or without pembrolizumab in a variety of advanced solid tumors including cholangiocarcinoma (ClinicalTrials.gov ID: NCT01174121).

While immunotherapy has revolutionized the treatment of many advanced malignancies over the past several years, the jury is still out in regards to its future role for patients with ICC. Adoptive immunity strategies involving infusing cytotoxic tumor-infiltrating lymphocytes may offer some value, though more data are needed to confirm this. Thus far, peptide and dendritic cell vaccines have yet to demonstrate significant efficacy. Although the early results of single-agent checkpoint inhibitors in cholangiocarcinoma have been fairly disappointing, combinatorial strategies

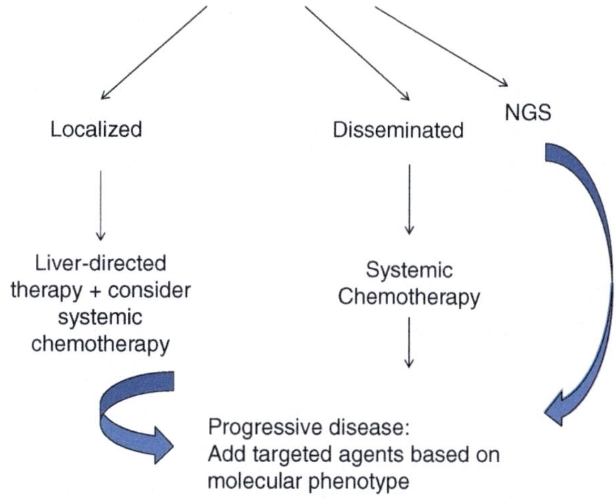

Fig. 13.1 Unresectable intrahepatic cholangiocarcinoma

with multiple checkpoint inhibitors and checkpoint inhibitors with targeted therapies are the next frontier of investigation and hold considerable promise.

In the past decade, there has been an abundance of therapeutic options for ICC and a rational, multidisciplinary, sequential approach is indicated (Fig. 13.1) Liver-directed therapies, systemic chemotherapy, and targeted therapies are changing the treatment paradigm of ICC and offer considerable promise towards improving the clinical outcome of this cancer.

References

1. Yamasaki S. Intrahepatic cholangiocarcinoma: macroscopic type and stage classification. J Hepato-Biliary-Pancreat Surg. 2003;10(4):288–91.
2. Spolverato G, Kim Y, Alexandrescu S, et al. Management and outcomes of patients with recurrent intrahepatic cholangiocarcinoma following previous curative-intent surgical resection. Ann Surg Oncol. 2016;23(1):235–43.
3. Liotta L, Quante M. Adjuvant chemotherapy with Capecitabine as new standard for resected cholangiocarcinomas – a look at the BILCAP trial. Z Gastroenterol. 2018;56(7):839–40.
4. Shinohara ET, Mitra N, Guo M, Metz JM. Radiation therapy is associated with improved survival in the adjuvant and definitive treatment of intrahepatic cholangiocarcinoma. Int J Radiat Oncol Biol Phys. 2008;72(5):1495–501.
5. Zheng X, Chen B, Wu JX, et al. Benefit of adjuvant radiotherapy following narrow-margin hepatectomy in patients with intrahepatic cholangiocarcinoma that adhere to major vessels. Cancer Manag Res. 2018;10:3973–81.
6. Lee J, Yoon WS, Koom WS, Rim CH. Efficacy of stereotactic body radiotherapy for unresectable or recurrent cholangiocarcinoma: a meta-analysis and systematic review. Strahlenther Onkol. 2018;195(2):93–102.
7. Jia AY, Wu JX, Zhao YT, et al. Intensity-modulated radiotherapy following null-margin resection is associated with improved survival in the treatment of intrahepatic cholangiocarcinoma. J Gastrointest Oncol. 2015;6(2):126–33.

8. Jiang W, Zeng ZC, Tang ZY, et al. Benefit of radiotherapy for 90 patients with resected intrahepatic cholangiocarcinoma and concurrent lymph node metastases. J Cancer Res Clin Oncol. 2010;136(9):1323–31.
9. Liu MY, Lo CH, Lin CS, et al. Stereotactic ablative radiotherapy for patients with unresectable or medically inoperable cholangiocarcinoma. Tumori. 2017;103(3):236–41.
10. Mahadevan A, Dagoglu N, Mancias J, et al. Stereotactic Body Radiotherapy (SBRT) for intrahepatic and hilar cholangiocarcinoma. J Cancer. 2015;6(11):1099–104.
11. Barney BM, Olivier KR, Miller RC, Haddock MG. Clinical outcomes and toxicity using stereotactic body radiotherapy (SBRT) for advanced cholangiocarcinoma. Radiat Oncol (London, England). 2012;7:67.
12. Shen Z-T, Zhou H, Li A-M, Li B, Shen J-S, Zhu X-X. Clinical outcomes and prognostic factors of stereotactic body radiation therapy for intrahepatic cholangiocarcinoma. Oncotarget. 2017;8(55):93541–50.
13. Tao R, Krishnan S, Bhosale PR, et al. Ablative radiotherapy doses lead to a substantial prolongation of survival in patients with inoperable intrahepatic cholangiocarcinoma: a retrospective dose-response analysis. J Clin Oncol. 2016;34(3):219–26.
14. Hong TS, Wo JY, Yeap BY, et al. Multi-institutional phase II study of high-dose hypofractionated proton beam therapy in patients with localized, unresectable hepatocellular carcinoma and intrahepatic cholangiocarcinoma. J Clin Oncol. 2016;34(5):460–8.
15. De Vreede I, Steers JL, Burch PA, et al. Prolonged disease-free survival after orthotopic liver transplantation plus adjuvant chemoirradiation for cholangiocarcinoma. Liver Transpl. 2000;6(3):309–16.
16. Zamora-Valdes D, Heimbach JK. Liver transplant for cholangiocarcinoma. Gastroenterol Clin N Am. 2018;47(2):267–80.
17. Goldstein RM, Stone M, Tillery GW, et al. Is liver transplantation indicated for cholangiocarcinoma? Am J Surg. 1993;166(6):768–71; discussion 771–62.
18. Pascher A, Jonas S, Neuhaus P. Intrahepatic cholangiocarcinoma: indication for transplantation. J Hepato-Biliary-Pancreat Surg. 2003;10(4):282–7.
19. Becker NS, Rodriguez JA, Barshes NR, O'Mahony CA, Goss JA, Aloia TA. Outcomes analysis for 280 patients with cholangiocarcinoma treated with liver transplantation over an 18-year period. J Gastrointest Surg. 2008;12(1):117–22.
20. Sapisochin G, Facciuto M, Rubbia-Brandt L, et al. Liver transplantation for "very early" intrahepatic cholangiocarcinoma: international retrospective study supporting a prospective assessment. Hepatology. 2016;64(4):1178–88.
21. Hong JC, Jones CM, Duffy JP, et al. Comparative analysis of resection and liver transplantation for intrahepatic and hilar cholangiocarcinoma: a 24-year experience in a single center. Arch Surg. 2011;146(6):683–9.
22. Hong JC, Petrowsky H, Kaldas FM, et al. Predictive index for tumor recurrence after liver transplantation for locally advanced intrahepatic and hilar cholangiocarcinoma. J Am Coll Surg. 2011;212(4):514–20; discussion 520–11.
23. Lunsford KE, Javle M, Gaber AO, Vauthey JN, Ghobrial RM. Liver transplantation for locally advanced intrahepatic cholangiocarcinoma – Authors' reply. Lancet Gastroenterol Hepatol. 2018;3(8):529–30.
24. Lunsford KE, Javle M, Heyne K, et al. Liver transplantation for locally advanced intrahepatic cholangiocarcinoma treated with neoadjuvant therapy: a prospective case series. Lancet Gastroenterol Hepatol. 2018;3(5):337–48.
25. Vogl TJ, Naguib NN, Nour-Eldin NE, et al. Transarterial chemoembolization in the treatment of patients with unresectable cholangiocarcinoma: results and prognostic factors governing treatment success. Int J Cancer. 2012;131(3):733–40.
26. Park SY, Kim JH, Yoon HJ, Lee IS, Yoon HK, Kim KP. Transarterial chemoembolization versus supportive therapy in the palliative treatment of unresectable intrahepatic cholangiocarcinoma. Clin Radiol. 2011;66(4):322–8.
27. Kim JH, Yoon HK, Sung KB, et al. Transcatheter arterial chemoembolization or chemoinfusion for unresectable intrahepatic cholangiocarcinoma: clinical efficacy and factors influencing outcomes. Cancer. 2008;113(7):1614–22.

28. Kiefer MV, Albert M, McNally M, et al. Chemoembolization of intrahepatic cholangiocarcinoma with cisplatinum, doxorubicin, mitomycin C, ethiodol, and polyvinyl alcohol: a 2-center study. Cancer. 2011;117(7):1498–505.
29. Herber S, Otto G, Schneider J, et al. Transarterial chemoembolization (TACE) for inoperable intrahepatic cholangiocarcinoma. Cardiovasc Intervent Radiol. 2007;30(6):1156–65.
30. Gusani NJ, Balaa FK, Steel JL, et al. Treatment of unresectable cholangiocarcinoma with gemcitabine-based transcatheter arterial chemoembolization (TACE): a single-institution experience. J Gastrointest Surg. 2008;12(1):129–37.
31. Burger I, Hong K, Schulick R, et al. Transcatheter arterial chemoembolization in unresectable cholangiocarcinoma: initial experience in a single institution. J Vasc Interv Radiol. 2005;16(3):353–61.
32. Schiffman SC, Metzger T, Dubel G, et al. Precision hepatic arterial irinotecan therapy in the treatment of unresectable intrahepatic cholangiocellular carcinoma: optimal tolerance and prolonged overall survival. Ann Surg Oncol. 2011;18(2):431–8.
33. Poggi G, Amatu A, Montagna B, et al. OEM-TACE: a new therapeutic approach in unresectable intrahepatic cholangiocarcinoma. Cardiovasc Intervent Radiol. 2009;32(6): 1187–92.
34. Aliberti C, Carandina R, Sarti D, et al. Chemoembolization with drug-eluting microspheres loaded with doxorubicin for the treatment of cholangiocarcinoma. Anticancer Res. 2017;37(4):1859–63.
35. Kuhlmann JB, Euringer W, Spangenberg HC, et al. Treatment of unresectable cholangiocarcinoma: conventional transarterial chemoembolization compared with drug-eluting bead-transarterial chemoembolization and systemic chemotherapy. Eur J Gastroenterol Hepatol. 2012;24(4):437–43.
36. Wu ZF, Zhang HB, Yang N, Zhao WC, Fu Y, Yang GS. Postoperative adjuvant transcatheter arterial chemoembolisation improves survival of intrahepatic cholangiocarcinoma patients with poor prognostic factors: results of a large monocentric series. Eur J Surg Oncol. 2012;38(7):602–10.
37. Salem R, Thurston KG. Radioembolization with 90Yttrium microspheres: a state-of-the-art brachytherapy treatment for primary and secondary liver malignancies. Part 1: technical and methodologic considerations. J Vasc Interv Radiol. 2006;17(8):1251–78.
38. Soydal C, Kucuk ON, Bilgic S, Ibis E. Radioembolization with (90)Y resin microspheres for intrahepatic cholangiocellular carcinoma: prognostic factors. Ann Nucl Med. 2016;30(1):29–34.
39. Shaker TM, Chung C, Varma MK, et al. Is there a role for Yttrium-90 in the treatment of unresectable and metastatic intrahepatic cholangiocarcinoma? Am J Surg. 2018;215(3): 467–70.
40. Saxena A, Bester L, Chua TC, Chu FC, Morris DL. Yttrium-90 radiotherapy for unresectable intrahepatic cholangiocarcinoma: a preliminary assessment of this novel treatment option. Ann Surg Oncol. 2010;17(2):484–91.
41. Reimer P, Virarkar MK, Binnenhei M, Justinger M, Schön MR, Tatsch K. Prognostic factors in overall survival of patients with unresectable intrahepatic cholangiocarcinoma treated by means of Yttrium-90 radioembolization: results in therapy-Naïve patients. Cardiovasc Intervent Radiol. 2018;
42. Ibrahim SM, Mulcahy MF, Lewandowski RJ, et al. Treatment of unresectable cholangiocarcinoma using yttrium-90 microspheres: results from a pilot study. Cancer. 2008;113(8):2119–28.
43. Hoffmann RT, Paprottka PM, Schon A, et al. Transarterial hepatic yttrium-90 radioembolization in patients with unresectable intrahepatic cholangiocarcinoma: factors associated with prolonged survival. Cardiovasc Intervent Radiol. 2012;35(1):105–16.
44. Al-Adra DP, Gill RS, Axford SJ, Shi X, Kneteman N, Liau SS. Treatment of unresectable intrahepatic cholangiocarcinoma with Yttrium-90 radioembolization: a systematic review and pooled analysis. Eur J Surg Oncol. 2015;41(1):120–7.
45. Shitara K, Ikami I, Munakata M, Muto O, Sakata Y. Hepatic arterial infusion of mitomycin C with degradable starch microspheres for unresectable intrahepatic cholangiocarcinoma. Clin Oncol (R Coll Radiol). 2008;20(3):241–6.

46. Jarnagin WR, Schwartz LH, Gultekin DH, et al. Regional chemotherapy for unresectable primary liver cancer: results of a phase II clinical trial and assessment of DCE-MRI as a biomarker of survival. Ann Oncol. 2009;20(9):1589–95.
47. Inaba Y, Arai Y, Yamaura H, et al. Phase I/II study of hepatic arterial infusion chemotherapy with gemcitabine in patients with unresectable intrahepatic cholangiocarcinoma (JIVROSG-0301). Am J Clin Oncol. 2011;34(1):58–62.
48. Tanaka N, Yamakado K, Nakatsuka A, Fujii A, Matsumura K, Takeda K. Arterial chemoinfusion therapy through an implanted port system for patients with unresectable intrahepatic cholangiocarcinoma–initial experience. Eur J Radiol. 2002;41(1):42–8.
49. Massani M, Nistri C, Ruffolo C, et al. Intrahepatic chemotherapy for unresectable cholangiocarcinoma: review of literature and personal experience. Updat Surg. 2015;67(4):389–400.
50. Ghiringhelli F, Lorgis V, Vincent J, Ladoire S, Guiu B. Hepatic arterial infusion of gemcitabine plus oxaliplatin as second-line treatment for locally advanced intrahepatic cholangiocarcinoma: preliminary experience. Chemotherapy. 2013;59(5):354–60.
51. Boehm LM, Jayakrishnan TT, Miura JT, et al. Comparative effectiveness of hepatic artery based therapies for unresectable intrahepatic cholangiocarcinoma. J Surg Oncol. 2015;111(2):213–20.
52. Konstantinidis IT, Groot Koerkamp B, Do RK, et al. Unresectable intrahepatic cholangiocarcinoma: systemic plus hepatic arterial infusion chemotherapy is associated with longer survival in comparison with systemic chemotherapy alone. Cancer. 2016;122(5):758–65.
53. Cercek A, D'Angelica M, Power D, et al. Floxuridine hepatic arterial infusion associated biliary toxicity is increased by concurrent administration of systemic bevacizumab. Ann Surg Oncol. 2014;21(2):479–86.
54. Shindoh J. Ablative therapies for intrahepatic cholangiocarcinoma. Hepatobiliary Surg Nutr. 2017;6(1):2–6.
55. Han K, Ko HK, Kim KW, Won HJ, Shin YM, Kim PN. Radiofrequency ablation in the treatment of unresectable intrahepatic cholangiocarcinoma: systematic review and meta-analysis. J Vasc Interv Radiol. 2015;26(7):943–8.
56. Bale R, Schullian P, Haidu M, Widmann G. Stereotactic radiofrequency ablation (SRFA) of intrahepatic cholangiocellular carcinomas: a minimal invasive alternative to liver resection. Wien Med Wochenschr. 2013;163(5–6):128–31.
57. Butros SR, Shenoy-Bhangle A, Mueller PR, Arellano RS. Radiofrequency ablation of intrahepatic cholangiocarcinoma: feasability, local tumor control, and long-term outcome. Clin Imaging. 2014;38(4):490–4.
58. Fu Y, Yang W, Wu W, Yan K, Xing BC, Chen MH. Radiofrequency ablation in the management of unresectable intrahepatic cholangiocarcinoma. J Vasc Interv Radiol. 2012;23(5): 642–9.
59. Haidu M, Dobrozemsky G, Schullian P, et al. Stereotactic radiofrequency ablation of unresectable intrahepatic cholangiocarcinomas: a retrospective study. Cardiovasc Intervent Radiol. 2012;35(5):1074–82.
60. Kim JH, Won HJ, Shin YM, Kim KA, Kim PN. Radiofrequency ablation for the treatment of primary intrahepatic cholangiocarcinoma. AJR Am J Roentgenol. 2011;196(2):W205–9.
61. Kim JH, Won HJ, Shin YM, Kim PN, Lee SG, Hwang S. Radiofrequency ablation for recurrent intrahepatic cholangiocarcinoma after curative resection. Eur J Radiol. 2011;80(3):e221–5.
62. Xu HX, Wang Y, Lu MD, Liu LN. Percutaneous ultrasound-guided thermal ablation for intrahepatic cholangiocarcinoma. Br J Radiol. 2012;85(1016):1078–84.
63. Giorgio A, Calisti G, DE Stefano G, et al. Radiofrequency ablation for intrahepatic cholangiocarcinoma: retrospective analysis of a single centre experience. Anticancer Res. 2011;31(12):4575–80.
64. Valle J, Wasan H, Palmer DH, et al. Cisplatin plus gemcitabine versus gemcitabine for biliary tract cancer. N Engl J Med. 2010;362(14):1273–81.
65. Eckel F, Schmid RM. Chemotherapy in advanced biliary tract carcinoma: a pooled analysis of clinical trials. Br J Cancer. 2007;96(6):896–902.

66. Rogers JE, Law L, Nguyen VD, et al. Second-line systemic treatment for advanced cholangiocarcinoma. J Gastrointest Oncol. 2014;5(6):408–13.
67. Lamarca A, Hubner RA, David Ryder W, Valle JW. Second-line chemotherapy in advanced biliary cancer: a systematic review. Ann Oncol. 2014;25(12):2328–38.
68. Borbath I, Ceratti A, Verslype C, et al. Combination of gemcitabine and cetuximab in patients with advanced cholangiocarcinoma: a phase II study of the Belgian Group of Digestive Oncology. Ann Oncol. 2013;24(11):2824–9.
69. Burris H, Mellinghoff I, Maher E, et al. Abstract PL04-05: the first reported results of AG-120, a first-in-class, potent inhibitor of the IDH1 mutant protein, in a phase I study of patients with advanced IDH1-mutant solid tumors, including gliomas. Mol Cancer Ther. 2015;14(12 Supplement 2):PL04–5.
70. Chen JS, Hsu C, Chiang NJ, et al. A KRAS mutation status-stratified randomized phase II trial of gemcitabine and oxaliplatin alone or in combination with cetuximab in advanced biliary tract cancer. Ann Oncol. 2015;26(5):943–9.
71. Chiorean EG, Ramasubbaiah R, Yu M, et al. Phase II trial of erlotinib and docetaxel in advanced and refractory hepatocellular and biliary cancers: Hoosier Oncology Group GI06-101. Oncologist. 2012;17(1):13.
72. Gruenberger B, Schueller J, Heubrandtner U, et al. Cetuximab, gemcitabine, and oxaliplatin in patients with unresectable advanced or metastatic biliary tract cancer: a phase 2 study. Lancet Oncol. 2010;11(12):1142–8.
73. Hezel AF, Noel MS, Allen JN, et al. Phase II study of gemcitabine, oxaliplatin in combination with panitumumab in KRAS wild-type unresectable or metastatic biliary tract and gallbladder cancer. Br J Cancer. 2014;111(3):430–6.
74. Javle M, Lowery M, Shroff RT, et al. Phase II study of BGJ398 in patients with FGFR-altered advanced cholangiocarcinoma. J Clin Oncol. 2018;36(3):276–82.
75. Jensen LH, Lindebjerg J, Ploen J, Hansen TF, Jakobsen A. Phase II marker-driven trial of panitumumab and chemotherapy in KRAS wild-type biliary tract cancer. Ann Oncol. 2012;23(9):2341–6.
76. Lee J, Park SH, Chang HM, et al. Gemcitabine and oxaliplatin with or without erlotinib in advanced biliary-tract cancer: a multicentre, open-label, randomised, phase 3 study. Lancet Oncol. 2012;13(2):181–8.
77. Leone F, Marino D, Cereda S, et al. Panitumumab in combination with gemcitabine and oxaliplatin does not prolong survival in wild-type KRAS advanced biliary tract cancer: a randomized phase 2 trial (Vecti-BIL study). Cancer. 2016;122(4):574–81.
78. Malka D, Cervera P, Foulon S, et al. Gemcitabine and oxaliplatin with or without cetuximab in advanced biliary-tract cancer (BINGO): a randomised, open-label, non-comparative phase 2 trial. Lancet Oncol. 2014;15(8):819–28.
79. Paule B, Herelle MO, Rage E, et al. Cetuximab plus gemcitabine-oxaliplatin (GEMOX) in patients with refractory advanced intrahepatic cholangiocarcinomas. Oncology. 2007;72(1–2):105–10.
80. Philip PA, Mahoney MR, Allmer C, et al. Phase II study of erlotinib in patients with advanced biliary cancer. J Clin Oncol. 2006;24(19):3069–74.
81. Rubovszky G, Lang I, Ganofszky E, et al. Cetuximab, gemcitabine and capecitabine in patients with inoperable biliary tract cancer: a phase 2 study. Eur J Cancer. 2013;49(18):3806–12.
82. Sohal DP, Mykulowycz K, Uehara T, et al. A phase II trial of gemcitabine, irinotecan and panitumumab in advanced cholangiocarcinoma. Ann Oncol. 2013;24(12):3061–5.
83. Vogel A, Kasper S, Weichert W, et al. Panitumumab in combination with gemcitabine/cisplatin (GemCis) for patients with advanced KRAS WT biliary tract cancer: a randomized phase II trial of the Arbeitsgemeinschaft Internistische Onkologie (AIO). J Clin Oncol. 2015;33(15_suppl):4082.
84. Bengala C, Bertolini F, Malavasi N, et al. Sorafenib in patients with advanced biliary tract carcinoma: a phase II trial. Br J Cancer. 2010;102(1):68–72.

85. El-Khoueiry AB, Rankin CJ, Ben-Josef E, et al. SWOG 0514: a phase II study of sorafenib in patients with unresectable or metastatic gallbladder carcinoma and cholangiocarcinoma. Investig New Drugs. 2012;30(4):1646–51.
86. Lee JK, Capanu M, O'Reilly EM, et al. A phase II study of gemcitabine and cisplatin plus sorafenib in patients with advanced biliary adenocarcinomas. Br J Cancer. 2013;109(4):915–9.
87. Moehler M, Ehrlich A, Ruckes C, et al. 2322 safety and efficacy of Afatinib with gemcitabine/cisplatin in chemo-naïve patients with metastatic biliary tract cancer: an open-label, uncontrolled phase Ib trial. Eur J Cancer. 2015;51:S440.
88. Moehler M, Maderer A, Schimanski C, et al. Gemcitabine plus sorafenib versus gemcitabine alone in advanced biliary tract cancer: a double-blind placebo-controlled multicentre phase II AIO study with biomarker and serum programme. Eur J Cancer. 2014;50(18):3125–35.
89. Neuzillet C, Seitz J-F, Fartoux L, et al. Sunitinib as second-line treatment in patients with advanced intrahepatic cholangiocarcinoma (SUN-CK phase II trial): safety, efficacy, and updated translational results. J Clin Oncol. 2015;33(3_suppl):343.
90. Ramanathan RK, Belani CP, Singh DA, et al. A phase II study of lapatinib in patients with advanced biliary tree and hepatocellular cancer. Cancer Chemother Pharmacol. 2009;64(4):777–83.
91. Santoro A, Gebbia V, Pressiani T, et al. A randomized, multicenter, phase II study of vandetanib monotherapy versus vandetanib in combination with gemcitabine versus gemcitabine plus placebo in subjects with advanced biliary tract cancer: the VanGogh study. Ann Oncol. 2015;26(3):542–7.
92. Yi JH, Thongprasert S, Lee J, et al. A phase II study of sunitinib as a second-line treatment in advanced biliary tract carcinoma: a multicentre, multinational study. Eur J Cancer. 2012;48(2):196–201.
93. Zhu AX, Meyerhardt JA, Blaszkowsky LS, et al. Efficacy and safety of gemcitabine, oxaliplatin, and bevacizumab in advanced biliary-tract cancers and correlation of changes in 18-fluorodeoxyglucose PET with clinical outcome: a phase 2 study. Lancet Oncol. 2010;11(1):48–54.
94. Ahn DH, Li J, Wei L, et al. Results of an abbreviated phase-II study with the Akt inhibitor MK-2206 in patients with advanced biliary cancer. Sci Rep. 2015;5:12122.
95. Bekaii-Saab T, Phelps MA, Li X, et al. Multi-institutional phase II study of selumetinib in patients with metastatic biliary cancers. J Clin Oncol. 2011;29(17):2357–63.
96. Bridgewater J, Lopes A, Beare S, et al. A phase 1b study of Selumetinib in combination with Cisplatin and Gemcitabine in advanced or metastatic biliary tract cancer: the ABC-04 study. BMC Cancer. 2016;16:153.
97. Goyal L, Zheng H, Yurgelun MB, et al. A phase 2 and biomarker study of cabozantinib in patients with advanced cholangiocarcinoma. Cancer. 2017;123(11):1979–88.
98. Ioka T, Ikeda M, Fukutomi A, et al. 2382 a proof-of-concept study of MEK inhibitor trametinib monotherapy in patients with biliary tract cancers. Eur J Cancer. 2015;51:S464.
99. Iyer RV, Pokuri VK, Groman A, et al. A multicenter phase II study of gemcitabine, Capecitabine, and bevacizumab for locally advanced or metastatic biliary tract cancer. Am J Clin Oncol. 2018;41(7):649–55.
100. Valle JW, Wasan H, Lopes A, et al. Cediranib or placebo in combination with cisplatin and gemcitabine chemotherapy for patients with advanced biliary tract cancer (ABC-03): a randomised phase 2 trial. Lancet Oncol. 2015;16(8):967–78.
101. El-Khoueiry AB, Rankin C, Siegel AB, et al. S0941: a phase 2 SWOG study of sorafenib and erlotinib in patients with advanced gallbladder carcinoma or cholangiocarcinoma. Br J Cancer. 2014;110(4):882–7.
102. Jensen LH, Fernebro E, Ploen J, Eberhard J, Lindebjerg J, Jakobsen AKM. Randomized phase II crossover trial exploring the clinical benefit from targeting EGFR or VEGF with combination chemotherapy in patients with non-resectable biliary tract cancer. J Clin Oncol. 2015;33(15_suppl):4071.

103. Lubner SJ, Mahoney MR, Kolesar JL, et al. Report of a multicenter phase II trial testing a combination of biweekly bevacizumab and daily erlotinib in patients with unresectable biliary cancer: a phase II consortium study. J Clin Oncol. 2010;28(21):3491–7.
104. Shroff RT, Yarchoan M, O'Connor A, et al. The oral VEGF receptor tyrosine kinase inhibitor pazopanib in combination with the MEK inhibitor trametinib in advanced cholangiocarcinoma. Br J Cancer. 2017;116(11):1402–7.
105. Sun W, Normolle DP, Bahary N, et al. A phase 2 trial of regorafenib as a single agent in patients with chemotherapy-refractory advanced and metastatic biliary adenocarcinoma/cholangiocarcinoma. J Clin Oncol. 2017;35(15_suppl):4081.
106. Luo X, Jia W, Huang Z, et al. Effectiveness and safety of sorafenib in the treatment of unresectable and advanced intrahepatic cholangiocarcinoma: a pilot study. Oncotarget. 2017;8(10):17246–57.
107. Lowery MA, O'Reilly EM, Harding JJ, et al. A phase I trial of binimetinib in combination with gemcitabine (G) and cisplatin (C) patients (pts) with untreated advanced biliary cancer (ABC). J Clin Oncol. 2015;33(15_suppl):e15125.
108. Bridgewater JA, Goodman KA, Kalyan A, Mulcahy MF. Biliary tract cancer: epidemiology, radiotherapy, and molecular profiling. Am Soc Clin Oncol Educ Book. 2016;35:e194–203.
109. Borger DR, Tanabe KK, Fan KC, et al. Frequent mutation of isocitrate dehydrogenase (IDH)1 and IDH2 in cholangiocarcinoma identified through broad-based tumor genotyping. Oncologist. 2012;17(1):72–9.
110. Javle M, Bekaii-Saab T, Jain A, et al. Biliary cancer: utility of next-generation sequencing for clinical management. Cancer. 2016;122(24):3838–47.
111. Goyal L, Govindan A, Sheth RA, et al. Prognosis and Clinicopathologic features of patients with advanced stage Isocitrate Dehydrogenase (IDH) mutant and IDH wild-type intrahepatic cholangiocarcinoma. Oncologist. 2015;20(9):1019–27.
112. Zhu AX, Borger DR, Kim Y, et al. Genomic profiling of intrahepatic cholangiocarcinoma: refining prognosis and identifying therapeutic targets. Ann Surg Oncol. 2014;21(12):3827–34.
113. Lowery MA, Abou-Alfa GK, Burris HA, et al. Phase I study of AG-120, an IDH1 mutant enzyme inhibitor: results from the cholangiocarcinoma dose escalation and expansion cohorts. J Clin Oncol. 2017;35(15_suppl):4015.
114. Abdel-Wahab R, Ali SM, Borad MJ, et al. Variations in DNA repair genomic alterations and tumor mutation burden in biliary tract cancer (BTC) subtypes. J Clin Oncol. 2018;36(4_suppl):263.
115. Ame JC, Spenlehauer C, de Murcia G. The PARP superfamily. BioEssays. 2004;26(8):882–93.
116. Turk AA, Deming DA, Lubner SJ, et al. A phase I study of veliparib (Vel) in combination with oxaliplatin (Ox) and capecitabine (Cap) in advanced solid tumors. J Clin Oncol. 2018;36(4_suppl):314.
117. Gibney GT, Weiner LM, Atkins MB. Predictive biomarkers for checkpoint inhibitor-based immunotherapy. Lancet Oncol. 2016;17(12):e542–51.
118. Chalmers ZR, Connelly CF, Fabrizio D, et al. Analysis of 100,000 human cancer genomes reveals the landscape of tumor mutational burden. Genome Med. 2017;9(1):34.
119. Dijkstra KK, Voabil P, Schumacher TN, Voest EE. Genomics- and transcriptomics-based patient selection for cancer treatment with immune checkpoint inhibitors: a review. JAMA Oncol. 2016;2(11):1490–5.
120. Chong DQ, Zhu AX. The landscape of targeted therapies for cholangiocarcinoma: current status and emerging targets. Oncotarget. 2016;7(29):46750–67.
121. Kim ST, Jang KT, Lee J, et al. Molecular subgroup analysis of clinical outcomes in a phase 3 study of gemcitabine and Oxaliplatin with or without Erlotinib in advanced biliary tract cancer. Transl Oncol. 2015;8(1):40–6.
122. Lavingia V, Fakih M. Impressive response to dual BRAF and MEK inhibition in patients with BRAF mutant intrahepatic cholangiocarcinoma-2 case reports and a brief review. J Gastrointest Oncol. 2016;7(6):E98–E102.

123. Loaiza-Bonilla A, Clayton E, Furth E, O'Hara M, Morrissette J. Dramatic response to dabrafenib and trametinib combination in a BRAF V600E-mutated cholangiocarcinoma: implementation of a molecular tumour board and next-generation sequencing for personalized medicine. Ecancermedicalscience. 2014;8:479.
124. Subbiah V, Kreitman RJ, Wainberg ZA, et al. Efficacy of dabrafenib (D) and trametinib (T) in patients (pts) with BRAF V600E–mutated anaplastic thyroid cancer (ATC). J Clin Oncol. 2017;35(15_suppl):6023.
125. Al-Shamsi HO, Anand D, Shroff RT, et al. BRCA-associated protein 1 mutant cholangiocarcinoma: an aggressive disease subtype. J Gastrointest Oncol. 2016;7(4):556–61.
126. Kwak TW, Kim DH, Jeong Y-I, Kang DH. Antitumor activity of vorinostat-incorporated nanoparticles against human cholangiocarcinoma cells. J Nanobiotechnol. 2015;13:60.
127. Topalian SL, Hodi FS, Brahmer JR, et al. Safety, activity, and immune correlates of anti-PD-1 antibody in cancer. N Engl J Med. 2012;366(26):2443–54.
128. Brahmer JR, Tykodi SS, Chow LQ, et al. Safety and activity of anti-PD-L1 antibody in patients with advanced cancer. N Engl J Med. 2012;366(26):2455–65.
129. Wolchok JD, Chiarion-Sileni V, Gonzalez R, et al. Overall survival with combined Nivolumab and Ipilimumab in advanced melanoma. N Engl J Med. 2017;377(14):1345–56.
130. Koster BD, de Gruijl TD, van den Eertwegh AJ. Recent developments and future challenges in immune checkpoint inhibitory cancer treatment. Curr Opin Oncol. 2015;27(6):482–8.
131. Goeppert B, Frauenschuh L, Zucknick M, et al. Prognostic impact of tumour-infiltrating immune cells on biliary tract cancer. Br J Cancer. 2013;109(10):2665–74.
132. Galon J, Costes A, Sanchez-Cabo F, et al. Type, density, and location of immune cells within human colorectal tumors predict clinical outcome. Science. 2006;313(5795):1960–4.
133. Fukunaga A, Miyamoto M, Cho Y, et al. CD8+ tumor-infiltrating lymphocytes together with CD4+ tumor-infiltrating lymphocytes and dendritic cells improve the prognosis of patients with pancreatic adenocarcinoma. Pancreas. 2004;28(1):e26–31.
134. Wang Y, Ding M, Zhang Q, et al. Activation or suppression of the immune response mediators in biliary tract cancer (BTC) patients: a systematic review and meta-analysis. J Cancer. 2017;8(1):74–84.
135. Chen DS, Mellman I. Elements of cancer immunity and the cancer–immune set point. Nature. 2017;541:321.
136. Herbst RS, Soria J-C, Kowanetz M, et al. Predictive correlates of response to the anti-PD-L1 antibody MPDL3280A in cancer patients. Nature. 2014;515:563.
137. Bonneville R, Krook MA, Kautto EA, Miya J, Wing MR, Chen HZ, et al. Landscape of microsatellite instability across 39 cancer types. JCO Precis Oncol. 2017;2017.
138. Silva VW, Askan G, Daniel TD, et al. Biliary carcinomas: pathology and the role of DNA mismatch repair deficiency. Chin Clin Oncol. 2016;5(5):62.
139. Diaz LA, Marabelle A, Delord J-P, et al. Pembrolizumab therapy for microsatellite instability-high (MSI-H) colorectal cancer (CRC) and non-CRC. J Clin Oncol. 2017;35(15_suppl):3071.
140. Aruga A. Vaccination of biliary tract cancer patients with four peptides derived from cancer-testis antigens. Oncoimmunology. 2013;2(7):e24882.
141. Yoshitomi M, Yutani S, Matsueda S, et al. Personalized peptide vaccination for advanced biliary tract cancer: IL-6, nutritional status and pre-existing antigen-specific immunity as possible biomarkers for patient prognosis. Exp Ther Med. 2012;3(3):463–9.
142. Shimizu K, Kotera Y, Aruga A, Takeshita N, Takasaki K, Yamamoto M. Clinical utilization of postoperative dendritic cell vaccine plus activated T-cell transfer in patients with intrahepatic cholangiocarcinoma. J Hepatobiliary Pancreat Sci. 2012;19(2):171–8.
143. Kida A, Mizukoshi E, Tamai T, et al. Immune responses against tumor-associated antigen-derived cytotoxic T lymphocyte epitopes in cholangiocarcinoma patients. Liver Int. 2018;38(11):2040–50.

Index

T. M. Pawlik et al. (eds.), *Intrahepatic Cholangiocarcinoma*,
https://doi.org/10.1007/978-3-030-22258-1

R

S

T

The manufacturer's authorised representative in the EU is Springer Nature Customer Service Centre GmbH, Europaplatz 3, 69115 Heidelberg, Germany. If you have any concerns regarding our products, please contact ProductSafety@springernature.com

Printed and bound by CPI Group (UK) Ltd, Croydon, CR0 4YY
24/07/2026
02175923-0001